PERSPECTIVES ON THE MITRAL VALVE

PERSPECTIVES ON THE MITRAL VALVE

JOHN B. BARLOW, M.D.

Professor of Cardiology
University of the Witwatersrand
and Johannesburg Hospital
Johannesburg, South Africa

F. A. DAVIS COMPANY • PHILADELPHIA

NOTE: As new scientific information becomes available through basic and clinical research, recommended treatments and drug therapies undergo changes. The author(s) and publisher have done everything possible to make this book accurate, up-to-date, and in accord with accepted standards at the time of publication. However, the reader is advised always to check product information (package inserts) for changes and new information regarding dose and contraindications before administering any drug. Caution is especially urged when using new or infrequently ordered drugs.

Library of Congress Cataloging-in-Publication Data

Barlow, John B., 1924–
   Perspectives on the mitral valve.

   Includes bibliographies and index.
   1. Mitral valve—Diseases. I. Title. [DNLM:
1. Heart Valve Diseases. 2. Mitral Valve.
WG 262 B258p]
RC685.V2B37 1987   616.1′25   86–8834
ISBN 0–8036–0617–6

DEDICATION

To all students of medicine
Who listen, look, touch, and reflect:
May they hear, see, feel, and comprehend.

FOREWORD

When I first met John Brereton Barlow at the South African Cardiac Society Congress (a meeting he organized and one to which he had invited me to speak), I was struck by his exquisitely sharp mind and clinical acumen. Following the meeting I got to know him better by visiting the University of the Witwatersrand, where he has been Chairman of the Department of Cardiology since 1961 and a force in cardiology for 25 years. The university's large hospital provides an extraordinary array of patients with all forms of valvular heart disease, an array simply not accessible to physicians in the United States. John Barlow, a master clinician, has drawn on his enormous and unique clinical experience and his keen observations of these experiences to produce the present book on mitral valve disease.

Born in Cape Town in 1924, John Barlow graduated from medical school in 1951. He trained in medicine, surgery, and pediatrics at Baragwanath Hospital in Soweto for 3 years and then spent 3 years training in London, mainly with Dr. John Shillingford and Sir John McMichael. Under McMichael he was exposed to the view that current dogma must always be carefully examined, and he has done so with valuable results.

Barlow entered the international cardiology scene in 1963 with publication of his article "The significance of late systolic murmurs" (American Heart Journal 66:443–452, 1963). The presence of a late systolic murmur and the accompanying mid- or late systolic click(s) subsequently have been known as *the Barlow syndrome*. It was Barlow who demonstrated that the apical late systolic murmur, whether pansystolic with late accentuation or entirely confined to late systole, denotes mitral regurgitation. Previously, the murmur and the associated systolic click(s) had been considered extracardiac in origin.

Since 1963, Barlow has expanded his research and published on many new topics. Known around the world for his precise descriptions and definitions of mitral valve mechanisms, in this book John provides the reader with an excellent resource, magnificently illustrated on these topics, and then goes beyond to his new work. Always the serious and careful observer, John brings our attention to new clinical findings concerning the hemodynamics of cardiac chamber inter-relationships and related topics such as submitral left ventricular aneurysm, pulmonary arterial hypertension, hypertrophic cardiomyopathy, and tricuspid valve disease.

Because of his extensive patient-care responsibilities, teaching commitments, and national and international cardiologic activities, Barlow was hesitant to undertake this book. He did, of course, accept the challenge, and I am pleased and gratified that he did, for his sharp eye, inquiring mind, and strong will have brought enlightenment to a large variety of topics.

WILLIAM C. ROBERTS, M.D.

PREFACE

I have given considerable thought as to what meaningful contribution I could make in a book on the somewhat vast subject of mitral valve disease. The mitral valve is directly or indirectly involved in numerous pathological conditions affecting the heart; however, I would not want to be repetitious of the many excellent descriptions of most aspects of mitral valve disease that appear in textbooks and scientific papers.

I have to be cognizant, however, of having had an opportunity to practice cardiology in an environment where the broad spectrum of clinical material combined with the sophisticated means of investigation and treatment is unique or, to say the least, most unusual compared with that found elsewhere in the world. In addition to cases of all ages with congenital heart disease, cardiomyopathy, hypertension, pericarditis, and the many other cardiovascular disorders that are encountered everywhere, I have had ample opportunity to gain substantial experience with the Third World diseases, such as virulent rheumatic carditis and advanced infective endocarditis, which are prevalent in Black children and young adults, as well as with the First World scourge of coronary artery disease, which devastates the adult Asiatic and White sections of the population of my country. Although rheumatic heart disease remains prevalent elsewhere in Africa and in countries in the Asian Pacific region, economic and other factors in most of those areas have limited the accuracy of diagnosis, access to surgery, and thus the availability of pathological examination. South Africa is unique among the Third World countries in that it possesses a hospital service with sophisticated means of investigation and treatment at its disposal—a service that is available for the most part to all population groups at small cost to the patient.

I decided, therefore, that there may be a message in my recording in this book some of the lessons I have learned and opinions I have formed after practicing clinical cardiology in this environment. An *opinion* on any topic is necessarily based on a balance between one's own experiences and what one learns from the observations and teachings of others. Working in a country that is geographically somewhat isolated, there are limited opportunities to attend scientific meetings, visit prestigious departments, and have personal discussions with international authorities. It is therefore obligatory to attempt to meet the ongoing and enormous challenge of keeping abreast with the surfeit of scientific literature. The clinical commitments for the department of cardiology and cardiac surgery in this institution have been, and remain, vast. The staff-to-patient ratio is considerably lower than in academic units in the United States or the United Kingdom, and time does not allow us, for example, to catheterize more than 10 percent of patients referred for valve replacement. Nonetheless, we indeed visit leading institutions, and we are cognizant of their diagnostic policies, their methods of investigation, and their surgical results. It is my firm belief that the overall service meted out to patients with heart disease in this institution compares favorably.

I have entitled this book *Perspectives on the Mitral Valve* but re-emphasize that no attempt is made to review all aspects relating to this subject. My aim is to discuss features related to mitral valve disease that, in my view, are important, require clarification, or have hitherto received insufficient emphasis. In writing such a book, I have found it prudent to confine most of my comments to subject matter on which I have personal experience. There is therefore much emphasis on physical examination and general clinical assessment. Although I have extensive experience with the preoperative assessment, immediate postoperative complications, and the long-term follow-up of patients subjected to cardiac surgery, it has been obligatory for me to enlist the assistance of my surgical colleagues, R. H. Kinsley and M. J. Antunes, for chapters that have predominantly surgical content. Similarly, because I have little practical experience of echocardiography, I have had to rely to a large extent on the opinions and expertise of colleagues working in that field. Wendy Pocock, an astute clinical cardiologist with whom I have had a long association, has contributed to the writing of most chapters.

The book is neither a monograph nor a comprehensive reference book on the mitral valve. It is directed at those individuals—whether students or trained cardiologists—who adhere to the belief that a careful clinical assessment remains most important; at those who have an interest in the mitral valve and related diseases; but especially at those who concede that it is invariably the doctor, as an observer, interpreter, or operator, who makes the errors and who may need to improve his or her expertise. Almost invariably my own mistakes have been due to failure to elicit or interpret correctly an important symptom, sign, or other piece of information. Irrespective of how it is obtained, all data should be assessed in the context of the specific patient. For example, a small pressure difference at cardiac catheterization, a soft systolic murmur, or normal QRS voltages on the electrocardiogram are, alone or in combination, compatible with critically tight calcific aortic stenosis! Failure to detect vegetations on echocardiography does not exclude infective endocarditis. Was the postexercise ECG indeed a "false positive" for ischemia or was it typical of a so-called nonspecific T wave change? Is the chest radiograph of that patient with pulmonary hypertension "normal" or does it, in fact, show conclusive evidence of chronic pulmonary thromboembolic disease? This book purports to remind some readers, and perhaps to teach others, that it is mandatory for every clinician to judge each situation for him- or herself and always to query—even to challenge—the apparently obvious.

I am concerned about the highly prevalent custom of accepting without question statements, results, or conclusions as indisputable fact, as the truth, or as authentic just because they have been written, regarded as objective evidence, or based on so-called hard data. Conclusions drawn by reputable investigators, obtained from "hard data," and documented in prestigious scientific journals cannot *always* be correct; otherwise there could never exist directly contradictory conclusions drawn by others in an identical context. If I had been able to believe and accept some of the "hard data" and "objective evidence" that has been provided by a number of "reputable" investigators, I would not have to contend with the many unresolved problems that continue to confront me. I would know the optimal time for valve replacement and the type of prosthetic valve that should be inserted. I would know the indications for left ventricular aneurysmectomy, intracoronary streptokinase, and percutaneous coronary angioplasty. I would also know whether left ventricular function is abnormal in patients with primary mitral valve prolapse and whether there is true obstruction to left ventricular outflow in hypertrophic cardiomyopathy. I would have few doubts about the indications for surgery in the latter condition or, for that matter, about what operation should be performed. Accurate assessment of left ventricular function by echocardiography would also confront me with few problems!

In the context of a hospital environment, authoritative documents such as the report on a chest radiograph, echocardiogram, or cardiac catheterization; the histology of a biopsy; a radionucleotide study; as well as the learned opinion of the most senior consultant and the operative report of a cardiac surgeon are often offered as "hard data." It is surely a sobering experience for all clinicians when it not infrequently transpires that one, more than one, or all of these were found to be incorrect after they had been importantly, even disastrously, misleading?

Although a great deal has been written relating to this subject, I have intentionally quoted references only when highly pertinent. Furthermore, while articles or books listed under "Further Reading" may not always represent the best reviews of the relevant subject, I recommend them because they relate, sometimes in disagreement, to the theme of my argument. This book reflects the experience of a clinical cardiologist after serving for three decades a multiracial patient population of all ages in an academic institution. I hope that it reaches some receptive readers and achieves some of its aims.

JOHN B. BARLOW, M.D.

ACKNOWLEDGMENTS

I could not have completed this book without the immense assistance of Dr. Wendy Pocock, and I am grateful to her and to the other chapter co-authors for their varied contributions. Oria Cohen was invaluable for her typing, and Ruth Melrose for her organisation of the illustrations. I acknowledge Alastair Webb and his staff in the photographic section of this Department of Medicine, and Barbara Bryden of Baragwanath Hospital for the photographic reproductions.

Dr. Jeff King fulfilled many of my clinical, administrative, and teaching commitments during my preoccupation with the book. He is a principal "unsung hero" of the endeavour, whereas others, including my family, exhibited patience or lent encouragement.

I am indebted to Dr. William C. Roberts for his recommendation to Dr. Sylvia K. Fields of F. A. Davis that I be invited to undertake the project. Sylvia Fields and the F. A. Davis Company, in turn, provided splendid cooperation and supportive guidance.

CONTRIBUTORS

MANUEL J. ANTUNES, M.D. (LM), M. Med., F.A.C.C.
Acting Head, Department of Cardiothoracic Surgery, University of the Witwatersrand and Johannesburg Hospital, Johannesburg, South Africa

ROBIN H. KINSLEY, M.B., B.Ch. (Witwatersrand), F.C.S. (SA), F.A.C.C.
Consultant Cardiothoracic Surgeon, and formerly Head, Department of Cardiothoracic Surgery, University of the Witwatersrand and Johannesburg Hospital, Johannesburg, South Africa

JEFFREY B. LAKIER, M.D.
Senior Staff Physician, Division of Cardiovascular Medicine, Henry Ford Hospital, Detroit, Michigan

THEO E. MEYER, M.B., B.Ch. (Pret), F.C.P. (SA)
Consultant Cardiologist, University of the Witwatersrand and Baragwanath Hospital, Johannesburg, South Africa

WENDY A. POCOCK, M.B., B.Ch. (Witwatersrand), F.R.C.P.
Consultant Cardiologist, University of the Witwatersrand and Johannesburg Hospital, Johannesburg, South Africa

PINHAS SARELI, M.D. (Hadassah)
Consultant Cardiologist, University of the Witwatersrand and Baragwanath Hospital, Johannesburg, South Africa

CONTENTS

FUNCTIONAL ANATOMY OF THE MITRAL VALVE

with MANUEL J. ANTUNES

This review of the functional anatomy of the mitral valve is included as a refresher and as an immediate reference for our diverse readers. Cardiologists will be aided in their understanding of the mechanism whereby the numerous pathological processes affect one or more of the valve components. It will also be beneficial to surgeons, to whom a thorough knowledge of the anatomy and function of the valve is essential before attempting to restore normal function to a diseased mitral valve.

Our description of mitral valve functional anatomy is based on studies by Ranganathan and colleagues,[1,2] Perloff and Roberts,[3] and others.[4,5] It is also based on our own experience derived from the intraoperative examination of more than a thousand mitral valves, the dissection of many specimens of normal hearts, and the clinical assessment of patients with mitral valve disease.

ANATOMY OF THE MITRAL VALVE

The mitral valve has two leaflets, which separate the left atrial and left ventricular cavities (Fig. 1-1). The leaflets are attached at their bases to an ill-defined fibromuscular ring, the anulus fibrosus, and by their free edges to the chordae tendineae. The latter originate from one of two digital extensions of the ventricular myocardium, the papillary muscles. Normal valve function depends on the mechanical integrity of all components of the mitral apparatus, including the left atrial and ventricular walls.

PAPILLARY MUSCLES

The left ventricle has two papillary muscles, an anterior (anterolateral) one and a posterior (posteromedial) one, which arise at the junction of the apical and middle thirds of the ventricular free wall. The anterior papillary muscle originates from the anterior wall of the ventricle at its lateral border, and the posterior muscle arises from the posterior wall, at its junction with the ventricular septum. The two have equal functional importance and similar volume, but vary in shape. They usually bifurcate

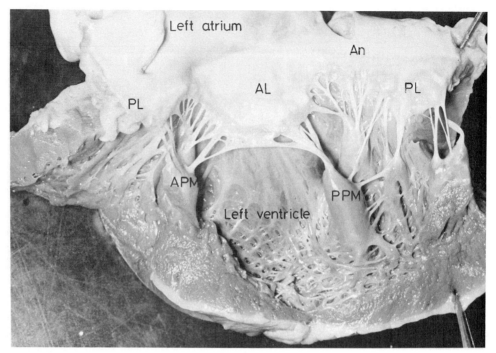

FIGURE 1-1. View of the mitral valve interposed between the opened left atrium and left ventricle. AL = anterior leaflet; An = anulus; APM = anterior papillary muscle; PL = posterior leaflet; PPM = posterior papillary muscle.

into two, very closely related structures, although the anterior papillary muscle may be single. Invariably, the two halves of each papillary muscle face each other in a convex (anterior) and matching concave (posterior) surface. During ventricular contraction, there is an intimate contact of the two halves. Occasionally, four or five papillary muscles originate from the ventricular wall as independent columns. The apices of the papillary muscles bifurcate or trifurcate into smaller digital terminations (heads) from which the chordae tendineae originate (Fig. 1-2A). The bases are formed by the confluence of a variable number of muscular trabeculae (Fig. 1-2B). The bodies are not infrequently attached to the left ventricular free wall by muscular or tendinous chordae (false chordae). Similar chordae interconnect the two main papillary muscles and their different divisions.

The papillary muscles receive their **nerve supply** from direct continuations of the anterior and posterior branches of the left bundle branch of His, which run up the papillary muscles and form the Purkinje mesh in the subendocardium. Connecting fibers between the two main branches are contained in the substance of the false chordae, which run between the two papillary muscles as well as between them and the ventricular wall.

The **blood supply** to the papillary muscles is provided by septal branches of both the right and left coronary arteries. The anterior muscle is almost invariably supplied by the second septal branch of the left anterior descending (interventricular) artery and usually also by a branch of the left circumflex artery. The posterior muscle is supplied by one of the septal branches of the posterior descending (interventricular) artery. The latter is most commonly a branch of the right coronary artery. The posterior papillary muscle almost always receives another branch directly from the circumflex artery. Hence, each papillary muscle is usually supplied by at least two arteries, which are interconnected within the body of the muscle. Within the papillary muscle, each artery divides into two branches, which run centrally and subendocardially. Although in most cases multiple anastomoses interconnect these

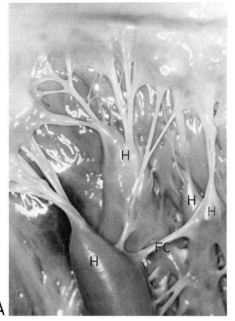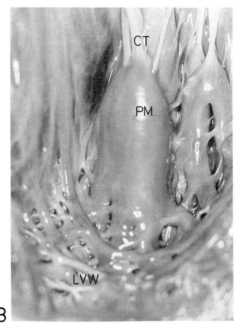

FIGURE 1-2. Magnified view of the posterior papillary muscle showing its heads (*A*) and the base (*B*). CT = chordae tendineae; H = heads; LVW = left ventricular wall; PM = papillary muscle; FC = false chorda.

branches, the supply may be from a single central artery. The papillary muscles are the last structures in the heart to be perfused by arterial blood and consequently their apices are most vulnerable to ischemia and anoxia.

LEAFLETS

The two mitral valve leaflets, anterior (septal or aortic) and posterior (mural or ventricular), insert as a continuous veil around the entire circumference of the mitral orifice. The anterior leaflet is roughly triangular in shape with a round apical contour. It is thin and translucent at the base, but there is a crescentic, thicker, opaque area bordering the free edge, the **rough zone** (Fig. 1-3). The chordae tendineae which insert on the ventricular surface of the rough zone are responsible for the increased thickness. The width of this zone is about one-third that of the leaflet. The posterior leaflet is narrower than the anterior, but it has a longer attachment to the anulus and thus the total surface area of the two leaflets is virtually identical. The free edge of the posterior leaflet is indented by one or two "clefts," giving it a scalloped appearance. The lateral (commissural) scallops are often small, creating an impression of accessory leaflets. The leaflet also has a rough zone, slightly narrower than that of the anterior leaflet to which it apposes during closure. This rough zone is wider than the corresponding **clear zone** (ratio 1.4:1). The dimensions of the leaflets and scallops and of their respective rough and clear zones, extracted from published reports[2,6] and modified according to our own observations, are shown in Table 1-1.

Although many believe that the valve leaflets consist only of collagen-reinforced endothelium with no neurovascular pedicle, this concept does not appear to be correct. Striated muscle cells, nonmyelinated nerve fibers, and blood vessels have been observed in animals[7-9] extending two-thirds into the leaflet tissue towards the free edge. Substantial numbers of muscle fibers, cardiac muscle, have been demonstrated in the human mitral valve. These fibers, which appear to be of atrial origin, are probably activated in conjunction with the atrial wall and may contribute to

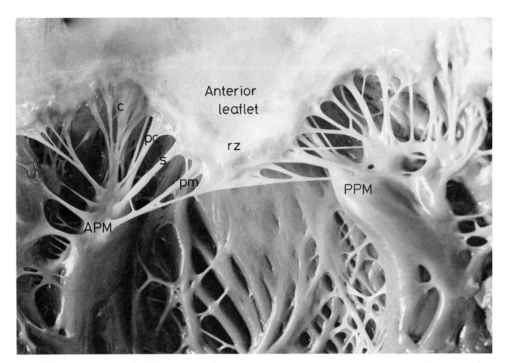

FIGURE 1-3. Anterior mitral valve leaflet with its chordae tendineae and papillary muscles. APM = anterior papillary muscle; c = commissural chordae; pc = paracommissural chordae; pm = paramedial chordae; PPM = posterior papillary muscle; s = strut chordae; rz = rough zone.

TABLE 1-1. Dimensions of the Mitral Valve Leaflets (mm)

		WIDTH	
	LENGTH	CLEAR ZONE	ROUGH ZONE
Anterior leaflet	2.5–4.5	1.2–2.0	0.6–1.2
Posterior leaflet			
lateral scallop	1.0–1.8		
central scallop	2.0–4.0	0.4–0.9	0.5–1.2
medial scallop	0.8–1.6		

mitral valve function.[9,10] They are more numerous in children and are a constant feature of the structure of the anterior leaflet, but they are extremely rare in the posterior leaflet.

The two leaflets are joined by the anteromedial and posterolateral commissures and are thus always in continuity.

CHORDAE TENDINEAE

Although the chordal system has been extensively studied, it remains the most controversial component of the mitral apparatus. There are wide variations in number and form of the chordae and their attachments. The chordae tendineae are fibrous structures that originate from the heads of the papillary muscles, although some arise directly from the ventricular wall. After a short course most of them branch, but a small number may insert without branching into the leaflets. Insertion into the posterior leaflet occurs at any point between the free edge and the base (Fig. 1-4). It has

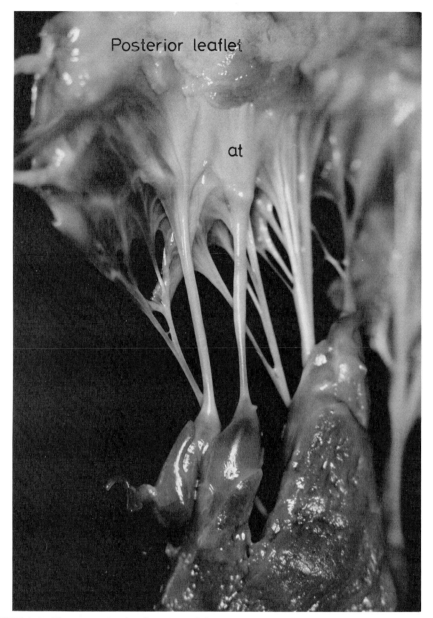

FIGURE 1-4. The posterior leaflet viewed from its ventricular surface, which is covered by the triangular attachments (at) of the chordae tendineae.

been widely accepted that the ventricular surface of the anterior leaflet beyond the rough zone is devoid of chordae. This is at variance with our experience of diseased valves, and we have not infrequently found thick chordae, which may originate from either papillary muscle, inserting near the centre of the ventricular surface of the anterior leaflet, well inside the clear zone (Fig. 1-5). Furthermore, we have observed some valves in which the entire anterior leaflet surface, from the free edge to the base, was occupied by the insertion of chordae.

In the past, the classification of first-, second-, and third-order chordae tendineae, which insert respectively into the free edge, ventricular surface, and basal segment of the leaflets, has generally been used. There are from 17 to 29 first-order chordae (average 25), of which 5 to 13 (average 9) insert into the anterior leaflet, 8

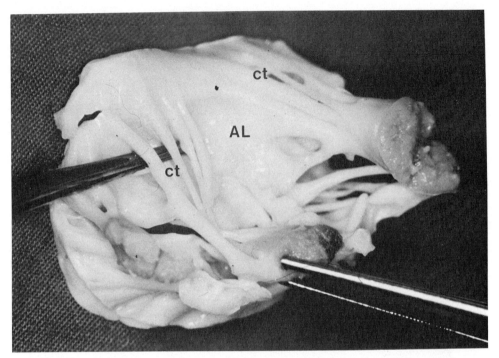

FIGURE 1-5. Mitral valve specimen removed during surgery for valve replacement demonstrating chordae tendineae (ct) inserting well beyond the rough zone, into the body of the anterior leaflet (AL).

to 20 (average 14) into the posterior leaflet, and 2 into the commissural areas. This classification of first-, second-, and third-order chordae is of limited value to the surgeon. The sites of chordal insertion into the free edge and rough zone of both leaflets have greater functional significance, and a classification based on this is of more practical value.

Commissural Chordae

A single chorda divides into smaller chordae, which insert in a fanlike manner into the free edge of the commissural region of each leaflet (Fig. 1-6). The arrangement is similar for each commissure but with a wider lateral spread in the posteromedial commissural area. The central chorda of each commissural group contributes to the identification of the commissure, because it points directly to it in the vast majority of cases. To our knowledge, second- and third-order commissural chordae have not been reported, nor have they been observed by us. Rarely, we have noted complete absence of chordae tendineae of one of the commissures.

Leaflet Chordae

From each papillary muscle, three groups of chordae insert into each half of the body of the anterior leaflet, namely paramedial, central (strut), and paracommissural chordae (see Fig. 1-3). These chordae insert in an oblique manner into the rough zone of the anterior leaflet. Typically, each chorda divides into three branches, which insert directly, or after further branching, into the free edge, intermediate area, and limit of the rough zone. These three branches act together as a functional unit. The strut chordae are the thickest and arise at the summit of the papillary muscle. They appear

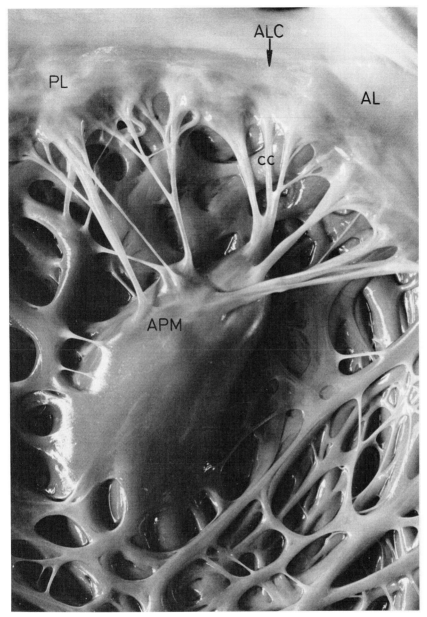

FIGURE 1-6. Anatomy of the commissural chordae (cc) inserting in the area of the anterolateral commissure (ALC). Note the fanlike distribution of these chordae. AL = anterior leaflet; APM = anterior papillary muscle; PL = posterior leaflet.

to constitute the "cornerstone" of the chordal system of the anterior leaflet, and their insertion corresponds to the critical areas of leaflet closure described by Brock[11] in 1952.

The posterior leaflet chordae reach the free edge and the ventricular surface of the leaflet in a parallel alignment and have a broad fan-shaped base of insertion. Like the anterior leaflet, the posterior has chordae that insert into the free edge and rough zone, but in addition, the posterior leaflet has basal and cleft chordae. The former originate from either the ventricular wall or papillary muscles and attach to the base of the body of the posterior leaflet. The latter originate from the papillary muscles and insert into the margins and adjacent areas of the posterior leaflet scallops.

There are wide variations in the number of chordae tendineae attaching to a leaflet. Most of these "variations from normal"[12] are characterized by the absence of one or of a group of chordae, leaving a portion of the leaflet unprotected. Becker and de Wit[12] observed that 90 percent of patients with nonrheumatic and nonischemic mitral valve prolapse had abnormalities of the chordae, mostly in the form of an irregular or deficient arrangement or branching pattern.

ANULUS FIBROSUS

Two fibrous trigones form part of the mitral valve ring or anulus (Fig. 1-7). The right fibrous trigone or central fibrous body is the most prominent element of the cardiac skeleton and is located between the mitral, tricuspid, and aortic orifices. The left fibrous trigone, situated between the left margins of the mitral and aortic valves, has a similar structure but is less prominent. The two trigones are connected medially by collagen fibers that constitute part of the common portion of the aortic and mitral valve rings. On either side, the two fibrous bodies continue as a band of resistant connective tissue that runs superficially in a subendocardial position and partially surrounds the mitral valve orifice. This structure gradually fades out so that the posterior half or third of the mitral anulus is devoid of collagen fibers and is ill defined. Thus, the base of the posterior leaflet attaches directly to the left atrial and ventricular endocardium. The two trigones serve as insertion points for the cardiac muscle fibers and as fixed points for the myocardial contraction.

The posterior mitral anulus is in proximity to the circumflex coronary artery, which runs in the posterior atrioventricular groove. Only a few millimeters separate

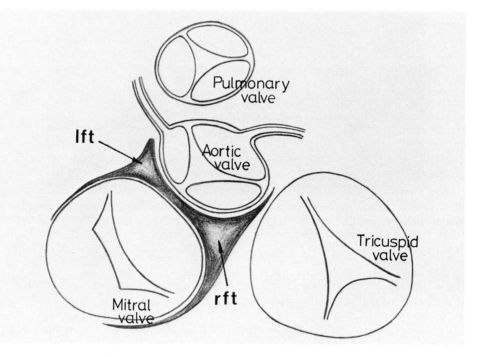

FIGURE 1-7. Fibrous skeleton of the heart. The left fibrous trigone (lft) and the right fibrous trigone (rft) are situated between the mitral and aortic valve orifices and constitute part of the anulus fibrosus of the mitral valve. Its collagen fibers do not encircle the valve orifice completely, leaving part of the posterior anulus unprotected from dilatation.

the endocardium and the vessel in this region, and surgical disruption is a potential hazard. The relationship of the anterior anulus to the conduction bundle is not as close, and damage to the conducting system during mitral valve surgery is extremely rare.

LEFT ATRIUM AND LEFT VENTRICLE

The papillary muscles are digital extensions of the left ventricular free wall, sharing its vascularization and innervation. The posterior leaflet is in direct continuity with the ventricular and atrial endocardium and is affected by the changes in structure and function of the relevant chambers. The muscular, vascular, and nervous components of the anterior leaflet are intimately related to the corresponding structures of the left atrial wall. Whatever role they might have must be related to the function of the left atrium.

MITRAL VALVE FUNCTION

Some confusion has resulted from difficulty in defining the precise timing of opening and closure of the mitral valve. It is beyond the scope of this dissertation to discuss in detail the functional anatomic factors that may cause opening or closing movements of the leaflets independent of pressure events. From a clinical standpoint, we regard the timing of closure of the mitral valve to occur at pressure crossover (Fig. 1-8) and regard the leaflet edges as apposing at that time. Similarly, we define the point of opening as the time of crossover of the descending left ventricular pressure and the left atrial V wave (Fig. 1-8). These two pressure crossover points also mark the onset and offset of the left ventricular isovolumetric contraction and relaxation phases, respectively.

Anatomical integrity and coordinated interaction of all the components of the mitral valve are necessary to maintain competence. In the following section, the relative contribution of each component to the function of the valve are discussed.

CLOSURE OF THE MITRAL VALVE

Leaflets

Closure of the mitral valve, after the beginning of ventricular contraction, is achieved by the apposition of the two leaflets. A slow movement towards closure occurs in diastole as the leaflets float together at the end of rapid ventricular filling. With atrial systole, which momentarily increases forward flow through the mitral valve, the leaflets have a reopening movement. The leaflets are approximated by vortices (eddy currents) generated behind their ventricular surfaces. Ventricular contraction provides the last impetus for closure of the valve. The greater width (base to free edge) of the anterior leaflet gives it increased mobility, which makes it the major contributor to closure of the valve. The posterior leaflet, by virtue of its larger circumference, has a supportive role. It moves anteriorly during systole, as does the ventricular wall behind it, and acts as the "wall" against which the anterior leaflet locks. The leaflets come into contact at their corresponding rough zones. The apposing surfaces, stabilized by the action of the chordae tendineae, and the anulus are relatively fixed points. The remaining leaflet substance billows into the left atrium because of the high left ventricular pressure. The left ventricular pressure is directed not only to the anular area of each leaflet but against the opposite sides of the mitral seal, tending to hold it in place (see Chap. 7, Fig. 7-6A). This buttressing, or "keystone" effect,

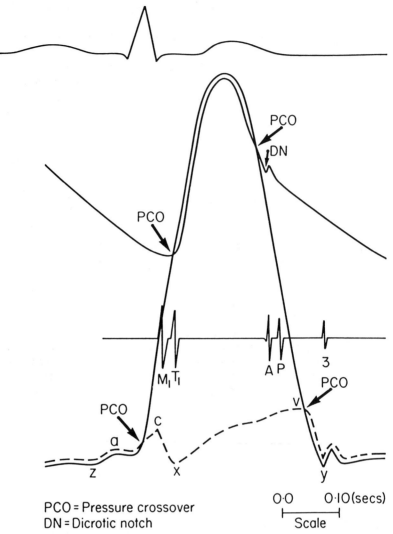

PCO
DN
PCO
PCO

M_1 T_1

A P

3
PCO

v

a
c

z
X
y

PCO = Pressure crossover
DN = Dicrotic notch

0·0   0·10(secs)
Scale

FIGURE 1-8. Diagrammatic representation of simultaneous left atrial, left ventricular, and aortic pressures with electrocardiogram and phonocardiogram. Pressure crossover (PCO) between the left atrium and ventricle occurs immediately after the onset of ventricular systole and is synchronous with mitral valve closure. The mitral component of the first sound (M_1) occurs when the apposed leaflets billow towards the left atrial cavity at the time of the left atrial C wave. The mitral valve opens when the left ventricular pressure falls below that of the left atrial V wave.

greatly reduces the tension on the chordae and papillary muscles. The larger the area of mutual contact, the firmer is the seal. The combined surface area of the two leaflets is nearly twice that of the relaxed mitral valve orifice, which indicates the large area of coaptation. As a result of anular contraction, the valve orifice is smaller during ventricular systole compared with the relaxed state in early ventricular diastole, and the surface of leaflet available for coaptation is much enhanced. The area of the anterior leaflet may become greater than that of the mitral orifice, and it is possible for the orifice to be closed by this leaflet alone.

An essential requirement for normal valve function is unrestricted movement at commissural level. The characteristic mode of insertion of the commissural chordae facilitates the mobility of the leaflets in this region. Whereas the lateral portions of the leaflets hinge on the commissural chordae, the central portion of the anterior leaflet between the two strut chordae appears to move with its basal attachment acting as fulcrum.

The functional contribution, if any, of the muscle fibers in the mitral leaflets is uncertain. It appears that the anterior leaflet has the capacity to shorten when its muscle fibers contract with the atrial wall during atrial systole. This action may contribute to maintaining the orifice open when the tendency is for closure, because of anular contraction at that time. Shortening of the anterior leaflet may also reduce the extent of its bulging into the atrium immediately after pressure crossover and hence during the isovolumetric phase of ventricular systole.

Left Atrial Wall and Anulus

The continuity between the posterior leaflet and the atrial wall is such that left atrial enlargement will cause that leaflet to be displaced posteriorly, with an effective reduction of the coaptation area with the anterior leaflet. This posterior displacement, by impairing the keystone effect, will increase the tension on the chordae tendineae. Moreover, the mobility of the leaflet is lost as it becomes stretched over its basal attachment.

The portion of the anulus to which the anterior mitral leaflet attaches is part of the fibrous skeleton of the heart, which has very limited movement. The posterior anulus, on the other hand, is devoid of fibrous tissue and is surrounded by the myocardium of the left atrium and ventricle, contraction of which constitutes the functional anatomical basis for anular movement. During ventricular systole a slight medial and dorsal movement of the fibrous anterior segment is produced by traction from the muscle bound posterior anulus. Contraction of this posterior segment results in an approximation of the posterior leaflet towards the anterior one, which effectively reduces the area that the leaflets must bridge to maintain competence. Maximal size of the anulus occurs in late ventricular diastole coinciding with the P wave of the electrocardiogram and therefore just prior to the onset of atrial systole. There is then a reduction of 20 to 40 percent of the original area of the mitral orifice (Fig. 1-9). One half to two thirds of this anular narrowing occurs during atrial systole and the remainder during ventricular contraction. Factors such as arrhythmias, the absence of atrial contraction, duration of the P-R interval, ventricular end-diastolic volume, and ejection fraction will influence the extent of anular narrowing. Marked atrial and ventricular enlargement will also decrease the respective contribution of atrial and ventricular systole to the diminution of the valvular ring.

Papillary Muscles and Chordae Tendineae

The papillary muscles share the innervation of the contiguous left ventricular wall and have their appropriate position in the contraction sequence. According to the observations of Tsakiris and associates,[13,13a] maximal shortening and elongation of the papillary muscles in dogs occurred 65 ± 6 milliseconds later than that of the muscle fibers of the left ventricular wall. Hence, papillary muscle contraction commenced after the start of ventricular ejection. During isovolumetric contraction and the early part of the ejection phase, the papillary muscles were still elongating. Conversely, they were still shortening during and immediately after the isovolumetric relaxation phase. The papillary muscles were thus shortest when the mitral valve was open, and they were lengthening at the time of valve closure. Papillary muscle elongation during isovolumetric ventricular contraction may facilitate mitral valve closure because the distance between the left ventricular free wall and the mitral leaflets is then bridged in order to allow coaptation. This functional role is in accord with the cineangiocardiographic observation that premature ventricular contractions result in mitral valve regurgitation when they occur in early or mid-diastole before

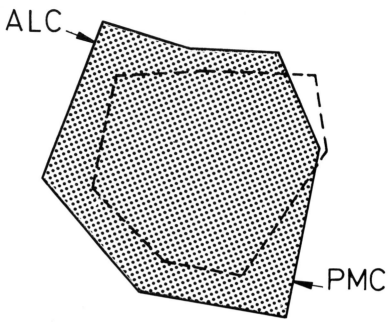

FIGURE 1-9. Movements of the mitral anulus during the cardiac cycle. The shaded area represents the size of the orifice in late diastole, just prior to the onset of atrial systole. The area enclosed by the broken line represents the surface area of the orifice at the end of ventricular systole. There is a reduction in orifice size of 35 percent between the two phases. ALC = anterolateral commissure; PMC = posteromedial commissure. (Adapted from Tsakiris et al,[13] with permission.)

adequate lengthening of the papillary muscles has taken place. Early in the ventricular ejection phase, the papillary muscles contract isometrically. This isometric contraction is necessary to maintain leaflet edge apposition during the rapid pressure and volume changes of the ejection period. Shortening of the papillary muscles during the late ejection phase contributes to the prevention of leaflet prolapse as the distance between the valve and the apex diminishes.

Anatomical and functional integrity of the chordae tendineae is essential to maintain valve competence, since they intervene between the papillary muscles and the leaflets. Rough zone chordae play a more important role in preventing leaflet prolapse than do commissural chordae. Amongst the former, strut chordae are essential pillars of the mitral valve mechanism. The role of the basal chordae of the posterior leaflet still requires clarification. They may be important in providing continuity between the left ventricular free wall and the posterior leaflet and anulus.

Left Ventricular Free Wall

The importance of atrial and ventricular contractility in narrowing the mitral anulus and hence contributing to the maintenance of valve competence has been discussed. Mitral regurgitation is known to occur with left ventricular dilatation. However, this is probably related more to the geometrical characteristics of the papillary muscles and to decreased contractility of the anulus than to the circumferential size of the latter. The papillary muscles arise from the ventricular wall, close to its apical zone. When they contract, they pull the chordae tendineae vertically, thus allowing the leaflets to appose. This action is facilitated by the juxtaposition of the two halves of the papillary muscles during systole. If this vertical alignment of the papillary muscles is lost owing to dilatation of the ventricle, the traction on the chordae tendineae is lateralized, thus mechanically inappropriate, and leaflet apposition may not be maintained.

Opening of the Mitral Valve

In addition to the traditional concept of passive opening of the mitral valve based on a pressure difference, functional anatomical factors contribute to optimal flow through the valve orifice. Shortening of the papillary muscles during and after the isovolumetric ventricular relaxation period encourages the separation of the two leaflets. Moreover, an unrestricted flow of blood into the ventricle is facilitated by relaxation of the anulus. The extent of dilatation will depend partly on the duration of diastole, but maximal size of the orifice is present just before atrial systole. Eccentric change in the shape of the anulus, caused principally by movement of its posterior portion, shifts the less mobile posterior leaflet away from the centre of the mitral orifice and contributes further to unimpeded flow. The functional role of the reduction in size of the leaflets caused by intrinsic contraction during late diastole requires confirmation. The muscle fibers in the anterior mitral leaflet appear to be atrial in origin and would thus be activated simultaneously with those of the left atrium. Contraction of these fibers may remove the leaflets from the path of blood at the time when flow into the left ventricle is augmented by atrial systole.

Movements of the ventricular wall during early diastole may also play a role in the opening of the mitral valve. Traditionally, it was accepted that the left ventricular volume does not change between aortic valve closure and the diastolic crossover point of the left ventricular and left atrial pressures. However, an increase in left ventricular volume in dogs has been observed in this phase by Ruttley and associates,[14] and this may be caused by the pre-inflow relaxation of the left ventricular free wall. Distinct shape changes accompany the increment in the cavitary volume during this early diastolic phase.[15] An increase in the base-to-apex distance of the left ventricle has been demonstrated by Fabian and Abrams[16] and was attributed to a degree of aortic regurgitation in early diastole. Hence, the changes in ventricular shape have been presumed to be the result of the volume changes rather than the cause. Whatever the mechanism, these alterations in the shape of the left ventricle could contribute, in part, to the early separation of the mitral valve leaflets before the diastolic pressure crossover point.

REFERENCES

1. LAM, JHC, RANGANATHAN, N, WIGLE, ED, AND SILVER, MD: *Morphology of the human mitral valve. I. Chordae tendineae: A new classification.* Circulation 41:449–458, 1970.

2. RANGANATHAN, N, LAM, JHC, WIGLE, ED, AND SILVER, MD: *Morphology of the human mitral valve. II. The valve leaflets.* Circulation 41:459–467, 1970.

3. PERLOFF, JK, AND ROBERTS, WC: *The mitral apparatus. Functional anatomy of mitral regurgitation.* Circulation 46:227–239, 1972.

4. EDWARDS, JE, AND BURCHELL, HB: *Pathologic anatomy of mitral insufficiency.* Proc Staff Meet Mayo Clin 33:497–509, 1958.

5. DU PLESSIS, LA, AND MARCHAND, P: *The anatomy of the mitral valve and its associated structures.* Thorax 19:221–227, 1964.

6. RUSTED, IE, SCHEIFLEY, CH, AND EDWARDS, JE: *Studies of the mitral valve. I. Anatomic features of the normal mitral valve and associated structures.* Circulation 6:825–831, 1952.

7. COOPER, T, NAPOLITANO, LM, FITZGERALD, MJT, MOORE, KE, DAGGET, WM, WILLMAN, VL, SONNENBLICK, EH, AND HANCON, CR: *Structural basis of cardiac valvular function.* Arch Surg 93:767–771, 1966.

8. WILLIAMS, TH: *Mitral and tricuspid valve innervation.* Br Heart J 26:105, 1964.

9. SONNENBLICK, EH, NAPOLITANO, LM, DAGGET, WM, AND COOPER, T: *An intrinsic neuro-muscular basis for mitral valve motion in the dog.* Circ Res 21:9–15, 1967.

10. BUCCINO, LRA, SONNENBLICK, EH, COOPER, T, AND BRAUNWALD, E: *Direct positive inotropic effect of acetylcholine on myocardium.* Circ Res 19:1097–1108, 1966.

11. BROCK, RC: *The surgical and pathological anatomy of the mitral valve.* Br Heart J 14:489–513, 1952.

12. BECKER, AE, AND DE WIT, APM: *Mitral valve apparatus. A spectrum of normality relevant to mitral valve prolapse.* Br Heart J 42:680–689, 1979.

13. TSAKIRIS, AG, VON BERNUTH, G, RASTELLI, GC, BOURGEOIS, MJ, TITUS, JL, AND WOOD, EH: *Size and motion of the mitral valve annulus in anesthetized intact dogs.* J Appl Physiol 30:611–618, 1971.

13a. TSAKIRIS, AG, GORDON, DA, PADIYAR, R, AND FRECHETTE, D: *Relation of mitral valve opening and closure to left atrial and ventricular pressure in the intact dog.* Am J Physiol 234(2):H146–151, 1978.

14. RUTTLEY, MS, ADAMS, DF, COHN, PF, AND ABRAMS, HL: *Shape and volume changes during "isovolumetric relaxation" in normal and asynergic ventricles.* Circulation 50:306–316, 1974.

15. ALTIERI, PI, LEIGHTON, RF, AND WILT, SM: *The segmental early relaxation phenomenon (SERP): A normal type of left ventricular wall motion.* Clin Res 21:397, 1973.

16. FABIAN, CE, AND ABRAMS, HL: *Reflux through normal aortic valves.* Invest Radiol 3:178–183, 1968.

BIBLIOGRAPHY

ORMISTON, JA, SHAH, PM, TEI, C, AND WONG, M: *Size and motion of the mitral valve annulus in man. I. A two-dimensional echocardiographic method and findings in normal subjects.* Circulation 64:113–120, 1981.

ORMISTON, JA, SHAH, PM, TEI, C, AND WONG, M: *Size and motion of the mitral valve annulus in man. II. Abnormalities in mitral valve prolapse.* Circulation 65:713–719, 1982.

ROBERTS, WC: *Morphologic features of the normal and abnormal mitral valve.* Am J Cardiol 51:1005–1028, 1983.

STEFFENS, TG, AND HAGAN, AD: *Role of chordae tendineae in mitral valve opening: Two-dimensional echocardiographic evidence.* Am J Cardiol 53:153–156, 1984.

VERED, Z, MELTZER, RS, BENJAMIN, P, MOTRO, M, AND NEUFELD, HN: *Prevalence and significance of false tendons in the left ventricle as determined by echocardiography.* Am J Cardiol 53:330–332, 1984.

WESTABY, S, KARP, RB, BLACKSTONE, EH, AND BISHOP, SP: *Adult human valve dimensions and their surgical significance.* Am J Cardiol 53:552–556, 1984.

2

THE CARDIAC CYCLE AND BRIEF COMMENTS ON CLINICAL EXAMINATION

THE CARDIAC CYCLE AND HEART SOUNDS

Fundamental to the learning of auscultation, and to the understanding of virtually all other aspects of clinical cardiology, is a sound knowledge of the configuration of the atrial, ventricular, and arterial pressure tracings and their time relationships to the opening and closing of the heart valves, to the heart sounds, and also to the simultaneously recorded electrocardiogram (Fig. 2-1). Although there is ongoing discussion on the mechanism of production of some heart sounds, certain principles can be accepted and form a basis for the practice of clinical cardiology. In the normal heart, contraction takes place in the order of the right atrium, left atrium, left ventricle, and finally right ventricle. Because of pressure, volume, and anatomical differences between events on the left and right sides of the heart, there are changes in the timing and intensity of sound events. Nevertheless, the principles of sound production in the right side of the heart are similar to those in the left. For purposes of simplification, pressure and sound events in the left side of the heart will be considered on their own and in some detail.

During the upstroke of the R wave of the simultaneous electrocardiogram, the left ventricular pressure starts rising and then crosses the left atrial pressure, at which point the mitral valve closes and the isovolumetric phase of left ventricular contraction commences. It is possible that a soft component of the first sound (M) occurs at pressure crossover, but this has little clinical significance.[1] As the left ventricular pressure continues to rise, the coapted and "closed" mitral leaflets billow back into the left atrium producing the left atrial C wave, at the peak of which the chordae and leaflets of the mitral valve come under maximal tension and produce the major left-sided (mitral) component of the first heart sound (M1). The intensity and timing of the mitral component of the first heart sound could be affected by several factors:

1. M1 will be louder if the *leaflets are relatively wide open* at the onset of ventricular contraction, and therefore have a longer excursion before apposing and billowing into the atrium to the point at which M1 occurs. A short PR interval, mitral stenosis, and a left atrial myxoma provide the clinical set-up for that to occur.

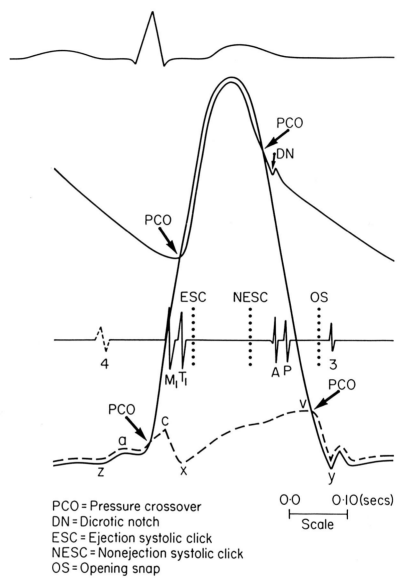

Cardiac cycle with abnormal heart sounds

PCO = Pressure crossover
DN = Dicrotic notch
ESC = Ejection systolic click
NESC = Nonejection systolic click
OS = Opening snap

FIGURE 2-1. Diagrammatic representation of left-sided (aortic, left ventricular, and left atrial) pressure and sound events. See text.

2. A relatively *rapid rise of left ventricular pressure* such as occurs during good left ventricular function, emotion, exercise, or tachycardia will also increase the intensity of M1.

3. The *functional anatomical status of leaflets and chordae.* If the chordae are relatively elongated and the leaflets mobile and voluminous, then maximum billow of the leaflets will be greater and more delayed than would normal leaflets. This would increase the intensity and slightly delay M1. Hence, and contrary to usual teaching, M1 may be loud in pure mitral regurgitation. Rigid and immobile leaflets, whether associated with mitral stenosis or predominant mitral regurgitation, will result in a soft M1. If part of a leaflet is flail, the billowing back of the leaflets into the left atrium will be asynchro-

nous and two components of the mitral first sound may be recorded and be clinically audible. The relative inadequacy of incompetent leaflets to halt the "regurgitant" flow tends to decrease the intensity of M1 despite mobile leaflets.

The rate of rise of ventricular pressure may be observed to increase after the peak of the left atrial C wave, especially if the leaflets are voluminous, and the mitral valve is competent or nearly so (see Chapter 5). Prior to the peak of the C wave, the billowing back of the mitral leaflets results in a slightly larger left ventricular cavity than if the contracting left ventricle had had a rigid mitral mechanism.

The left ventricular pressure continues to rise until it exceeds the aortic pressure and opens the aortic valve, thus ending the isovolumetric contraction phase and starting the left ventricular ejection phase. The opening of the aortic valve is silent under normal circumstances. With a bicuspid aortic valve, aortic stenosis with mobile cusps, and possibly with a dilated ascending aorta, an aortic ejection click may be audible.

Left-sided clicking sounds, probably arising from mitral chordae, may occur at any time during the ejection phase but are commonly in mid-late systole. Although the mitral valve mechanism may have only minimal pathology to cause these sounds, they are regarded as abnormal. In order to differentiate them from aortic or pulmonary ejection sounds, these chordal sounds are referred to as nonejection systolic clicks.

The ejection period of left ventricular contraction continues until the ventricle relaxes. Thereafter, the left ventricular pressure decreases until it falls below the aortic pressure, at which time the aortic valve closes. The apposed aortic leaflets billow towards the left ventricular cavity, causing the dicrotic notch on the aortic pressure trace and resulting in the aortic component of the second heart sound. The aortic component (A2) will be relatively loud if the closing pressure is high, as in systemic hypertension, or if the ascending aorta is dilated, which allows increased transmission of the sound. It will be relatively soft if the closing pressure is low, as in hypotension from any cause and including aortic stenosis, if the leaflets are rigid (as in calcific aortic stenosis) or if they fail to coapt (as in hemodynamically significant aortic regurgitation). With closure of the aortic valve, the isovolumetric phase of left ventricular relaxation starts and continues until the declining left ventricular pressure crosses the left atrial V wave, at which time the mitral valve opens. Opening of the normal mitral valve is silent, but a mitral "opening snap" may be heard if the leaflets are fibrosed but retain a degree of mobility. A mitral opening snap may be present with predominant mitral regurgitation, and the occurrence of this sound is not, in itself, an indication of tight mitral stenosis. It simply indicates that the mitral leaflets are abnormal and that a degree of mobility, especially of the anterior leaflet, is retained.

The descending limb of the left atrial V wave and the declining left ventricular pressure now fall to the y points of these descents. At this point the rapid filling phase ends and vibrations are set up, either in the left ventricular wall or in the chordae of the mitral valve, which result in a third heart sound. The left ventricular myocardium is now less compliant and some rise in pressure may occur to the so-called anular ascent wave or H wave. Left ventricular filling is now slower, and the leaflets move towards closure. The mechanism of the early diastolic sound of constrictive pericarditis is similar to that of a third heart sound, but the former sound occurs earlier because of very rapid filling of the small ventricular cavity. It is also louder and of a higher pitch because of the sudden decrease in compliance of the left ventricle as it is resisted by the thickened and restricted pericardium. In constrictive pericarditis, there is a rapid rise of the anular ascent wave, now the beginning of the so-called plateau of the diastolic pressure (Fig. 2-2).

It is rare for any other sounds to occur during diastole until the onset of left atrial systole of the next complex. Occasionally, however, clicks with variable timing

---

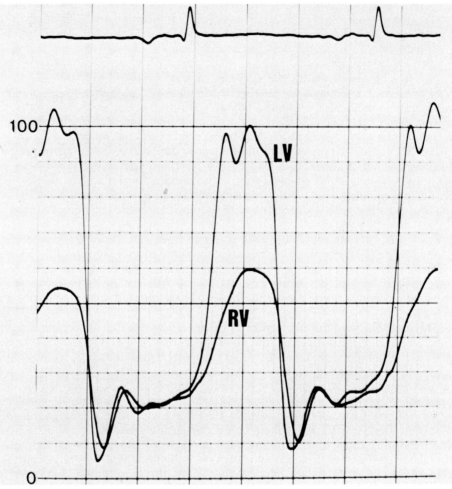

FIGURE 2-2. Simultaneous right (RV) and left (LV) ventricular pressures (mmHg) in a 16-year-old girl with tuberculous constrictive pericarditis showing similar pressures in diastole and the typical "dip and plateau" pattern.

are heard in diastole and have been recorded in mitral valve prolapse. In my experience, these are usually similar in timing to a third heart sound but are of much higher pitch. I have observed them in some patients with calcific aortic stenosis and postulate that they result from calcification of mitral chordae. I therefore consider that they have a similar mechanism of origin as a third heart sound.

In the normal heart with a normal PR interval, atrial systole contributes to a low-pitched component of the first heart sound that may be both audible and recordable on a phonocardiogram. This sound occurs with or immediately after the Q wave of the next QRS complex and should not be confused with the audible atrial sound, which precedes the Q wave and which, in my experience, is never present in normal hearts. An atrial sound will occur earlier, in relation to the onset of the P wave of the electrocardiogram, when the left ventricle is relatively less compliant and therefore the pathological state "worse." An early atrial sound can be heard and recorded later and thus closer to the first heart sound (Fig. 2-3) when hypertension is treated or when there is improvement of left ventricular function in ischemic heart disease. An audible atrial sound is an extremely sensitive sign of left ventricular dysfunction. It is often present in the early stages of acute myocardial infarction when other evidence of infarction, such as the electrocardiogram, may be indefinite. With improve-

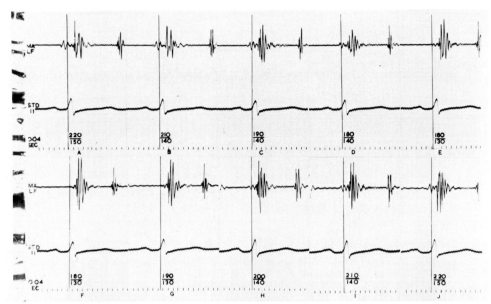

FIGURE 2-3. Serial phonocardiograms (*A–J*) taken during acute reduction of the blood pressure in a patient with malignant hypertension. An injection of 5 mg of pentolinium tartrate (Ansolysen) was given intravenously after the control tracing (*A*) had been taken. Records *B–F* were taken as the blood pressure fell, with the patient sitting in a semi-upright position in a cardiac bed. Records *G–J* were taken as the patient was gradually lowered into a recumbent position and as the blood pressure rose. The atrial sound approaches and disappears into the first sound as the pressure falls and moves out into a presystolic position as the pressure rises. (From Kincaid-Smith, P and Barlow, JB: *The atrial sound in hypertension and ischemic heart disease.* Br Heart J 21:479–490, 1959, with permission.)

ment of cardiac status, the atrial sound moves towards the major component of the next first heart sound, until it becomes indistinguishable from a so-called atrial component of the first sound (Fig. 2-4). An atrial sound is obviously more easily audible if the PR interval is relatively long. Soft atrial sounds may be recorded with an abnormally long PR interval or third-degree heart block (Fig. 2-5) in an otherwise normal heart and are occasionally audible during diastole. These sounds should not be con-

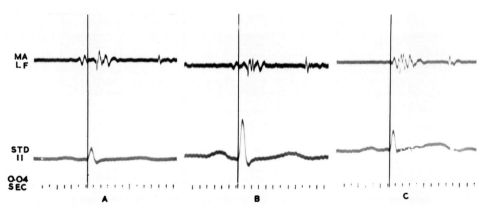

FIGURE 2-4. Serial phonocardiograms taken at 10-day intervals following an acute myocardial infarction in a patient with normal blood pressure. The atrial sound moves towards the first sound (*B*) and becomes incorporated as an atrial component of the first sound (*C*). (From Kincaid-Smith, P and Barlow, JB: *The atrial sound in hypertension and ischemic heart disease.* Br Heart J 21:479–490, 1959, with permission.)

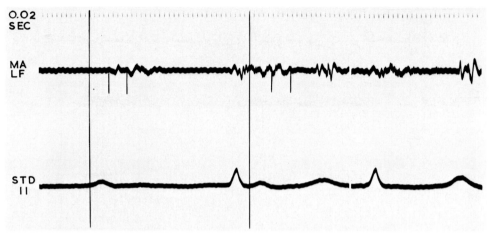

FIGURE 2-5. Phonocardiogram in a patient with complete heart block demonstrating two components of the atrial sound. A long vertical line is drawn through the beginning of the P wave, and the short vertical lines show the commencement of the two components of the atrial sound. It can be seen that the second component disappears when atrial contraction occurs during ventricular systole. The tracing on the right shows a flat base line between the first and second heart sounds when no P wave is present. (From Barlow, JB: *Some observations on the atrial sound.* S Afr Med J 34:887–892, 1986, with permission.)

fused with the short mid-diastolic murmur, first described by Rytand,[2] in cases of complete heart block and some calcification of the mitral anulus.

Sound events arising in the right side of the heart have similar mechanism to those in the left. Billowing following closure of the tricuspid leaflet coincides with the peak of the right atrial C wave and the onset of the second major component of the first heart sound. This tricuspid component (T1) can be heard at the lower sternal border in most normal subjects. It is slightly delayed and louder with an atrial septal defect and is an important physical sign of that entity. T1 is usually very delayed and loud in Ebstein's anomaly because of the markedly voluminous tricuspid leaflet in that condition. The loud delayed tricuspid component of the first heart sound in Ebstein's anomaly is sometimes referred to as a "sail sound."

Pulmonary ejection sounds occur with mild abnormalities of that valve, pulmonary stenosis, or dilatation of the pulmonary artery. Prominent pulmonary ejections clicks are heard in pulmonary hypertension from any cause. Idiopathic dilatation of the pulmonary artery is associated with a relatively late pulmonary ejection click, and it is probable that these cases have an abnormal pulmonary valve with minimal stenosis.

Nonejection clicks, due to tricuspid valve billow, have been recorded. A tricuspid opening snap may be associated with rheumatic tricuspid valve disease, and it is difficult to differentiate these clinically from mitral opening snaps. Earlier movement and increased intensity of a tricuspid opening snap during inspiration has occasionally been demonstrated phonocardiographically. A right-sided early diastolic sound of constrictive pericarditis may certainly occur (Fig. 2-6) and is often more prominent than the left-sided early diastolic sound. I consider that the physiological third heart sound is invariably of left-sided origin, but Leatham and colleagues[3] have postulated that a right-sided physiological third heart sound may also occur and that when both right- and left-sided sounds are present they mimic a short mid-diastolic murmur. Pathological third heart sounds arising on the right side of the heart are common when right ventricular pathology is present. A right-sided atrial sound is an important clinical sign of acute pulmonary embolism. The sound becomes louder and earlier with inspiration (Fig. 2-7), which would be expected since the right ventricle is relatively overloaded at that time.

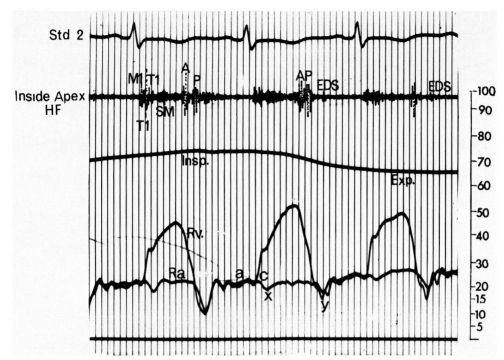

FIGURE 2-6. Simultaneous external phonocardiogram; right atrial (Ra) and right ventricular (Rv) pressures (mmHg) recorded in a young woman with constrictive pericarditis. The right-sided early diastolic sound (EDS) coincides with the y point of the atrial and ventricular pressures and is louder during inspiration (Insp). A typical "dip and plateau" pattern is shown in the pressure tracings. M1, T1 = mitral and tricuspid components of the first heart sound; A, P = aortic and pulmonary components of the second heart sound; SM = systolic murmur of tricuspid regurgitation. Exp = expiration. Time lines, 0.04 second.

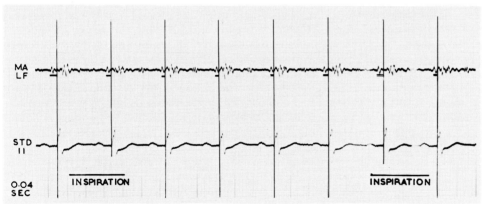

FIGURE 2-7. Phonocardiogram showing the effect of respiration on the timing of the right atrial sound in cor pulmonale in a patient who had had an acute pulmonary embolus. The atrial sound is more widely separated from the first sound in inspiration than in expiration. The maximum effect is seen in early inspiration. The time marking refers to the smaller subdivisions only just visible. The larger clear markings are at 0.2-second intervals. MA = mitral area; LF = low-frequency. (From Kincaid-Smith, P and Barlow, JB: *The atrial sound in hypertension and ischemic heart disease.* Br Heart J 21:479–490, 1959, with permission.)

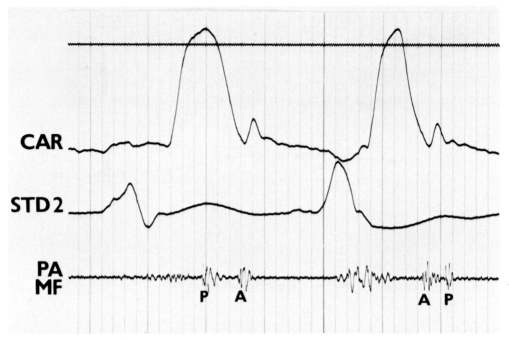

FIGURE 2-8. Simultaneous external carotid tracing (CAR), electrocardiogram, and phonocardiogram recorded at the pulmonary area (PA) in a 66-year-old woman with ischemic heart disease and left bundle branch block (LBBB). The second heart sound is completely reversed (so-called paradoxical splitting) in the first complex (LBBB). With an atrial ectopic beat and aberrant conduction (RBBB pattern) the second heart sound is widely split. The dicrotic notch of the carotid tracing identifies the aortic component of the second sound.

Another of Leatham's major contributions to clinical auscultation was his emphasis on the importance of assessment of the two components of the second sound.[4] Variations in intensity, position, and therefore the character of the "splitting" of the second sound (Fig. 2-8) are the "key to auscultation" of the heart. Patterns of abnormal variations of the second heart sound are summarized diagrammatically in Figure 2-9. Although reversed (paradoxical) splitting of the second heart sound is well recognized in hemodynamically significant aortic stenosis and in some patients with complete left bundle branch block, little attention has been given to a modified form of this (Fig. 2-10), which we have called partial reversed splitting.[5] It is, understandably, more common than reversed splitting but not as easy to detect. The pulmonary component occurs after the aortic component in inspiration but precedes it in expiration. Thus, the second sound is fairly narrowly reduplicated during both phases of respiration. In moderate aortic stenosis, reversed splitting has a fairly constant relationship to respiration. In patent ductus arteriosus and hypertrophic cardiomyopathy, the partial reversed splitting is very variable and the second sound sometimes appears single, whereas at other times it is fairly widely reduplicated during any phase of respiration. The depth of respiration, mild straining, and other factors seem to affect the splitting of the second sound in both hypertrophic cardiomyopathy and patent ductus. Nevertheless, the abnormal behavior of the second sound is an important clinical sign in both these conditions.

CARDIAC MURMURS

All heart murmurs should be related to the cardiac cycle and, in most instances, are readily understandable on the basis of turbulence being produced at a valve or at an

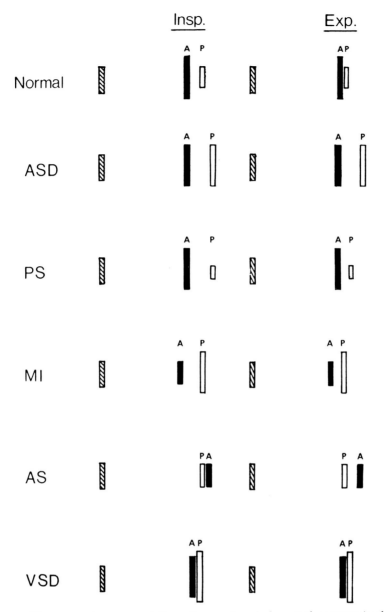

FIGURE 2-9. Diagrammatic representation of normal and abnormal patterns in the respiratory variation of the second heart sound. A = aortic component; P = pulmonary component; ASD = atrial septal defect; PS = pulmonary stenosis; MI = mitral incompetence; AS = aortic stenosis; VSD = ventricular septal defect.

abnormal communication between two chambers, two vessels, or a chamber and a vessel with a pressure difference. Functional anatomical factors may prevent a murmur from lasting throughout the time interval during which the pressure difference exists. Examples are the short "atypical" systolic murmur of a small muscular ventricular septal defect and the late systolic murmur of mild mitral regurgitation associated with mitral valve prolapse. In both instances, "regurgitation" from the left ventricle is limited by functional anatomical factors. Murmurs will be discussed more fully under specific conditions in later chapters.

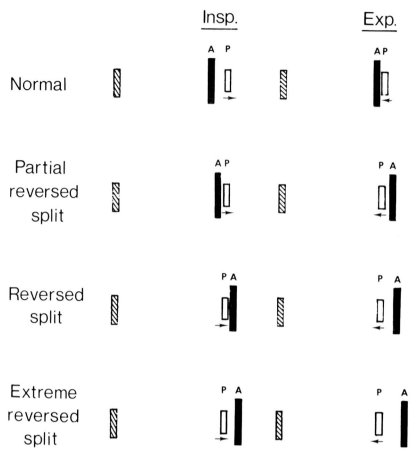

FIGURE 2-10. Reversed and partially reversed splitting of the second heart sound. *Arrows* indicate the direction of movement of P during expiration and inspiration.

CARDIAC CATHETERIZATION

Our understanding of normal and abnormal hemodynamics and of clinical cardiology in general has been made possible by cardiac catheterization. It was responsible for our learning to recognize many forms of cardiac disease, to clarify their severity, and to assess the results of surgical treatment. In my experience, there has often been difficulty in deciding which patients should be subjected to cardiac catheterization. Cardiac catheterization is a relatively minor invasive procedure but has a risk, albeit small in most cases, of morbidity and mortality. The large majority of patients with clinical evidence and sometimes echocardiographic confirmation of secundum atrial septal defect, patent ductus arteriosus, hemodynamically significant mitral stenosis or regurgitation, mitral valve prolapse, aortic stenosis, and many other conditions can be treated correctly and with confidence, whether medically or surgically, without catheterization data. In our unit many valve replacements for rheumatic heart disease or bacterial endocarditis in black patients are emergency procedures, and these patients are seldom catheterized. We have not found it mandatory to catheterize more than 10 percent of all patients referred for elective valve replacement. The cardiac surgeons with whom I work expect an accurate diagnosis prior to surgery and, although they are academically orientated, it is of little interest to them in what manner the diagnosis is obtained. Clearly, they cannot perform optimal coronary artery bypass grafts without having seen technically excellent selective coronary arteriograms; but this does not apply to valve replacements, provided they have the assurance that the relevant valve lesion is hemodynamically significant. Most valvular lesions can be very accurately assessed clinically and, in some instances, confirmed on echocardiography. The contribution to the individual patient of conclusions drawn from cardiac catheterization data is determined by the expertise of the operator and, more importantly, by the operator's interpretation of the results in the context of the patient's situation. For example, there may be only a small pressure difference across the aortic valve in tight calcific aortic stenosis with marked left ventricular dysfunction; gradients across both valves in combined aortic and mitral stenosis are considerably decreased if the patient has been dehydrated by overenthusiastic diuretic therapy; the assessment of the severity of mitral regurgitation, both on the left atrial pressures and on the cineangiogram, depends to a large extent on the size of the left atrial cavity.

Roberts[6] made a plea for routine preoperative cardiac catheterization. One of his reasons was the importance of the surgeon's knowing whether associated coronary artery disease is present in patients over 50 years of age, in most Western countries. I have reservations about that. If a 65-year-old man has tight aortic stenosis with breathlessness, syncope, and even angina, is it always relevant to know whether he has some coronary artery stenosis? Our operative results in such patients have been excellent with aortic valve replacement alone. If the left ventricle is small and the aortic stenosis very tight, then significant coronary artery disease is unlikely. If the aortic stenosis is less tight and the left ventricle dilated, aortic valve replacement is still indicated. Even if associated coronary artery disease is demonstrated in such cases, a decision that combined aortic valve replacement and coronary artery bypass grafting will give a better result should depend on many factors, and much hard data are still unavailable. It is readily conceded that preoperative catheterization data can be highly contributory as a "base-line of information to which postoperative data can be compared,"[6] but this is most applicable when a medical center is systematically addressing itself to a research project such as the assessment of a new prosthetic valve, of postoperative myocardial function, or of any other meaningful project. I consider it relevant to clarify whether catheterization is indicated for the benefit of a specific patient or whether the data obtained will be available, and ever used, for an improved understanding of that and similar patients' cardiac disease. I believe that it is often unnecessary in fulfilling a routine clinical commitment to individual patients.

REPORTING INTRACARDIAC PRESSURES AT CARDIAC CATHETERIZATION

Much information can be obtained from the wave form of the intracardiac pressure tracings, and it is my plea that these be described in more detail, both for routine cardiac catheterization reports as well as for the scientific literature. Reporting only the peaks of the A and V waves of an atrial tracing omits important information relating to the depths of the x and y descents, as well as the level of the so-called slow filling wave during mid-diastole. Furthermore, a report, for example, of a right ventricular pressure as 40/3–15 mmHg does not make it clear which points on the pressure tracing are being reported. Some cardiologists believe that the end-diastolic pressure in a ventricular tracing should be measured after the A wave or immediately before the rise in the ventricular pressure, but those levels depend on the PR interval and will necessarily be higher when the PR interval is short.

If atrial tracings were routinely reported as a,c,v/x,y,z and ventricular tracings as peak systole/y,z,a, then the reader would know, in nearly all instances, the configuration of the wave forms and would be able to visualize a gradient across an atrioventricular valve (Fig. 2-11). We take the z point as the pressure immediately before the A wave if sinus rhythm is present, or immediately before the rising ventricular pressure in atrial fibrillation.

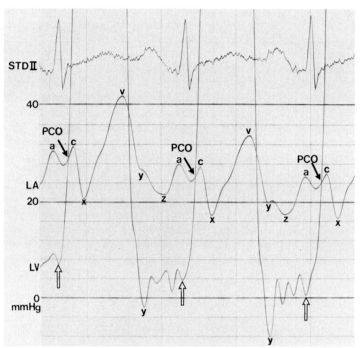

FIGURE 2-11. Simultaneous left atrial (LA) and left ventricular (LV) pressures in a 53-year-old woman with tight pliable mitral stenosis in sinus rhythm. *Open arrows* mark onset of ventricular systole. PCO = pressure crossover.

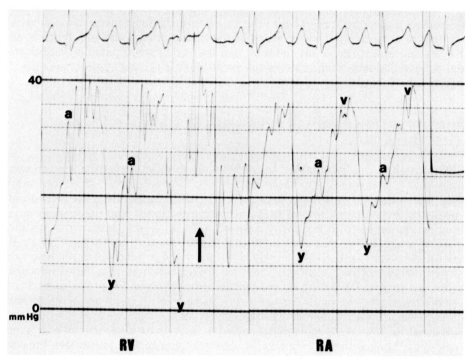

FIGURE 2-12. Withdrawal pressure tracing from right ventricle (RV) to right atrium (RA) in a 26-year-old man with a traumatic ventricular septal defect and marked tricuspid regurgitation. *Arrow* indicates transition between the chambers. The right atrial tracing is "ventricularized," and there is loss of the x descent.

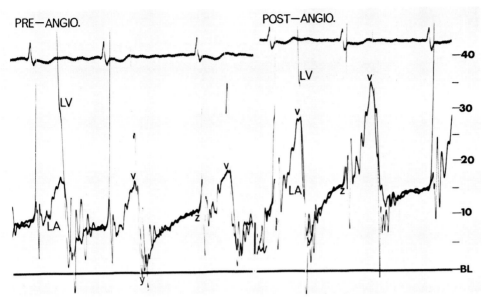

FIGURE 2-13. Simultaneous left atrial (LA) and left ventricular (LV) pressures in a 53-year-old man with severe mitral regurgitation due to ruptured chordae tendineae. There is a steep rise in the anular ascent wave, with higher end-diastolic and V wave pressures postangiography (POST-ANGIO). PRE-ANGIO = preangiography.

Abnormalities or variations of the pressure tracings are of much diagnostic significance. The right atrial x descent disappears in marked tricuspid regurgitation (Fig. 2-12). When the anular ascent wave is prominent, such as in acute mitral regurgitation with a relatively noncompliant ventricle (Fig. 2-13) or constrictive pericarditis (see Fig. 2-2), this reading can be reported specifically. A marked tachycardia often makes it difficult to assess the pressure tracings in diastole. In such instances, it is useful to create a ventricular extrasystole with the catheter in order to observe the wave form during the compensatory pause. This may be very contributory, for example, in patients with severe aortic regurgitation and premature mitral valve closure (Fig. 2-14).

HISTORY AND CLINICAL EXAMINATION

Only a few general comments on history taking and clinical examination will here be made. There will be more detailed discussion in later chapters when specific conditions are considered.

HISTORY TAKING

Racial and cultural differences and language problems must always be borne in mind when obtaining a history. The use of an interpreter makes history taking more time consuming and tedious, and the information obtained is often inaccurate or misleading because of important omissions and subtle nuances of language. There may be basic differences in customs and concepts as to what constitutes good manners, which may conflict with accurate history taking. It has been my experience, for example, that many Black patients in Africa, especially children, will answer a question in the affirmative because the patient considers that it is polite so to do.

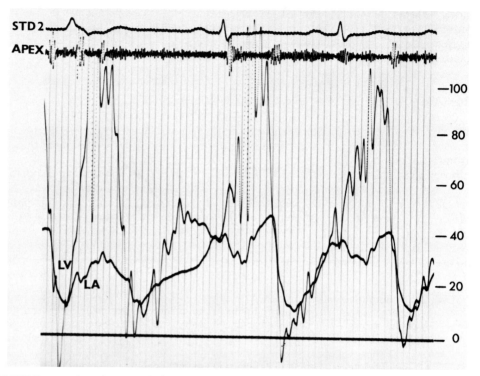

FIGURE 2-14. Simultaneous left atrial (LA) and left ventricular (LV) pressures in a 57-year-old man with gross aortic regurgitation due to prolapse of the right coronary cusp. There is premature closure of the mitral valve in early diastole, and the left ventricular diastolic pressure clearly exceeds that of the left atrium in the longer diastole following an ectopic beat.

With the exception of patients who consult a doctor for a routine examination, for insurance purposes, or for an examination prior to employment, most patients are symptomatic and are concerned about themselves. The doctor should bear this in mind and always try to alleviate the patient's anxiety. The clinical examination, in fact, begins while the history is being taken. Dyspnea, anxiety, and pain are usually readily apparent. Symptoms of heart disease are somewhat limited in number and should be relatively easy to assess, but a few comments are pertinent.

Dyspnea

This is a most important and probably the most common symptom of heart disease. Although the majority of patients are aware of being dyspneic, a few confuse it with tiredness. Occasionally, even while patients are observed to be tachypneic owing to pulmonary venous hypertension, they may deny an awareness of breathlessness. Breathlessness from heart disease can usually be differentiated from hyperventilation because of the constant relationship to exercise and aggravation by lying flat (orthopnea). Patients who complain of dyspnea but are unaware of any difference whether they sit up or lie flat usually have hyperventilation. Paroxysmal nocturnal dyspnea remains somewhat mystical, and, to my knowledge, the mechanism has not been satisfactorily explained. The phrase is often misused and it should not be applied to the orthopneic patient who goes to sleep on five pillows, wakes up breathless in the recumbent position, and improves rapidly on sitting up. Patients with true paroxysmal nocturnal dyspnea are comfortable when they go to sleep and may even have been unaware of dyspnea on exercise. Increased intravascular fluid volume during recumbency and sleep as well as an emotional dream may be factors that contribute to the episode. A sudden increase in return of blood to the right side of the heart after muscular contraction during sleep is probably important. Paroxysmal nocturnal dyspnea is essentially a symptom that reflects left-sided heart disease.

Chest Pain

The most important and probably the most frequent cause of severe chest pain that persists for more than a few seconds or minutes is myocardial ischemia. Both pericardial and esophageal pain can be central and severe. Pericardial pain may vary with position, be aggravated by swallowing, and have an association with a pyrexial disease or other condition (including acute orchitis); the onset and offset of the pain are usually atypical for myocardial ischemia. Esophageal pain may follow a dietary indiscretion or have other gastrointestinal associations. The severe pain of an acute dissecting aneurysm of the aorta (Fig. 2-15) is difficult to differentiate from acute myocardial ischemia, and dissection is sometimes accompanied by myocardial ischemia (Fig. 2-16) as a result of involvement of a coronary ostium or from acute aortic regurgitation. The chest pain associated with mitral valve prolapse and other so-called atypical chest pain syndromes can usually be distinguished from ischemic pain. Angina pectoris itself may be "atypical," and few cardiologists would claim that the distinction is always easy. A number of patients with myocardial ischemia

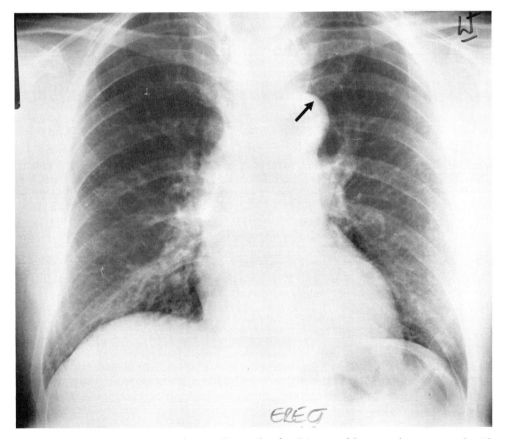

FIGURE 2-15. Posteroanterior chest radiograph of a 56-year-old man who presented with severe chest pain due to acute aortic dissection *(arrow)*. Several years previously, a nonejection systolic click and a retrosternal thyroid (clearly visible on the radiograph) had been detected.

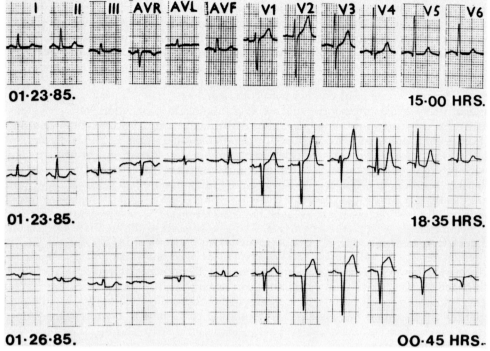

FIGURE 2-16. Serial electrocardiograms of the same patient as in Figure 2-15, who developed an extensive anterior myocardial infarction while under observation in the coronary care unit. Necropsy confirmed that this was due to dissection of the left main coronary artery. At no stage did he have aortic regurgitation.

deny ever having had chest pain. On direct questioning they will admit to a "gripping," "pressing," or "constricting" sensation, but deny that it is a pain.

Palpitations

This is essentially an awareness, usually unpleasant, of the heart's pumping action in the chest. Some patients are aware of virtually every ectopic beat, whereas others are completely oblivious of tachyarrhythmias. Patients may have difficulty in finding and counting their own pulses, an assessment of which would be contributory in elucidating the nature of the palpitations. It is important to establish whether they are regular or irregular, the approximate rate, the duration, and the mode of onset and offset. It is sometimes helpful to ask them to reflect the rate and irregularity of the palpitations by tapping a finger on the table.

Syncope

This is a transient loss of consciousness for a cardiovascular reason and is caused essentially by cerebral ischemia. It has to be distinguished from epilepsy and other neurological causes of loss of consciousness. A diagnostic problem arises in elderly people, many of whom have a combination of postural hypotension, vertebrobasilar disease, and cardiac arrhythmias. Syncope is an alarming and serious symptom, and much effort should be made to determine the cause. When a conduction defect or transient tachyarrhythmia is responsible, the symptom is a warning of a life-threatening situation. The most common cause of syncope, especially in places such as restaurants, aircraft, and at social functions, is the so-called vasovagal attack. This is usually preceded by nausea, sweating, and an awareness of impending loss of consciousness. The pulse is always weak and of small volume, but bradycardia is not invariable. Vasovagal attacks with a pulse rate of 70 beats per minute may occur. The frequency of vasovagal attacks in "public places" such as restaurants is of interest. It seems probable that these episodes result from overaction of the parasympathetic and are preceded by anxiety with concomitant activity of the sympathetic. The attack often occurs after a dinner and alcohol consumption when the subject has relaxed and is no longer anxious. A contributory factor may be dilatation of vessels and diversion of blood flow to the skin and abdominal viscera.

It is important to remember that acute myocardial infarction, commonly inferior infarction, may present in a similar manner to a benign vasovagal attack, especially in the elderly.

EXAMINATION OF THE CARDIOVASCULAR SYSTEM

Physical signs outside of the cardiovascular system may be important clues to the diagnosis. Most doctors are aware of the characteristics of Down's syndrome, but the features of Turner's syndrome or supra-aortic stenosis (Fig. 2-17) are sometimes overlooked. Patients with coarctation of the aorta, usually men, often have muscular upper extremities. An atrial septal defect is usual in the Holt-Oram syndrome (Fig. 2-18). Skeletal features of a narrow posteroanterior chest diameter due to the "straight-back" syndrome or a depressed sternum may be overlooked. These skeletal malformations are often a cause of loud pulmonary systolic murmurs, widely split heart sounds, and even tricuspid mid-diastolic murmurs. They may also be associated with mitral valve prolapse. Many tall patients have long fingers, but laxity of joints, as occurs in Marfan's syndrome, should be sought.

Before the cardiovascular system is examined, every patient should be examined for cyanosis, anemia, edema, and clubbing. Clubbing of the fingers without cyanosis suggests infective endocarditis or atrial myxoma, a much less common

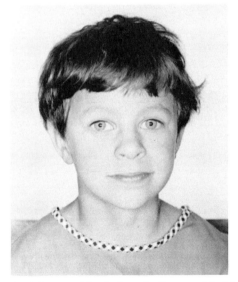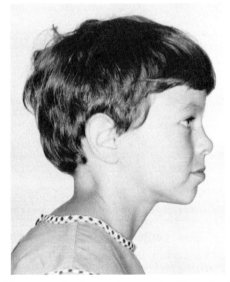

FIGURE 2-17. The facies of a 7-year-old girl with supravalvular aortic stenosis. (From Lachman, AS, Orsmond, GS, Zion, MM, Pocock, WA, and Barlow, JB: *Supravalvular aortic stenosis: A complex and variable entity.* S Afr Med J 46:23–28, 1972, with permission.)

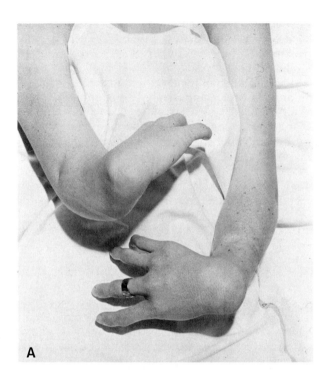

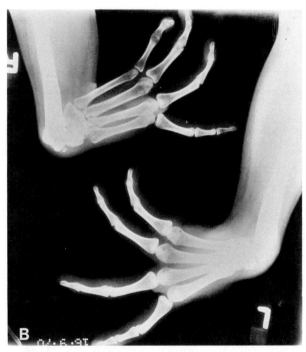

FIGURE 2-18. *A and B,* typical upper limb deformities of the Holt-Oram syndrome in a 19-year-old woman with a small atrial septal defect of the primum type and moderate mitral regurgitation.

entity. A patient without lung disease who has marked central cyanosis and clubbing (Fig. 2-19), but with a cardiovascular system that is normal on examination, will almost certainly have a congenital pulmonary arteriovenous fistula (Fig. 2-20). The only other possibilities are isolated drainage of the superior or inferior vena cava to the left atrium, but these are extremely rare and evidence of left ventricular enlargement may be apparent. Edema in infants manifests in the face and periorbital tissues and in the ambulant adult as bilateral swelling of the lower extremities. Mild edema in adult patients who have been lying in bed is first apparent on the posteromedial aspect of the thighs, and edema will be detected at that site before it is discernible over the sacrum. Anemia in nonpigmented or mildly pigmented patients can be detected clinically by assessing the color of the creases in the hyperextended palms. This sign is noncontributory in deeply pigmented patients, and the examiner has to rely on the color of the mucus membranes and conjunctivae. Jaundice is rare in cardiac disease but may occur with any cause of marked hepatic distension such as severe congestive cardiac failure, tricuspid regurgitation, or constrictive pericarditis. Cardiac "cirrhosis" is a misnomer. There is never destruction of the liver architecture nor regeneration of liver nodules. At worst, there is fibrosis around the central vein. Cardiac "cirrhosis," however severe, is always reversible if the hepatic venous hypertension can be relieved by appropriate treatment of the cardiac condition. Clubbing of the fingernails is detected not only by loss of the angle between the nail and the finger but also by the softness of the nail bed. My colleague, Leo Schamroth, who has had clubbing of the fingers himself, described a sign that we in Johannesburg call "Schamroth's sign." If the dorsal surfaces of the terminal phalanges of comparable fingers are placed together, a distinct aperture, usually diamond-shaped, is formed at the bases of the nailbeds. An early sign of clubbing is obliteration of this "window" (Fig. 2-21). In my experience, clubbing always disappears after successful treatment of infective endocarditis.

A nonproductive and irritating cough is an important sign of pulmonary venous hypertension. Patients seldom complain of the cough but concede on direct

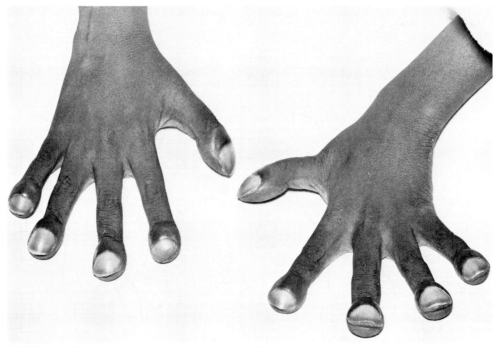

FIGURE 2-19. Marked clubbing in a 6-year-old boy who had severe cyanosis due to a congenital pulmonary arteriovenous fistula.

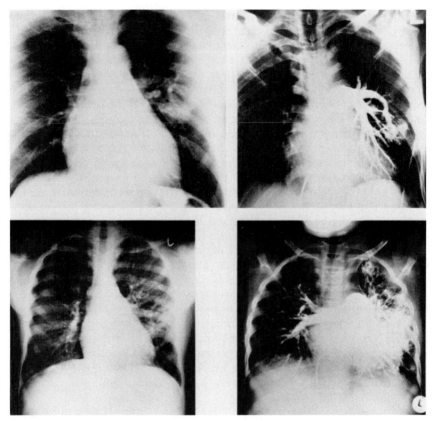

FIGURE 2-20. Posteroanterior chest radiographs and pulmonary angiograms of two patients with congenital pulmonary arteriovenous fistulae.

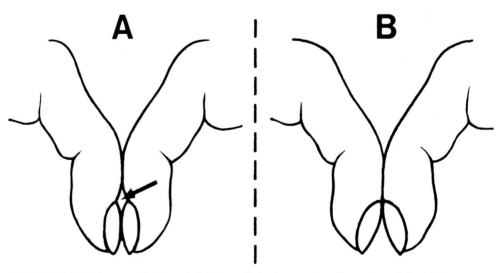

FIGURE 2-21. Schamroth's sign of clubbing of the fingers. For discussion of *A* and *B*, see text. (From Schamroth, L: *Personal experience.* S Afr Med J 50:297–300, 1976, with permission.)

questioning that they are aware of it and that it is worse when they lie flat. A dry cough may be the only physical sign of pulmonary venous hypertension.

THE PULSE

The pulse should be examined prior to the clinician knowing or suspecting the diagnosis. It is easy, for example, for the examiner to assess the pulse as "slow rising" if he or she knows that the patient suffers from tight aortic stenosis. All the pulses should be palpated and evaluated for volume and character. Cases of coarctation of the aorta, Takayashu's disease (Fig. 2-22), or previous aortic saddle embolus are missed because of failure to do this. Students are traditionally taught to assess the pulse for rate, rhythm, volume, character, and the state of the vessel wall.

Pulse Rate

Abnormalities of pulse rate should be assessed in the context of the situation. An anxious child or young adult may have a marked sinus tachycardia throughout the

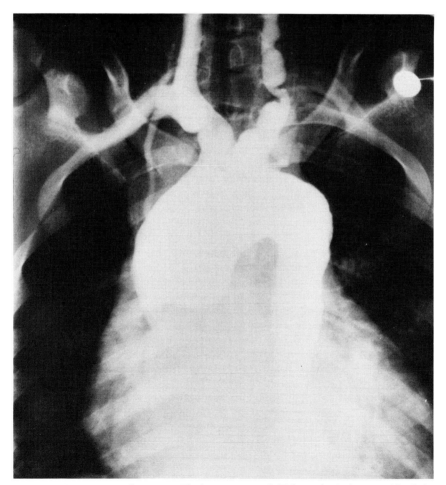

FIGURE 2-22. Aortogram of a young Black woman with Takayashu's disease. The left carotid artery shows marked irregularities in the lumen, and there is no opacification of the left subclavian artery. The ascending aorta is dilated, and the lumen of the descending aorta is irregular.

examination. A sustained sinus tachycardia, not due to anxiety, may be indicative of myocardial dysfunction, myocarditis, or pericardial effusion. Sinus tachycardia out of proportion to the pyrexia may be an early indication that the heart is involved in a viral illness or rheumatic fever. An unusually slow pulse (below 50 beats per minute), often associated with a marked sinus arrhythmia, is encountered in highly trained athletes.

Rhythm

Sinus arrhythmia in children and physically fit subjects is seldom difficult to detect. Requesting the patient to stop breathing without straining eliminates this irregularity of rhythm due to respiration. The true cardiac rate may be underestimated if the possibility of so-called dropped beats is not borne in mind. These result from underfilling of the left ventricle associated with an early ventricular ectopic beat or an irregular tachyarrhythmia such as atrial fibrillation. Dropped beats are best detected by simultaneous auscultation of the heart and palpation of the pulse.

Pulse Volume and Character

These are most meaningfully assessed together because they necessarily interrelate. The small-volume pulse of hypotension or mitral regurgitation is rapid rising, whereas the pulse in aortic stenosis is also of relatively small volume but is slow rising. The slow-rising pulse of calcific aortic stenosis in the elderly is often easier to detect in the carotid or femoral pulse. However, this important physical sign may be difficult to evaluate especially when the arterial walls are sclerotic and noncompliant. With left ventricular failure and aortic stenosis, the slow rise diminishes and is more difficult to detect. Tight subaortic stenosis in children or young adults may have an extremely small volume pulse, which is not always detectably slow rising.

Pulsus alternans is an uncommon sign in which the rhythm is regular but a relatively weaker beat alternates with a stronger one. It reflects severe left ventricular dysfunction and may be present for days, weeks, or longer, or it may occur for only a few beats after being initiated by a ventricular extrasystole. It is occasionally a notable feature after aortic or mitral valve replacement. The reason for pulsus alternans' manifesting so prominently after such surgery is not understood. Pulsus bigeminus also has alternating weaker and stronger beats, but this is due to a regularly occurring ventricular extrasystole and thus alternate relative underfilling and overfilling of the left ventricle. These two pulse abnormalities should not be confused.

Pulsus paradoxus should be suspected when there is an inspiratory reduction of arterial pressure exceeding about 6 mmHg. This is an arbitrary figure, however, and the significance is greater if the pulse pressure is small and less if the patient is hyperventilating. I consider it mandatory to request the patient to breathe deeply before a paradoxus is adjudged absent. In severe constrictive pericarditis (Fig. 2-23) or pericardial effusion, disappearance or diminution of the pulse during inspiration (Fig. 2-24A) can often be detected by palpation. In patients with lesser hemodynamic impairment, the patient should be asked to breathe deeply and the drop in systolic pressure during inspiration confirmed on a sphygmomanometer. Detection of pulsus paradoxus is important, and causes include bronchial asthma, acute severe pulmonary embolism, right ventricular infarction, cardiac tamponade, constrictive pericarditis, and left ventricular failure. Of all the causes of pulsus paradoxus, cardiac tamponade is the one most important to diagnose and to diagnose immediately. There are situations in which pulsus paradoxus will not be present despite severe tamponade. Aortic regurgitation is one of these, which I have personally experienced on several occasions, principally in cases of aortic dissection. Clearly, left ventricular filling does not decrease with inspiration during diastole, because of the aortic regur-

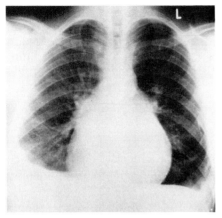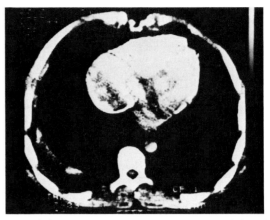

FIGURE 2-23. Posteroanterior chest radiograph *(left)* and computed tomograph (CT) *(right)* of a 26-year-old man with constrictive pericarditis. A thin line of calcification is visible on the left cardiac border, which the CT shows to be extensive and encasing the entire heart.

gitation. Reputedly, a large atrial septal defect is another condition, but I do not recall having observed that personally. It is understandable, however, that the free communication between the left and right sides of the heart at atrial level will equalize ventricular filling. A patient on mechanical ventilation, most importantly after cardiac surgery, will also not show a typical pulsus paradoxus despite cardiac tamponade.

The Jugular Venous Pulse

Assessment of the jugular venous pulse is extremely important, because it is essentially a reflection of the right atrial pressure. The first and most contributory observation is to determine whether or not the pressure is abnormally high. When the patient is reclining at about 45°, venous pulsation either may not be visible or may be seen for just a centimetre above the sternomanubrial angle. Distension of the external jugular vein, provided there is no local mechanical obstruction, can give a reflection of the mean right atrial pressure, but it is generally more accurate to assess pulsation of the internal jugular vein. The venous pulse can be identified by means of the so-called hepatojugular reflux, and the top level of the pulse can then be assessed. Although this sign is usually elicited by pressing on the liver, any abdominal compression will have the same effect. In addition to identifying the venous pulse, the hepatojugular reflux provides a clinical test for detecting incipient or mild congestive cardiac failure. Ducas and associates[7] found that abdominal compression applied in a standard way caused an increase in the height of the jugular venous pressure of at least 4.0 cm in patients with impaired ventricular function. Other methods often recommended to differentiate venous from arterial pulsation are of minor contribution or even misleading. For example, it is not correct to state that venous pulsation is not palpable because the systolic wave of tricuspid regurgitation is easily felt. The clinician should always be certain that he or she has found the top level of the venous pulsations. With constrictive pericarditis or gross right ventricular failure, the pressure may be so high that the patient has to sit at 90° or even to stand for the top level to be detected. A raised jugular venous pressure which reflects the right atrial pressure will always be associated with a distended liver, and systolic pulsation of the liver is invariable when severe tricuspid regurgitation is present. A very high venous pressure may cause puffiness of the face and congestion of the conjunctivae, especially when the patient lies flat. Proptosis has been observed in several patients with marked tricuspid regurgitation.

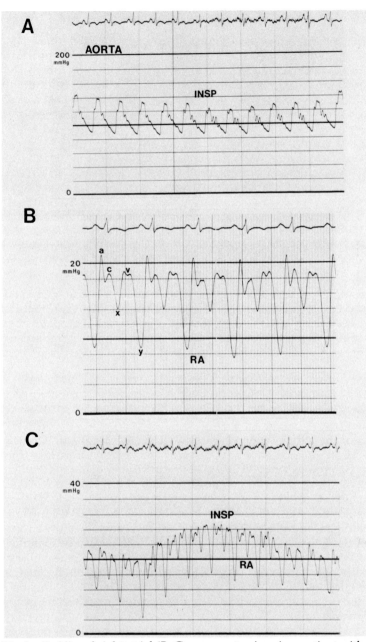

FIGURE 2-24. Aortic (*A*) and right atrial (*B*, *C*) pressure tracings in a patient with severe constrictive pericarditis. During inspiration (INSP), the aortic systolic pressure decreases by 20 mmHg (pulsus paradoxus). The right atrial (RA) pressure is considerably elevated and shows the typical configuration of constriction (*B*) with a positive Kussmaul's sign (*C*).

The right internal jugular pulsation is often easier to assess than the left. Sometimes the left is more distended and has diminished pulsation than the right because of partial obstruction due to an unfolded aorta. Distended jugular veins that are nonpulsatile cannot be explained on a cardiac basis and are due to mechanical obstruction such as occlusion of the superior vena cava.

Evaluation of the wave form of the jugular venous pulse may be contributory but is of less importance than to determine whether or not the level is raised. The A wave of the right internal jugular pulse precedes the arterial pulse and can be identified by palpating the left carotid artery in order to time the wave. Extremely prominent A waves may occur with tricuspid stenosis and right atrial myxoma. Any cause of resistance to right ventricular filling may result in an abnormally large A wave. Conditions causing such decreased compliance of the right ventricle include pulmonary stenosis, pulmonary hypertension, hypertrophic cardiomyopathy and subendocardial fibrosis. Giant A waves occurring synchronously with the carotid pulse are seen in nodal rhythm when the right atrium contracts against a closed tricuspid valve. Intermittent giant A waves, usually called "cannon" waves, depend on the same mechanism and will be seen in complete heart block and in some cases of ventricular tachycardia and ventricular extrasystoles.

The wave form of constrictive pericarditis is variable in relation to the prominence of the A wave and the depth, or absence, of the x descent. The invariable and characteristic feature of the jugular venous wave form of constrictive pericarditis is a rapid y descent (Fig. 2-24B), the nadir of which (y point) coincides with an early diastolic sound on auscultation and with a diastolic thrust of the right ventricle on palpation. This impulse is frequently mistimed as occurring in systole. It is felt best over or just to the left of the lower sternum. An inspiratory increase in the level of the jugular venous pressure (Kussmaul's sign) (Fig. 2-24C) reflects the impedance to filling of the right ventricle and is an important sign of pericardial constriction or effusion. Immediately after the y point, the systemic venous pressure rises rapidly to the start (see Fig. 2-6) of the diastolic plateau (H wave). The jugular veins and the liver thus expand at this time, and such expansion is clinically palpable, as demonstrated recently by Manga and colleagues.[8] This palpable impulse thus occurs fractionally later than the right ventricular diastolic impulse and the early diastolic sound.

Obese patients, those with thick muscular necks, or those in distress because of dyspnea or pain make clinical evaluation of the jugular pulse more difficult, but it should always be possible to assess whether the venous pressure is raised. The level of the jugular venous pressure is one of the most crucial signs in clinical cardiology. Provided that the hepatojugular reflux is used, it is also one of the easiest to elicit. The jugular venous pulse should not be assessed while patients are wearing tight corsets, belts, or other clothing that will produce continuous abdominal compression, as a falsely high level will then be produced. The venous pulse of patients with bronchial asthma or bronchospasm of any cause will be appreciably raised throughout the prolonged and necessarily forced expiration. Observations for a level that reflects right atrial pressure must then be made during the relatively brief period of inspiration.

THE PRECORDIUM

Inspection

The apex beat is easily seen in most children and young adults. It is also meaningful to inspect the precordium for abnormal pulsations. A right ventricular heave is often easily observed and is always abnormal. A pulsation visible over the left precordium may be due to a left ventricular aneurysm, marked left ventricular dyskinesis, transmitted pulsation from an aortic aneurysm, a left atrial lift resulting from gross mitral regurgitation, a diastolic thrust of constriction, or the tricuspid "rock" of gross tricuspid regurgitation. All these impulses are more accurately evaluated when combined with palpation.

Palpation

After checking that the trachea and therefore the mediastinum are not markedly displaced, the apex beat should be localised with the tip of a finger. The outward movement of the apex beat is, for practical purposes, synchronous with the first heart sound. Provided that the chest is not hyperinflated from obstructive airway disease, the apex beat, pulmonary artery, and right ventricle can be felt in most patients. The examiner has to learn whether these impulses are normal or abnormally forceful. When no impulses are felt, this may also be an important observation. Absence of right ventricular pulsation in a cyanosed patient is compatible with Ebstein's anomaly or tricuspid atresia. Absence of any cardiac pulsation, particularly when the jugular venous pressure is raised and the chest shape normal, is suggestive of a pericardial effusion. Although the site of the apex beat should be palpated with the patient supine, it is meaningful to feel the apex beat in the left lateral position as well. Absence of a palpable apex beat when the patient is supine but an impulse when in the left lateral position is compatible with a hyperinflated chest and virtually excludes a pericardial effusion. Even if the apex is palpable in the supine position, its character can be assessed more accurately with the patient in the left lateral position. A heart responds to an increased workload or to myocardial disease by hypertrophy, dilatation, or a combination of these two reactions. Displacement of the apex beat reflects essentially dilatation. On the other hand, the apex of pure left ventricular hypertrophy, as occurs in compensated aortic stenosis or systemic hypertension, is not displaced but is abnormally forceful and sustained. The force of the apex beat should be assessed with the ball of the hand and not the tip of a finger. Left ventricular hypertrophy produces a downwards and outwards movement. When the left ventricle is dilated but not hypertrophied, the apex is displaced but not forceful. Right ventricular hypertrophy with mild or moderate dilatation is not detected at the apex, but a heave at the sternum, palpated with the ball of the hand, is readily apparent. Right ventricular hypertrophy alone (that is, with no dilatation, as occurs in severe pulmonary stenosis) often does not produce a discernibly forceful heave over the sternum. Right ventricular hypertrophy and dilatation due to pulmonary hypertension from any cause, but perhaps most marked with tight mitral stenosis, can also result in a very displaced and forceful apex beat. This abnormal heave due to the right ventricle is directed outwards but also upwards and can usually be differentiated from the downward apical impulse of left ventricular dilatation and hypertrophy. With hypertrophy and considerable dilatation confined to the right ventricle, the left ventricle is displaced posteriorly and is not clinically palpable.

Palpation of the second left interspace should be routinely undertaken to assess whether the pulmonary artery pulsation is absent, is normally palpable, or is abnormally forceful. The pulmonary artery should be palpated with the tips of the index and middle fingers.

Clinicians routinely palpate for so-called thrills. This may be contributory provided it is remembered that a thrill is nothing but a palpable murmur. A thrill reflects a loud murmur, which is always pathological. Innocent systolic murmurs never give rise to a thrill. A murmur with a thrill does not necessarily imply that a hemodynamically significant lesion is present. For example, a mitral "honk" may be extremely loud and associated with a thrill, yet the degree of mitral regurgitation is usually very mild.

Percussion

Although it is seldom meaningful to try to outline the cardiac borders by percussion, this procedure is very helpful in two conditions. First, if there is no impaired percussion note in the sternal area, then the chest is hyperinflated. The second important contribution of percussion is to detect the stony, dull note of a pericardial effusion. With large effusions this can be detected over the sternal area with the patient in the supine position. With smaller effusions, the patient must turn to the left lateral position, and the heart should be percussed outside the midclavicular line. A stony, dull note may then be detected. The apex beat will not be palpable in such instances.

Percussion of the liver is important in order to assess its upper border. The lower border is assessed more easily by palpation, but sometimes percussion is also useful, especially in obese patients or in patients whose abdomens are very tender.

AUSCULTATION OF THE HEART

Which Stethoscope?

Provided the stethoscope is of a reputable make, I do not consider that any single design is notably better than another. Personal preference is important. I have used only one model of stethoscope throughout my professional career. It is the Fleischer stethoscope made by Becton-Dickinson (so-called BD), which is probably no longer manufactured. I am familiar with sounds and murmurs through using this stethoscope and have never been convinced that I personally would "hear better" with any of the numerous other stethoscopes that I have temporarily tried. My advice to junior colleagues and students would be to buy a good stethoscope with the intention of keeping it or a similar model throughout their professional careers. It is important that the earpieces fit snugly and that the tubing is the correct length. Very short tubing will conduct the sound vibrations better, but it is not practicable to auscultate some patients, particularly obese women with large breasts, if the tubing is too short. Very long tubing will decrease the intensity of sounds and murmurs and is more liable to touch bedclothes, parts of the patient, and so forth, which in turn distorts or decreases sound and introduces extraneous sounds.

How to Auscultate

Despite new developments in the investigation of disease, auscultation remains the most practicable and sensitive tool by which many forms of heart disease can be assessed. Mild mitral regurgitation, a small ventricular septal defect, patent ductus arteriosus, acute viral pericarditis, and aortic regurgitation are some such conditions. Auscultation is highly contributory to the examination of patients with pulmonary hypertension, dissecting aneurysm of the aorta, mitral stenosis, aortic stenosis, atrial septal defect, and numerous other forms of congenital heart disease. Neither echocardiography nor cardiac catheterization is foolproof, and the benefit derived from these investigations depends on the skill and experience of the investigator who performs the procedures and interprets the results. The same limitations apply to auscultation. Cursory auscultation, which is undertaken by some doctors as a formality and partly to satisfy the patient, will contribute little or nothing. There are certain aspects of learning the skills of auscultation that are mandatory if the procedure is to be of real value and contribute to, or in fact clinch, the final diagnosis. These features warrant consideration.

The Concentration of the Auscultator

In general, one will only hear what one listens for. I do not deny that everybody, unless stone deaf, will hear a loud clap of thunder, a revolver shot, or the screeching of tires immediately prior to an accident, but these are exceptional circumstances. If two people alone in a room are carrying on a conversation, then each should hear the other without difficulty. When the room is crowded, with a general buzz of conversation, the words of any one speaker will only be heard if the listener concentrates specifically on that individual. It is difficult to absorb meaningfully the comments of two speakers at the same time and impossible to listen to three or four.

There are other examples of one's hearing those sounds for which one listens specifically. The human brain possesses the ability of selective auditory attention whereby background noises such as traffic sounds, the ticking of a clock, or the fan of a slide projector can be excluded from awareness and attention directed exclusively to the words of a lecturer. Auscultation of the heart seldom takes place in a completely silent environment. The auscultator must therefore learn to concentrate only on the heart sounds and murmurs of the patient. He or she must ignore completely conversations or other noises in the ward, the traffic outside, the sounds of a respirator, and so forth.

Theoretical Knowledge of Cardiac Sounds and Murmurs

It is far easier to identify a noise such as the barking of a dog if one has heard that sound before, if one is cognizant of its origin, and if one listens specifically for it. Similarly, an auscultator of the heart must be familiar with all the sounds and murmurs that are potentially audible, their variations, their pitch or intonation, and their intensity. Most importantly, the auscultator has to learn the timing and cadence that one sound has in relation to another. The cadence of a mid-systolic click in relation to the first and second heart sounds is analogous to the sounds produced by a server in tennis who strikes the ball (first sound), which clips the net (mid-late systolic click) and then hits the ground (second sound). Two sounds, such as the aortic and pulmonary components of the second sound, can be detected fairly easily by the human ear when 0.02 second apart. It is more difficult when 0.01 second apart but still possible if the softer sound occurs first. Two sounds less than 0.01 second apart appear single to the human ear. Components of the second sound 0.04 or 0.05 second apart appear fairly "widely" split. A physiological third heart sound is low pitched and usually occurs about 0.12 second after the aortic component of the second sound. The timing, frequency, and cadence of the sound should make it easy to distinguish from a widely split second heart sound, an opening snap of mitral stenosis, or the early diastolic sound of constrictive pericarditis.

I personally was able to become proficient in auscultation for two main reasons. During the late 1950s, I acquired the theoretical knowledge of the variations, timing, frequency, and other aspects of normal and abnormal heart sounds and murmurs from the writings of others, principally those of the English cardiologist Aubrey Leatham. The other reason was that, both at the Royal Postgraduate Medical School of London and afterwards when I returned to Johannesburg, I was able to confirm or modify my clinical auscultatory findings by phonocardiography. A phonocardiogram seldom records a sound or murmur that is not audible clinically. Its main contribution is to confirm accurately the timing and pitch of sounds and murmurs. The majority of students and doctors do not have such phonocardiographic facilities, but it is possible to learn auscultation either from a more experienced auscultator or by correlating auscultatory features with the echocardiogram, catheterization findings, and so forth. Since fewer expert auscultators are likely to be available in the future, young cardiologists will have an increasing problem. Doppler techniques have already contributed to diagnostic endeavour. If they prove a practicable or improved substitution for accurate clinical auscultation within the next decade, I shall be both pleased and surprised.

Timing of Heart Sounds and Murmurs

It is pertinent to discuss the timing of sounds and murmurs by auscultation. The main "time marker" is the first heart sound. Murmurs that precede it are diastolic, and those that occur after it are systolic. Other sounds have also to be identified. In most instances there is little problem in identifying the first and second heart sounds, because systole is shorter than diastole. Some difficulty may arise when the time intervals of systole and diastole approximate each other during a tachycardia above 120 beats per minute, particularly if the rhythm is regular. With any irregular rapid rhythm, such as atrial fibrillation, diastole varies in length, and sooner or later there will be a relatively long pause. It is usually stated that the heart should be timed by palpating the carotid pulse. I have seldom found this helpful, since it entails trying to correlate auscultatory events with sensory impulses that are occurring some distance away. On the other hand, the apex beat is nearly always palpable, especially with the patient in the left lateral position, and the first heart sound can be timed easily from this. The bell of the stethoscope should be placed lightly on or next to the visible or palpable apical impulse. For practical purposes (and with rare exceptions), the apical impulse is synchronous with the first heart sound. The second heart sound can then be identified either by gradually moving the stethoscope to the base or sometimes by the fact that the second sound is louder at the base than the first heart sound. The main cause of difficulty is a sustained sinus tachycardia with a gallop rhythm. However, once the first heart sound has been identified, then the timing of other sounds or murmurs should be fairly easy. Occasionally, it is of further assistance if the heart can be temporarily slowed. This may be accomplished by carotid sinus pressure or by asking the patient to inspire deeply and to hold his or her breath. The patient will invariably do a Valsalva maneuver, which on release often results in a reflex bradycardia.

Where and How to Listen

The patient should be warm, comfortable, and relaxed. With few exceptions, the precordium should be completely exposed. Auscultation with the endpiece of the stethoscope under the clothing of bashful women does not allow for accuracy. Auscultation should be the last part of the clinical examination, and the examiner at this time should already have made a provisional diagnosis or at least have a short differential diagnosis. The examiner has had an opportunity to correlate the history and any abnormal signs detected from the general examination, the pulse, and the jugular venous pressure, as well as from inspection, palpation, and percussion of the precordium. Auscultation should start in the supine position unless the patient is very orthopneic. The assessment is *never* complete without auscultation with the patient in the left lateral position. Auscultation with the patient sitting up, standing, and squatting is sometimes indicated, depending on the possible diagnosis. The essential aim of auscultation is to clinch the diagnosis. The time taken for auscultation, the sites at which the examiner listens, and whether the effects of deep respiration and of postural changes are assessed all depend on the context of the situation.

Low-pitched vibrations such as a third heart sound, an atrial sound, and a mid-diastolic murmur are best heard with the bell of the stethoscope lightly pressed against the chest wall. Higher-frequency vibrations, notably the two components of the first and of the second heart sounds, a mitral opening snap, and systolic clicks, are often better assessed with the diaphragm. A pericardial rub is sometimes difficult to distinguish from a murmur, but auscultation during very firm compression with the bell of the stethoscope usually renders nearly all murmurs inaudible, whereas the vibrations of a pericardial rub remain.

Auditory Acuity

I do not believe that decreased auditory acuity is a problem in the majority of doctors who have difficulty with auscultation. Because of my age, my auditory acuity for high-frequency sounds is presumably deteriorating. Nevertheless, I am still able to hear any soft aortic early diastolic murmur that is audible to others. On theoretical grounds, it might be expected that electronic stethoscopes would facilitate clinical auscultation. In my limited experience of these, there is much distortion of sound in addition to interference from extraneous sound.

REFERENCES

1. LAKIER, JB, FRITZ, VU, POCOCK, WA, AND BARLOW, JB: *Mitral components of the first heart sound.* Br Heart J 34:160–166, 1972.
2. RYTAND, DA: *An auricular diastolic murmur with heart block in elderly patients.* Am Heart J 32:579–598, 1946.
3. LEATHAM, A, SEGAL, B, AND SHAFTER, H: *Auscultatory and phonocardiographic findings in healthy children with systolic murmurs.* Br Heart J 25:451–459, 1963.
4. LEATHAM, A: *Splitting of the first and second heart sounds.* Lancet 2:607–614, 1954.
5. TUCKER, RBK, ZION, MM, POCOCK, WA, AND BARLOW, JB: *Auscultatory features of hypertrophic obstructive cardiomyopathy.* S Afr Med J 49:179–186, 1975.
6. ROBERTS, WC: *No cardiac catheterization before cardiac valve replacement—a mistake.* Am Heart J 103:930–933, 1982.
7. DUCAS, J, MAGDER, S, AND MCGREGOR, M: *Validity of the hepatojugular reflux as a clinical test for congestive heart failure.* Am J Cardiol 52:1299–1303, 1983.
8. MANGA, P, VYTHILINGUM, S, AND MITHA, AS: *Pulsatile hepatomegaly in constrictive pericarditis.* Br Heart J 52:465–467, 1984.

BIBLIOGRAPHY

BASTA, LL, WOLFSON, P, ECKBERG, DL, AND ABBOUD, FM: *The value of left parasternal impulse recordings in the assessment of mitral regurgitation.* Circulation 48:1055–1065, 1973.

BRAUNWALD, E: *Physical examination.* In BRAUNWALD, E (ED): *Heart Disease. A Textbook of Cardiovascular Medicine*, ed 2. WB Saunders, Philadelphia, 1984, pp 14–39, 40–67.

CONTI, CR: *What is a clinical cardiologist in 1984?* Am J Cardiol 54:229–230, 1984.

CRAIGE, E: *Phonocardiography and pulse tracings.* Int J Cardiol 4:1–13, 1983.

HADA, Y, TAKENAKA, K, ISHIMITSU, T, YAMAGUCHI, T, AMANO, K, TAKAHASHI, H, TAKIKAWA, R, AND SAKAMOTO, T: *Echophonocardiographic study of the initial low frequency component of the first heart sound.* J Am Coll Cardiol 2:445–451, 1983.

KAPOOR, WN, KARPF, M, WIEAND, S, PETERSON, JR, AND LEVEY, GS: *A prospective evaluation and follow-up of patients with syncope.* N Engl J Med 309:197–204, 1983.

LAKIER, JB, BLOOM, KR, POCOCK, WA, AND BARLOW, JB: *Tricuspid component of first heart sound.* Br Heart J 35:1275–1279, 1973.

MANNING, DM, KUCHIRKA, C, AND KAMINSKI, J: *Miscuffing: Inappropriate blood pressure cuff application.* Circulation 68:763–766, 1983.

NEWBURGER, JW, ROSENTHAL, A, WILLIAMS, RG, FELLOWS, K, AND MIETTINEN, OS: *Noninvasive tests in the initial evaluation of heart murmurs in children.* N Engl J Med 308:61–64, 1983.

OZAWA, Y, SMITH, D, AND CRAIGE, E: *Origin of the third heart sound. II. Studies in human subjects.* Circulation 67:399–404, 1983.

PERLOFF, JK: *The physiologic mechanisms of cardiac and vascular physical signs.* J Am Coll Cardiol 1:184–198, 1983.

SAPIRA, JD: *Quincke, de Musset, Duroziez, and Hill: Some aortic regurgitations.* South Med J 74:459–467, 1981.

SHEIKH, MU, LEE, WR, MILLS, RJ, AND DAIS, K: *Musical murmurs: Clinical implications, long-term prognosis, and echo-phonocardiographic features.* Am Heart J 108:377–386, 1984.

STEIN, PD, SABBAH, HN, AND LAKIER, JB: *Origin and clinical relevance of musical murmurs.* Int J Cardiol 4:103–112, 1983.

TRAILL, TA AND FORTUIN, NJ: *Presystolic mitral closure sound in aortic regurgitation with left ventricular hypertrophy and first degree heart block.* Br Heart J 48:78–80, 1982.

3

MITRAL LEAFLET BILLOWING AND PROLAPSE

with WENDY A. POCOCK

In the practice of medicine, clinicians observe what they seek. Similarly, in auscultation of the heart, examiners will hear those sounds and murmurs for which they systematically listen. It was the clarification over two decades ago of the auscultatory features of nonejection clicks and late systolic murmurs that started the whole "mitral valve prolapse saga." When we made our initial observations on these auscultatory features in 1962, we were studying patients with relatively loud clicks and murmurs. We originally considered that these auscultatory features were rare. As a result of more careful auscultation, prevalence studies, and the detection of mitral valve prolapse by cineangiocardiography and echocardiography, it has become apparent that the anomaly is common. Widespread interest in aspects relating to it has resulted in a scientific "information explosion."

In accordance with the policy of this book, it is not our intention to review or to discuss all aspects of mitral valve prolapse. Jeresaty's[57] comprehensive monograph written in 1979 and his review of the scientific literature have contributed greatly to our knowledge. In addition, mitral valve prolapse now features prominently in textbooks and in volumes surveying recent advances in the knowledge of cardiovascular medicine. Because of our own longstanding and continued interest in the subject, however, there are features that we wish to consider in some detail and problems, albeit partially unresolved, that we wish to emphasize.

SOME HISTORICAL BACKGROUND

At the end of the last century, Griffith,[1] and later Hall[2] in 1903, suggested that an apical late systolic murmur denoted mitral regurgitation. However, following the teachings of Lewis[3] and MacKenzie,[4] systolic murmurs unaccompanied by other evidence of heart disease were regarded as of little consequence. The British cardiologist William Evans[5] emphasized both during and after the Second World War that late systolic murmurs were innocent, and this view was widely accepted. The common association of a mid-late systolic click with a late systolic murmur had long been recognized. In 1913, Gallavardin[6] attributed such clicks to pleuropericardial adhesions, and the theory of an extracardiac origin became so firmly established that McKusick[7] regarded clicks as evidence for a similar origin of late systolic murmurs. An exception to the general trend of opinion was the renowned American cardiologist Paul White,[8] who suggested in 1937 that mid-systolic sounds might sometimes arise from abnormal chordae tendineae.

In 1957, while on the staff of the Royal Postgraduate Medical School of London, one of us (JBB) observed a single fibrosed mitral valve chorda tendinea at the necropsy of a patient who in life had had an isolated mid-systolic click. There were no associated pericardial adhesions, and the observation stimulated our interest in the origin and significance of late systolic murmurs and mid-late systolic clicks. In 1961, our compatriot John Reid[9] revived the postulate that these clicks and late systolic murmurs were of mitral valvular origin. Reid suggested that the clicks arose from the chordae, and he used the term "chordal snap." Shortly thereafter, we[10] observed mitral regurgitation on left ventricular cineangiocardiography in four patients who had murmurs confined to late systole on phonocardiography. A much larger number of patients with late systolic murmurs and clicks were not subjected to cardiac catheterization but were studied by means of vasoactive maneuvers; the effects of amyl nitrite, a Valsalva maneuver, and other hemodynamic alterations were compatible with the behavior of a regurgitant systolic murmur of mitral incompetence. The behavior of systolic clicks was also compatible with an intracardiac origin. Because these clicks were shown to move to early systole, or sometimes to be confined to early systole, we introduced the term "nonejection" systolic click[11] in order to differentiate them from aortic and pulmonary ejection clicks or sounds.

Although it was important to demonstrate that these apical nonejection clicks and late systolic murmurs have a mitral valve origin, it was not those observations alone that have caused such widespread interest. Humphries and McKusick[12] in 1962 commented on the association between a late systolic murmur on auscultation and T-wave changes on the electrocardiogram. Some of their patients had systolic clicks as well as a history of anterior chest pain. They recognized a "characteristic electrocardiographic-auscultation syndrome" which "mimicks the syndrome of angina pectoris due to coronary insufficiency" but considered that previous pericarditis was the likely explanation.[12] It was then published from this unit, although we used different terminology at that time, that the mitral valve anomaly was an integral part of the "auscultatory-electrocardiographic syndrome." A plethora of observations and studies of different aspects ensued, and the widespread interest continues. Both before and shortly after our own early papers, meaningful observations were made by other investigators. These included Criley, Cobbs, Hancock, Likoff, McKusick, Humphries, Segal, and Wooley in the United States; Aubrey Leatham in London; Kesteloot in Holland; Sloman in Australia; and Bosman, Reid, and Vogelpoel in South Africa; but there were many others. The significance of observations made by some of these workers was misinterpreted just as we misinterpreted, or failed to clarify, several of our own. We underestimated the prevalence of the auscultatory features and of the specific syndrome. We[13] recognized but failed to emphasize, as late as 1971, the importance in distinguishing the specific syndrome from other pathological processes affecting the complex mitral valve mechanism, most importantly occlusive coronary artery disease, which result in the same auscultatory features.

NOMENCLATURE

We remain indebted to Michael Criley for clarifying the left ventricular cineangiocardiographic appearances of our original patients with the specific syndrome.[11] Following discussions with Criley, we preferred for many years the adjective "billowing" to describe the posterior mitral leaflet abnormality that we had observed on left ventricular cineangiocardiography in the right anterior oblique position. In 1966, however, Criley and colleagues[14] introduced the term "prolapse" to describe the cineangiocardiographic observations. "Mitral valve prolapse" is now widely used irrespective of whether or not the valve anomaly is anatomically mild, echocardiographically demonstrable, or functionally normal. This has contributed to the general confusion, and it would seem to us that it is now more than a matter of semantics for the terms "billowing," "prolapse," "floppy," and "flail" to be defined. Such definitions should be based essentially on the functional anatomy, or pathology, of the mitral valve mechanism. Auscultatory, echocardiographic, cineangiocardiographic, and other clinical features should then be correlated with the probable functional anatomy. It is, after all, the functional anatomy of the mitral valve mechanism that we attempt to understand and to assess by all invasive or noninvasive investigations.

We recently expressed the view that the concept propounded by the French cardiac surgeon Alain Carpentier defines the essential and important differences between prolapse and billowing.[15] In this context, Carpentier restricts the use of the term "prolapse" to failure of the leaflet edges to appose normally. Such partial loss of apposition may occur with or without abnormal billowing of the bellies of the leaflets, and some, albeit mild or even minimal, mitral regurgitation will inevitably result. This concept of prolapse implies that the valve function is abnormal, which is, in fact, both appropriate and correct. Any cardiac valve, provided there is not a hole in a leaflet, remains competent while there is sustained coaptation of the leaflets. Prevention of apposition may occur, of course, if one or more leaflets are fibrosed or retracted. When leaflets are normal in size or larger, failure of sustained apposition will result in prolapse. Based on Carpentier's understanding of mitral valve prolapse (MVP), we consider that the following terminology, which reflects normal and abnormal mitral valve functional anatomy, should clarify much of the current confusion.[16]

The normal mitral leaflets billow slightly, after closure, into the left atrial cavity (Fig. 3-1A). Exaggeration of this (Fig. 3-1B), which may range from being marked and diffuse to mild and involving only one scallop or even part of a scallop,[17] should be termed a "billowing mitral leaflet" (BML). This BML may produce a nonejection click, but conclusive evidence of mild BML will not necessarily be detected on echocardiography or cineangiocardiography. If the BML progresses, failure of leaflet edge apposition may supervene and then there is "mitral valve prolapse" (MVP) (Fig. 3-1C). With the MVP, there has to be some mitral regurgitation, which is reflected clinically by a mitral systolic murmur. Because the BML is more marked, this may be confirmed on echocardiography, but that technique, whether M-mode or 2-D, detects systolic displacement of the body of a leaflet. If the BML is extreme with very voluminous leaflets and elongated chordae, the term "floppy" is appropriate. Some MVP is almost always present with a floppy valve (Fig. 3-1D), and the mitral regurgitation is often holosystolic. The floppy leaflets are readily detected on echocardiography. Echocardiography alone, however, seldom demonstrates the MVP nor therefore the mitral regurgitation, irrespective of whether the valve has a BML or is floppy. Echocardiographic confirmation of MVP entails essentially the demonstration that the leaflet edges are disengaged, and this is, in our experience, not apparent until the MVP is very severe or a leaflet becomes flail. Progression of the MVP with a floppy valve or with a BML may result in ruptured or at least grossly elongated chordae, and part of the leaflet will then be flail (Fig. 3-1E). Mitral regurgitation is now hemodynamically significant, and the displacement of the leaflet edge is readily apparent on echocardiography. Thus, although there is overlap and the dividing margins somewhat ill defined at present, "floppy" connotes the extreme of marked BML and "flail" that of severe MVP.

Based on Carpentier's concept of "prolapse," MVP may occur with very mild, and possibly undetectable, BML. This could result, for example, from rupture of a minor chorda (Fig. 3-1G) due to infective endocarditis on a normal or near-normal mitral valve. Progression to flail (Fig. 3-1H), still without BML, would occur after rupture of a major chorda tendinea or with multiple chordal rupture. Functionally

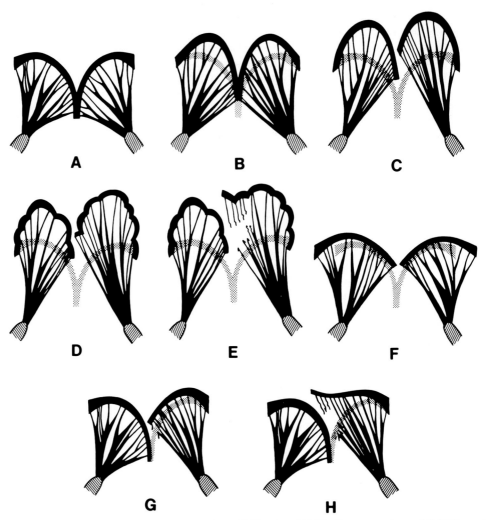

FIGURE 3-1. Diagrammatic representation of billowing (BML), floppy, prolapsed (MVP), and flail mitral valves. *A,* Normal mitral valve showing papillary muscles, chordae tendineae, and apposed leaflet edges. *B,* BML. The chordae are lengthened and the voluminous leaflets "billow" into the left atrium. In this and subsequent drawings, the positions of normal leaflets are superimposed with a stippled pattern. *C,* BML with MVP. The valve is incompetent. *D,* Floppy with MVP. *E,* Floppy and flail. Marked regurgitation is present. *F,* Recent-onset anular dilatation causes MVP with minimal BML, owing to loss of "keystone" effect. *G,* A ruptured minor chorda allows MVP without detectable BML. *H,* Flail with mild BML. (From Barlow and Pocock,[16] with permission.)

lengthened chordae due to recent onset papillary muscle dysfunction could also cause MVP, sometimes temporarily, with only mild BML. Another mechanism for MVP without BML would be recent-onset anular dilatation (Fig. 3-1F). The "keystone effect" of leaflet edge apposition would then be diminished, the chordae subjected to greater tension and stretch; and thus MVP may supervene. As discussed elsewhere (see Chapter 7), a principal cause of such acute onset of anular dilatation without BML is acute rheumatic carditis. It will be readily appreciated, however, that isolated anular dilatation is not as widely recognized as is the combination of a dilated anulus with either significant BML or a floppy valve. Considerable anular dilatation is a well-known feature of the so-called "floppy valve syndrome" with or without skeletal manifestations of Marfan's syndrome.

In this chapter we are concerned mainly with BML, which, whether a result of a degenerative process (that is, primary BML) or secondary to other valvular or myocardial pathology (secondary BML), may allow MVP to supervene in some instances, usually when the BML is relatively more severe. MVP without BML is necessarily a sequence of recent-onset secondary pathology, such as papillary muscle dysfunction, acute rheumatic carditis, or infective endocarditis, and will feature less prominently. We now consider it mandatory to differentiate BML, which on its own is a functionally normal valve in that it does not allow incompetence, from MVP, which entails lack of sustained leaflet edge coaptation and therefore some, albeit on occasion very mild or intermittent, mitral regurgitation.

AUSCULTATORY FEATURES OF BILLOWING MITRAL LEAFLETS AND PROLAPSE

Auscultation remains, in our experience, the most sensitive and specific method of detecting billowing of a mitral leaflet or leaflets (BML) and the presence of mitral valve prolapse (MVP). An isolated nonejection systolic click (NESC) reflects BML, albeit often extremely mild or localised to part of a scallop. The classical and generally accepted auscultatory signs of MVP include a late systolic murmur either with or without an accompanying NESC (Fig. 3-2). A holosystolic murmur may also reflect MVP, which is then liable to be relatively more severe. In addition, we firmly believe that an apical early, nonpansystolic murmur also denotes mitral regurgitation (Fig. 3-3). The configuration of systolic murmurs of mitral regurgitation depends largely on functional anatomical factors that affect the time of maximal regurgitation or limit incompetence to part of systole.

LATE SYSTOLIC MURMURS

The late systolic murmur of MVP is usually loudest at the apex and best heard with the patient in the left lateral position. The murmur is seldom louder than Grade 3, and the effect of respiration may be variable. The intensity is sometimes increased during inspiration, which suggests a functional anatomical alteration rather than a hemodynamic explanation. Phonocardiography confirms that the murmur is crescendo-decrescendo in shape with maximal accentuation near the middle of the murmur in most instances. The murmur extends to the aortic component of the second heart sound and vibrations may pass through that sound. When an NESC is an associated feature, this usually occurs at the beginning or shortly after the onset of the late systolic murmur. In order to illustrate the cadence of these features, 53 late systolic murmurs are represented diagrammatically (Fig. 3-4). Criley and co-workers[14] in 1966 showed on cineangiocardiography that the mitral regurgitation in patients with a late systolic murmur is confined to late systole.

Vasoactive maneuvers or other alterations affecting the functional anatomy of the mitral valve mechanism will affect the timing and intensity of late systolic murmurs. The murmur may become pansystolic with a ventricular extrasystole (Fig. 3-5); may grow louder but remain in late systole after phenylephrine injection (Fig. 3-6); but has a variable change in timing and intensity with alterations of blood pressure as well as end-diastolic left ventricular volume. Amyl nitrite inhalation (Fig. 3-7), the straining phase of the Valsalva maneuver (Fig. 3-8), and the adoption of the erect posture (Fig. 3-9)—all of which result in a decreased left ventricular end-diastolic volume—cause late systolic murmurs to move earlier in systole. In the former two instances, the murmur becomes softer, presumably because of the accom-

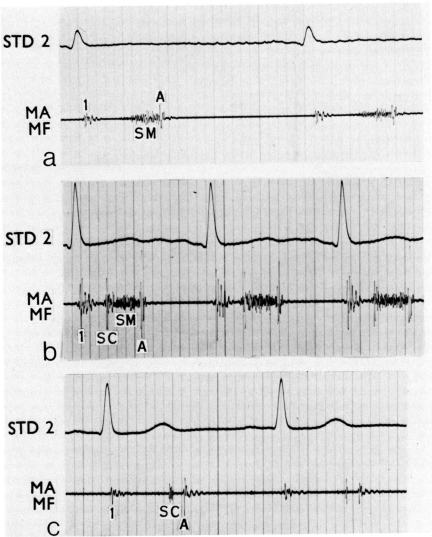

FIGURE 3-2. Phonocardiograms showing (*a*) isolated late systolic murmur (SM), (*b*) late systolic murmur and nonejection systolic click (SC), and (*c*) isolated nonejection click. Abbreviations for this and subsequent figures: MA = mitral area; MF = Medium frequency; A = Aortic component of the second heart sound. Time interval between the heavy vertical lines is 0.2 second.

panying hypotension. With the adoption of the erect posture, however, the murmur may become both louder and longer. This change may depend on the augmented force of ventricular contraction produced by increased sympathetic activity in that position as well as, in some instances, increased billowing and prolapse as a result of the decrease in left ventricular end-diastolic volume. A late systolic murmur of MVP may also become earlier, longer, and louder during acute anxiety or after the intravenous infusion of the sympathomimetic drug isoproterenol. It is noteworthy that phenylephrine, which produces systemic hypertension but has little inotropic action or effect on left ventricular end-diastolic volume, causes the late systolic murmur to become louder without significantly changing its configuration or timing (see Fig. 3-6).

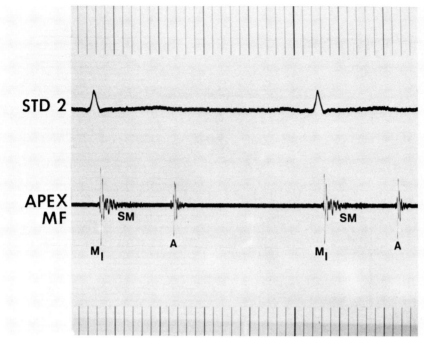

FIGURE 3-3. Phonocardiogram demonstrating a soft early apical systolic murmur in a middle-aged man. He also had an intermittent nonejection systolic click.

MUSICAL SYSTOLIC MURMURS

Like murmurs arising at other sites in the heart, mitral systolic murmurs may develop a musical intonation. The musical vibrations may occur throughout systole or be confined to early or late systole (Fig. 3-10). They frequently vary markedly in intensity and may be loudest during inspiration (Fig. 3-11). Musical murmurs may be extremely loud and audible to the patient as well as to persons nearby. In our experience, the musical intonation often disappears after days or weeks. These mitral "whoops" seldom have an ominous significance, and we have not observed them either to precede valve rupture or to develop more commonly during or after infective endocarditis. The response of musical late systolic murmurs to amyl nitrite and phenylephrine is similar to that of other late systolic murmurs (Figs. 3-12, 3-13).

EARLY SYSTOLIC MURMURS

The early nonpansystolic murmur of mitral regurgitation is decrescendo on a phonocardiogram. Confirmation that this early systolic murmur denotes mitral regurgitation has not always been convincing either by left ventricular angiography or, in our experience, by the use of phenylephrine. Circumstantial evidence of a mitral origin is sometimes provided by association with an NESC (Fig. 3-14). We have also been impressed by the observation that murmurs that are early systolic in the supine position may become late on standing, and that patients with an early systolic murmur at one examination may have a murmur confined to late systole at another. We consider that when an early systolic murmur is loudest at the apex, especially when associated with an NESC, it should be regarded as denoting mild mitral regurgitation and thus have similar significance to the more easily assessed late systolic murmur.

LATE SYSTOLIC MURMUR IN 53 PATIENTS

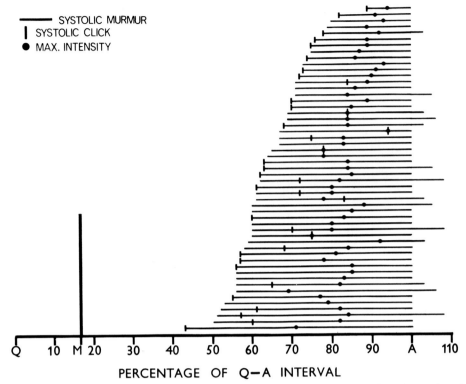

SYSTOLIC MURMUR
SYSTOLIC CLICK
MAX. INTENSITY

PERCENTAGE OF Q—A INTERVAL

FIGURE 3-4. Diagrammatic representation of late systolic murmurs in 53 patients showing the time of onset, maximal intensity, and end of each murmur expressed as a percentage of the QA interval. The mitral component of the first heart sound (M) is indicated, at an arbitrary distance of 0.06 second after Q, in order to demonstrate the cadence of the murmurs on clinical auscultation. The positions of the systolic clicks are represented by vertical lines. In two instances the clicks had marked spontaneous movement and are omitted from the diagram. It can be seen that clicks commonly occur at, or shortly after, the onset of the murmurs and that maximal intensity of the latter is usually near their midpoint. In 14 cases vibrations extended beyond A (aortic valve closure), and these are shown on the diagram. (From Barlow et al,[25] with permission.)

NONEJECTION SYSTOLIC CLICKS

Although most commonly occurring in mid-late systole (see Fig. 3-2), NESCs vary in intensity and timing either spontaneously (Fig. 3-15) or accompanying hemodynamic alterations (Fig. 3-16).

Criley and associates[14] were the first to demonstrate from their cineangiocardiographic studies that a billowing posterior mitral leaflet reached its peak at the time of the NESC. We have thought that the click resulted from elongated, and functionally unequal, chordae being put on stretch at the time of such maximal billow. This postulate is compatible with the recording in some instances of an incisura on the apex cardiogram (Fig. 3-17) that is synchronous with the click. The incisura reflects the tugging of chordae on papillary muscles at the time of peak billow of the mitral leaflets, which is, as will be discussed later, our explanation for the so-called systolic contraction ring of the left ventricle seen on cineangiocardiography. A carotid pulse wave retraction may also be recorded to coincide with the click. The falling pressure in the carotid artery would rise immediately after maximal billowing of the mitral leaflets because left ventricular ejection should then increase. We favor that an early

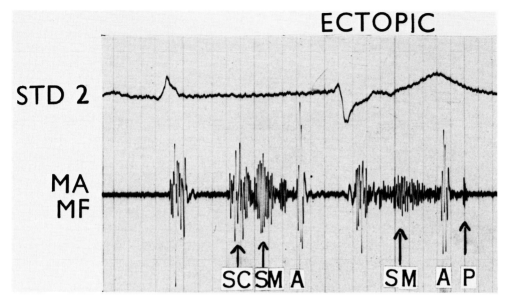

FIGURE 3-5. Nonejection systolic click and late systolic crescendo-decrescendo systolic murmur. The pansystolic nature of the murmur and the disappearance of the click are clearly demonstrated with the ectopic beat. (From Barlow, JB and Bosman, CK: *Aneurysmal protrusion of the posterior leaflet of the mitral valve.* Am Heart J 71:166–178, 1966, with permission.)

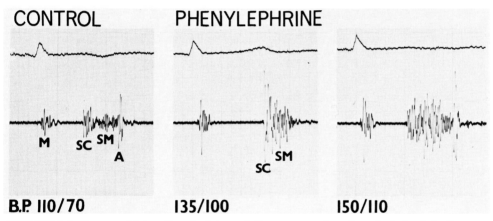

FIGURE 3-6. Increased intensity of a late systolic murmur after phenylephrine injection.

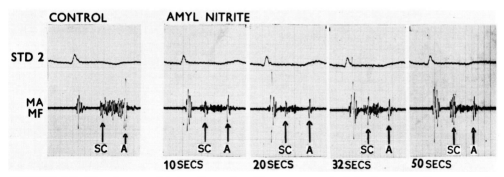

FIGURE 3-7. The decreased intensity and earlier movement of the late systolic murmur is shown in the recordings taken 10, 20, and 32 seconds, respectively, after inhalation of amyl nitrite. At 50 seconds, the murmur is still softer than in the control tracing. An earlier movement of the nonejection click can also be seen. The patient is an 8-year-old girl.

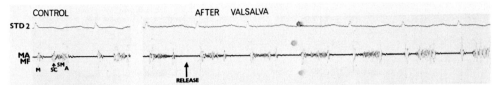

FIGURE 3-8. Effect of the Valsalva maneuver on the same patient as in Figure 3-7. Straining stopped at the arrow marked "release." The last complex during straining is seen and shows decreased intensity and earlier movement of the late systolic murmur. The delayed return of the murmur, and an intensity greater than that of the control period, can be seen in the last two cycles.

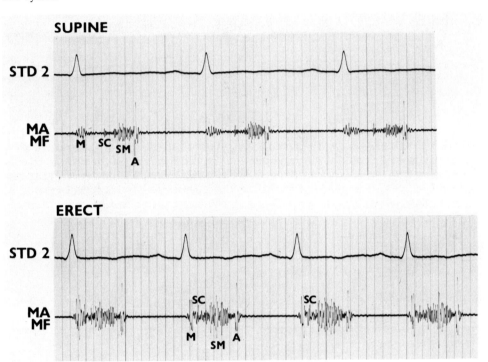

FIGURE 3-9. Increased intensity of a nonejection click and late systolic murmur with the adoption of the erect posture. The click has moved earlier in systole, and the murmur has become pansystolic. (From Barlow et al,[25] with permission.)

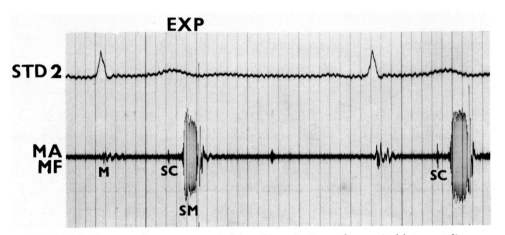

FIGURE 3-10. Phonocardiogram, recorded in mid-expiration, of a musical late systolic murmur in a 15-year-old girl. A nonejection click is also present. (From Barlow et al,[25] with permission.)

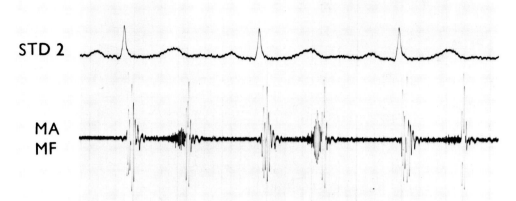

FIGURE 3-11. Musical late systolic murmur in a 7-year-old girl. The murmur was loudest during inspiration, as the child breathed. (From Barlow,[11] with permission.)

NESC, well exemplified by those occurring after mitral commissurotomy in relatively rigid valves with some shortened chordae, results from the functionally unequal chordae being put on stretch earlier in systole. Furthermore, the earlier movement of a mid-late NESC when left ventricular end-diastolic volume is decreased by amyl nitrite inhalation, the straining phase of the Valsalva maneuver, or the adoption of the standing position has been noted to coincide with an earlier and greater billowing of the posterior mitral leaflet. None of these observations negates the postulate of Dock[18] that an NESC arises in the leaflets themselves at the time of maximal bil-

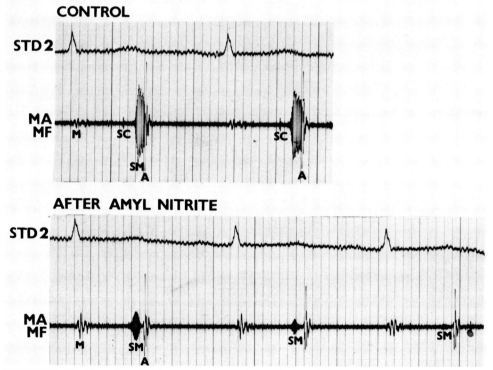

FIGURE 3-12. Showing the decreasing intensity and virtual disappearance of a musical late systolic murmur after amyl nitrite inhalation.

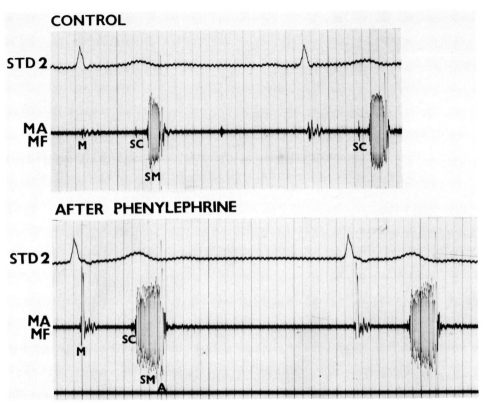

FIGURE 3-13. Increased intensity of a musical late systolic murmur after phenylephrine. This is the same patient as in Figures 3-10 and 3-12.

low. The fact that we have observed NESCs after the insertion of artificial chordae also does not disprove Dock's hypothesis.

Perhaps of more clinical importance than the alteration in the timing or intensity of an NESC or a mitral systolic murmur is an awareness that these auscultatory features may be audible only after a postural change. Repeated auscultation in the supine, left lateral, standing, and squatting positions may be necessary before the presence of an NESC or a mitral systolic murmur can be definitely excluded. The clinical significance of an inconstant NESC or a mitral systolic murmur will be considered later.

CINEANGIOCARDIOGRAPHIC AND ECHOCARDIOGRAPHIC EVIDENCE AND CORRELATIONS

The most sensitive and specific sign of a BML is an NESC, whereas the detection of MVP depends essentially on the presence of a mitral systolic murmur. Any correlation with, and confirmation by, angiocardiography or echocardiography will be more accurate only when the terms "billowing" and "prolapse" are differentiated.[16] Left ventricular angiocardiography was of value in earlier studies in order to confirm the mitral valve anatomical anomaly of billowing and the functional abnormality of incompetence. Angiocardiography remains useful in demonstrating a BML, which may be marked (Fig. 3-18), moderate, or confined to one scallop (Fig. 3-19); but it cannot, and should not, be used as an absolute diagnostic criterion, especially in patients with an isolated NESC. It will also confirm mitral regurgitation, should that

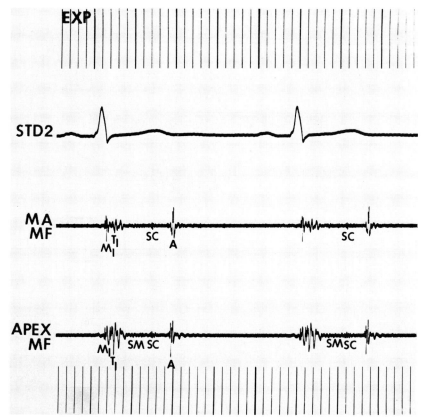

FIGURE 3-14. Soft early systolic murmur and nonejection click in a 28-year-old man who complained of palpitations due to numerous multifocal ventricular extrasystoles. T1 = Tricuspid component of first heart sound. (From Barlow, JB and Pocock, WA: *Challenge of the billowing mitral leaflet*. Cardiology Today 4:4, 1976, with permission.)

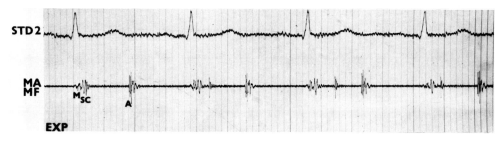

FIGURE 3-15. Spontaneous variation in the timing of a nonejection click during held expiration.

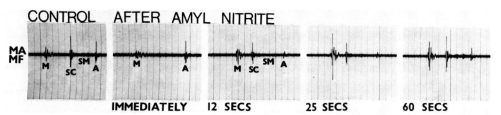

FIGURE 3-16. Phonocardiogram showing the earlier movement and decreased intensity of a systolic click. Immediately after inhalation of amyl nitrite, the click disappeared.

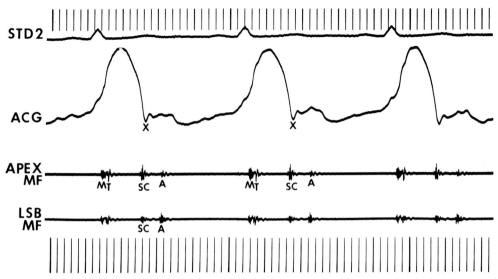

FIGURE 3-17. Simultaneous phonocardiograms and apex cardiogram *(ACG)* in a young woman demonstrating an incisura (marked X) occurring synchronously with the click.

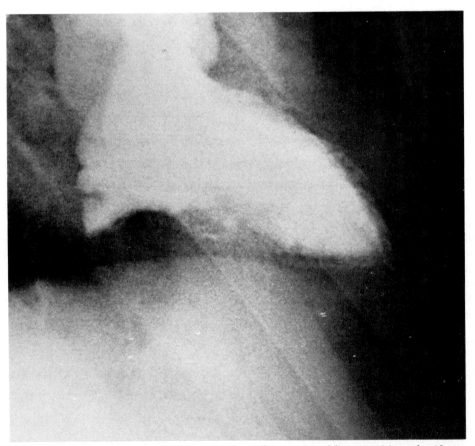

FIGURE 3-18. Left ventricular angiogram in the right anterior oblique position of a 40-year-old man with severe triple-vessel coronary artery disease and probable primary BML. Marked scalloping of the posterior leaflet is shown.

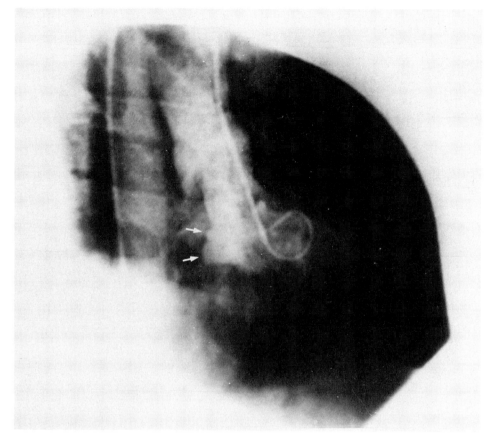

FIGURE 3-19. Frame during systole of left ventricular cineangiogram in a 48-year-old man with a nonejection systolic click who complained of atypical chest pain. Fairly mild billowing of the middle and posterior scallops of the posterior mitral leaflet are seen *(arrows).*

confirmation be necessary, in patients with late or holosystolic murmurs, but it will not demonstrate the lack of leaflet apposition, which is MVP.

Echocardiography has provided further objective evidence of the mitral valve anomaly, but criteria and conclusions have again been confused by terminology. Echocardiography, either M-mode or two-dimensional (2-D), may demonstrate a BML or a floppy leaflet. It will not demonstrate failure of leaflet edge coaptation, which is true MVP, until the MVP is severe or, in fact, until a leaflet is flail. The M-mode echocardiography study by Haikal and co-workers[19] compared patients with an NESC, 85 percent of whom had an associated late or holosystolic murmur, with controls. It was concluded that the accepted echocardiographic signs of late systolic posterior motion and holosystolic hammocking indicating so-called prolapse of the mitral leaflets, when combined as a single criterion, had a sensitivity of 85 percent and specificity of 99 percent. Two-dimensional echocardiography has reputedly contributed further to the diagnosis of so-called prolapse and is considered by Shah[20] and others to be superior to M-mode. Superior arching of the mitral leaflets above the level of the atrioventricular ring is the most reliable indication of billowing. When both the left ventricular long axis and the apical four-chamber view are used, diagnostic accuracy is increased.[21] Our experience of both types of echocardiography has been somewhat at variance with that reported but is in accord with Carpentier's concept of the functional anatomy of billowing and prolapse. We are seldom able to demonstrate a BML on echocardiography in patients with an isolated NESC, but we agree that it can usually be confirmed in the presence of a constant, as opposed to a

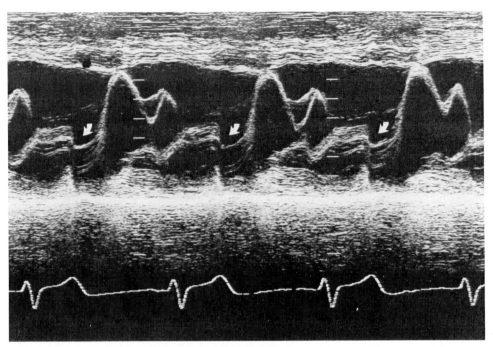

FIGURE 3-20. M-mode echocardiogram of an asymptomatic 25-year-old woman with a none-jection systolic click and loud late systolic murmur. *Arrows* demonstrate the late systolic billowing of the posterior mitral leaflet.

transient, late systolic murmur (Fig. 3-20). Such patients, exemplified by the large majority of those studied by Haikal and associates,[19] have relatively marked billowing, because this has allowed MVP to supervene. Patients with a BML and a holosystolic murmur have even greater billowing, which can invariably be shown on both M-mode (Fig. 3-21) and 2-D echocardiography.

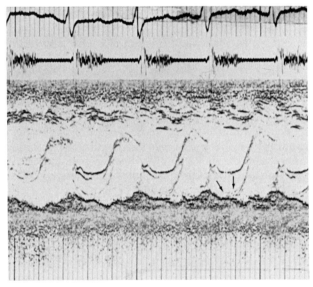

FIGURE 3-21. Pansystolic (so-called hammock shape) billowing of the posterior leaflet of a 27-year-old man with a mitral pansystolic murmur.

TABLE 3-1. Conditions Causing or Associated with MVP or Nonejection Click/Mitral Regurgitant Systolic Murmur

Primary mitral valve prolapse	von Willebrand's syndrome
Marfan's syndrome	Platelet abnormalities
Floppy valve syndrome	Migraine
Rheumatic endocarditis	Hypomagnesemia
Coronary artery disease	Osteogenesis imperfecta
Cardiomyopathy, congestive, hypertrophic	Inherited disorders of metabolism (Hunter-Hurler
Myocarditis	syndrome, Sanfilippo's syndrome, Fabry's
Trauma	disease, Sandhoff's disease)
Left atrial myxoma	Anxiety neurosis, neurocirculatory asthenia,
Polyarteritis nodosa, systemic lupus	autonomic dysfunction
erythematosus	Congenital prolonged QT syndrome
Left ventricular aneurysm	Athlete's heart
Ehlers-Danlos syndrome, pseudoxanthoma	Turner's syndrome
elasticum	Noonan's syndrome
Pulmonary emphysema	Congenital heart disease (atrial septal defect,
Relapsing polychondritis	ventricular septal defect, patent ductus
Muscular dystrophy	arteriosus, aortico-pulmonary window,
Wolff-Parkinson-White syndrome	complete-absence left pericardium,
Straight back syndrome	membranous subaortic stenosis, supravalvular
Thoracic skeletal abnormalities	aortic stenosis, Ebstein's anomaly, corrected
Neuro-ecto-mesodermal histodysplasia	transposition of great vessels, infundibular
Hyperthyroidism	pulmonary stenosis, Uhl's anomaly

SECONDARY BILLOWING MITRAL LEAFLETS AND PROLAPSE

The mitral valve mechanism is complex, and any condition affecting the papillary muscles, chordae tendineae, anulus, leaflets, or the size of the left ventricular cavity could result in a BML or MVP. Many conditions have been reported in association with or as causative of a BML and MVP (Table 3-1). When the BML or MVP is secondary or an associated entity, clearly the clinical and other features as well as the prognosis are determined as much or more by the underlying or associated condition as by the valve anomaly itself. This will be readily apparent, for example, if a primary BML occurs coincidentally with the congenital prolonged QT syndrome or if MVP is secondary to hypertrophic cardiomyopathy or occlusive coronary artery disease. In our experience, auscultatory features of a BML and MVP are extremely common, and a recent survey of our outpatient records shows that there is a prevalence of one in seven among patients attending our cardiac clinic. In many instances, these auscultatory features are an incidental finding in patients with ischemic heart disease, cardiomyopathy, systemic hypertension, or congenital heart disease, and they may be either secondary to the principal pathological condition or associated but unrelated features.

It is relevant now to discuss briefly some of the entities listed in Table 3-1 as causing or being associated with a BML or MVP. Other conditions, notably Marfan's or floppy valve syndrome, occlusive coronary artery disease, athlete's heart, and neurocirculatory asthenia will be discussed later in this chapter under primary, or idiopathic, BML and the specific syndrome related to that.

RHEUMATIC MITRAL VALVE DISEASE

It is readily understandable that chronic rheumatic mitral disease causing shortening of some chordae and partial billowing (Fig. 3-22E) and prolapse of a leaflet could result in an NESC and mitral regurgitation. Similar mechanisms could apply after

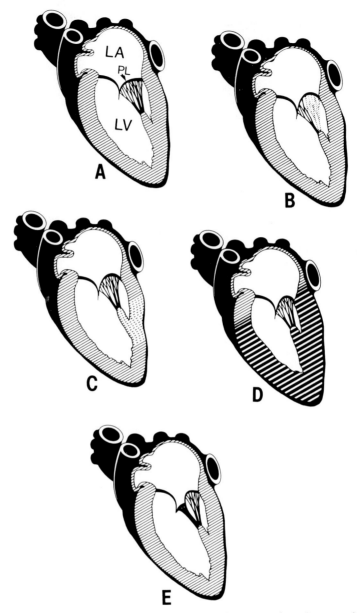

FIGURE 3-22. Diagrammatic representation of the mechanisms of production of anatomically or functionally lengthened chordae and billowing of the posterior leaflet (PL) during left ventricular (LV) systole. *A,* Normal heart. *B,* Primary BML. The chordae are lengthened allowing the slightly voluminous PL to billow into the left atrium *(LA). C,* Papillary muscle dysfunction. The chordae are functionally long, and there is billowing of the PL because of abnormal or no contraction of the papillary muscle and adjacent myocardium. *D,* Small LV cavity, functionally elongated chordae, and billowing of PL due to asymmetrical myocardial hypertrophy. *E,* Anatomically and functionally unequal chordae and partial PL billowing in chronic rheumatic mitral disease. (From Barlow, JB, Pocock, WA, and Obel, IWP: *Mitral valve prolapse—primary, secondary, both or neither?* Am Heart J 102:140–143, 1981, with permission.)

closed mitral commissurotomy and many ''postvalvotomy clicks'' are very variable in timing and intensity (Fig. 3-23). Prolapsing or flail leaflets may also complicate closed commissurotomy.

It is known that the pansystolic murmur of mitral regurgitation that appears during active rheumatic carditis often disappears when the carditis has subsided.

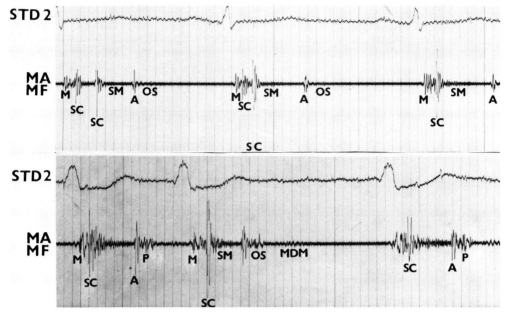

FIGURE 3-23. *Top,* Phonocardiogram of a 31-year-old woman in sinus rhythm showing spontaneous variation in timing and intensity of the postvalvotomy clicks. A soft pansystolic murmur (SM) and opening snap (OS) are present. *Bottom,* Phonocardiogram of a 56-year-old man with atrial fibrillation. The postvalvotomy click again varies in position and intensity. P = pulmonary component of second sound; MDM = mid-diastolic murmur. (From Barlow et al,[25] with permission.)

Under such circumstances, pansystolic murmurs may become confined to late systole before disappearing. Cobbs[22] challenged the classic teaching that mitral regurgitation that occurs with active rheumatic carditis and that later disappears is caused by inflammation of the leaflets. Kalbian[23] has postulated that temporary papillary muscle dysfunction, due to rheumatic coronary arteritis, would explain this phenomenon. In children with severe rheumatic mitral regurgitation, the mitral anulus is frequently very dilated as a result of involvement by the rheumatic process, which sometimes spares or only mildly affects the leaflets themselves. Earlier in the course of this pathological process, or with active rheumatic carditis of lesser severity, it is possible that the physiological decrease in size of the anulus during ventricular systole is partly or entirely lost, although only temporarily. Thus "anular dysfunction" may play an important role in transient rheumatic mitral regurgitation (see Fig. 3-1F).

PAPILLARY MUSCLE DYSFUNCTION

The concept of papillary muscle dysfunction due to occlusive coronary artery disease was propounded over two decades ago by Burch and associates[24] and has subsequently received wide acceptance. They realized that the systolic murmur of papillary muscle dysfunction was often not pansystolic but were reluctant to accept that an NESC could result from occlusive coronary artery disease. In 1968, we reported the association of an NESC or a late systolic murmur with ischemic heart disease (see Fig. 3-22C),[25] and it is now readily apparent that both these auscultatory features are common in that condition. Billowing and MVP secondary to hypertrophic cardiomyopathy probably result mainly from the asymmetrical ventricular hypertrophy affecting functional chordal length (see Fig. 3-22D), but papillary muscle dysfunction due to inadequate contraction may be a factor. Impaired myocardial contractility is the likely mechanism of papillary muscle dysfunction in congestive cardiomyopathy.

We have observed auscultatory features of BML or MVP in patients with poly-arteritis nodosa and disseminated lupus erythematosus. In addition, we have observed mitral systolic murmurs in patients with acute viral myocarditis, some of whom remain with an NESC after the acute episode has subsided. We are uncertain whether this is a causal or associated feature. Several young women, in our experience, were asymptomatic prior to acute viral myocarditis but had the symptoms and signs of the primary BML syndrome after recovery.

TRAUMA

We experienced an example of direct trauma causing MVP after radio-opaque dye had inadvertently been injected directly beneath the posterior leaflet of a 4-year-old child during cardiac catheterization. Nonpenetrating, or indirect, trauma is a well-recognized cause of mitral, tricuspid, or aortic valve rupture. We have personally examined several patients with MVP after severe indirect trauma and have learnt of others through postal communications.

CONGENITAL HEART DISEASE

BML and MVP may be associated with many forms of congenital heart disease (Table 3-1). Both are relatively common in patients with a secundum atrial septal defect, and mitral valve surgery has occasionally been necessary at the time of closure of the defect or afterwards. In most instances the BML is mild and detected by an isolated NESC, or it is an echocardiographic or cineangiocardiographic observation. Jane Somerville and co-workers[26] consider that the relatively small left ventricular cavity in patients with atrial septal defect is often responsible for the angiocardiographic appearances of a BML.

LEFT VENTRICULAR ANEURYSM

Auscultatory and other evidence of MVP associated with left ventricular aneurysms after myocardial infarction probably reflects a form of papillary muscle dysfunction. In some instances, mitral regurgitation may result from retraction of one leaflet, hence prevention of leaflet edge apposition, when a papillary muscle is involved in the dyskinetic segment and thus chordae are functionally shortened.

The nonischemic submitral ventricular aneurysms encountered in South African Blacks and other Negroid subjects affect the posterior anulus of the mitral valve, and MVP not uncommonly results.

LEFT ATRIAL MYXOMA

Although left atrial myxoma usually causes predominant obstruction of the mitral valve orifice, the tumor may damage the leaflets and exhibit significant mitral regurgitation. We have recorded NESCs in several patients with left atrial myxoma, presumably a result of functionally unequal chordae because of mechanical interference with the valve mechanism. In at least one instance the click disappeared after surgical removal of the neoplasm.

PRIMARY BILLOWING MITRAL LEAFLETS AND PROLAPSE

Primary, or idiopathic, BML is essentially a degenerative condition of the leaflets and chordae in which increased myxomatous tissue can be detected on histology. As has been emphasized by Roberts,[17] this results in redundant leaflet tissue, sometimes associated with excessive length of chordae tendineae. The process may be focal, involving only one scallop or even a portion of one scallop, or it may be diffuse, involving both leaflets (Figs. 3-24, 3-25). The increase in transverse dimension results in the circumference of the leaflets being larger than the circumference of the mitral valve anulus. Roberts[17] draws an analogy between the normal mitral valve, which when opened is flat and smooth with appearances similar to the mucosa of the ileum, whereas a BML has an undulating surface and simulates the mucosa of the jejunum.

The reason for the onset of this degenerative condition is ill understood. It may commence in childhood, but most pathologists have limited experience of the condition in children and young adults. On the other hand, according to Pomerance,[27] myxomatous degeneration is common in the elderly. The condition has a familial incidence in some cases and in others pectus excavatum or other abnormalities of the bony thorax suggest a generalized disorder of connective tissue.

PREVALENCE

The prevalence of BML and MVP in population surveys has depended, to an extent, on the nature of the population studied, as well as the relative significance of auscultation and echocardiography. The more recent surveys have given a prevalence ranging from 6.3 percent to nearly 18 percent. It is difficult to claim that such very high numbers denote pathology, and presumably subjects at one end of the normal curve of distribution are included.

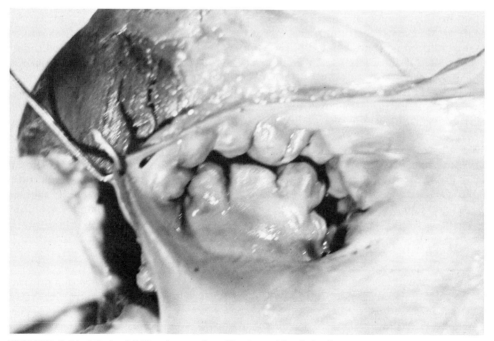

FIGURE 3-24. Marked billowing and scalloping of both leaflets of the mitral valve of a 9-year-old child who died of leukemia. A loud nonejection systolic click and T-wave changes on the electrocardiogram had been present.

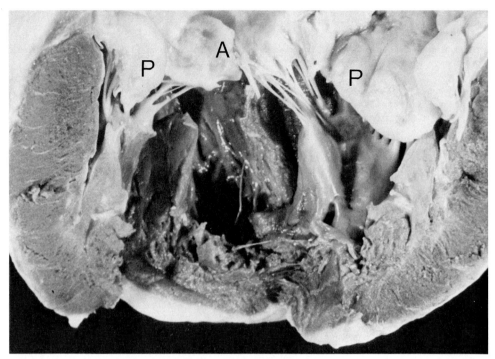

FIGURE 3-25. Mitral valve of a 24-year-old woman with BML syndrome, who died suddenly. There is marked billowing and interchordal hooding involving both the anterior (*A*) and posterior (*P*) leaflets. (From Pocock et al,[66] with permission.)

Our own data on the prevalence of BML and MVP surprised us. During a survey of 12,050 Black schoolchildren, aged 2 to 18 years, conducted primarily to determine the prevalence of rheumatic heart disease, we found auscultatory features of BML or MVP in 168 children (1.4 percent).[28] Because of the nature of that survey, many children with an isolated NESC or an early mitral systolic murmur could have been missed. Four years later, we elected to re-auscultate those 168 children in order to assess progression of their mitral valve abnormality. One hundred thirty-nine of the 168 children were available for re-examination. The same number of age- and sex-matched controls was also examined. Physical examination of all the children was undertaken by one of us (JBB) who was unaware as to whether a child was a "1972 subject" or a "1976 control." The study[29] therefore gave us information on the follow-up of the subject group and a prevalence of auscultatory features of BML and MVP in the control group. The auscultatory features of the 139 "subject" children in 1972 are shown in Figure 3-26 which also illustrates the status on re-examination in 1976. One hundred two children had had an isolated NESC, 26 an NESC with an associated late systolic murmur, 7 an isolated late systolic murmur, and 4 an NESC with an early nonpansystolic murmur, thought to denote mitral regurgitation. In 1976, 45 children had an isolated NESC, 16 an NESC and late systolic murmur, 2 an isolated late systolic murmur, 16 an NESC and early systolic murmur, 5 a pansystolic murmur (of whom 3 had an associated NESC), and as many as 55 (39.5 percent) were passed as normal. Only 1 of the 5 children with a pansystolic murmur had moderate mitral regurgitation, whereas in the remaining 4 the mitral regurgitation was assessed as mild.

The auscultatory features detected in the 139 age- and sex-matched controls are also shown in Figure 3-26. One hundred thirteen were normal, and one had the typical auscultatory features of a small ventricular septal defect. One child had an isolated late systolic murmur, and another had a pansystolic murmur of mitral regur-

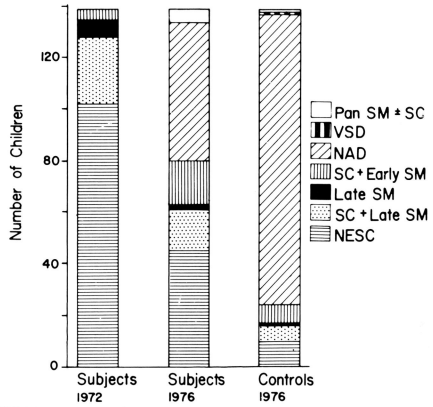

FIGURE 3-26. Histograms showing the auscultatory features of the 139 subjects in 1972 and on re-auscultation in 1976, together with the auscultatory features of the 139 control children. For full description, see text. Pan SM ± SC = pansystolic murmur ± nonejection systolic click; VSD = ventricular septal defect; NAD = no abnormality detected; SC + Early SM = nonejection systolic click and early systolic murmur; Late SM = late systolic murmur; SC + Late SM = nonejection systolic click and late systolic murmur; NESC = nonejection systolic click. (From Cohen et al,[29] with permission.)

gitation in the standing position, without an associated NESC. Twenty-three children had an NESC, 13 of whom had associated mitral systolic murmurs, late systolic in 6 and early systolic in 7.

The results of this blind, controlled study revealed that of the 139 control subjects examined, 10 (7.2 percent) had BML, and 13 (9.4 percent) with an NESC and mitral regurgitation had BML and MVP. If the 2 children with isolated mitral systolic murmurs are included, 15 (10.8 percent) had auscultatory features compatible with MVP. However, if the 7 subjects with an early mitral murmur are excluded, the prevalence of MVP is 5.8 percent. There is a high prevalence of rheumatic heart disease in the population group studied, but it seems improbable that these children had early rheumatic heart disease. The more than 10-fold increase in prevalence detected among the 139 controls in this study, compared with our larger survey of 12,050 children, requires explanation. Only 10 percent of the 12,050 children had been postured, and because of the nature of the survey, auscultation was necessarily hurried. In addition, the primary objective of that survey was the detection of rheumatic heart disease, and some of the auscultators were relatively inexperienced. In the second, smaller study, auscultation was detailed, prolonged, and undertaken in quiet and comfortable surroundings by an experienced auscultator who was listening specifically for auscultatory features of BML and MVP.

THE PRIMARY BILLOWING MITRAL LEAFLET (BARLOW'S) SYNDROME

Despite the large number of subjects, asymptomatic and otherwise completely normal, with auscultatory or echocardiographic evidence of primary BML, our extensive experience of patients complaining of chest pain, palpitations, dizziness, or syncope, who have auscultatory and sometimes echocardiographic or cineangiocardiographic features of a BML or MVP with no other cardiac abnormality, has convinced us of the existence of a specific syndrome. The term "syndrome" is justified, because there may be a large number of associated features including symptoms, electrocardiographic changes, arrhythmias, conduction defects, systemic emboli, autonomic disorders, and possibly myocardial dysfunction. The importance of making the diagnosis of primary BML syndrome, particularly in symptomatic patients, lies in the knowledge that in the large majority of cases, reassurance can and should be given that serious heart disease is not present, that the symptoms are of nuisance value only, and that the prognosis for life is excellent. Many symptomatic patients are anxious, and we concede that anxiety may be responsible for, or certainly may aggravate, some symptoms. For example, breathlessness is a common symptom, yet this cannot be explained organically. Similarly, the chest pain, which is often sharp, severe, localised, and fleeting, is difficult to explain on an organic basis, and some physicians do not believe that it is related to the mitral valve anomaly. A similar pain occurs in many patients, particularly anxious patients, without definite evidence of a BML. The large number of patients with primary BML who suffer from anxiety is noteworthy and is not always understood. In some, anxiety supervenes after an incorrect diagnosis of occlusive coronary artery disease has been made. In others, anxiety in a genuinely symptomatic patient may be caused or worsened by the insistence of medical attendants that there is no organic heart disease present or that there is another organic explanation for the symptoms. It is not "reassuring" to patients with disturbing symptoms, such as chest pain, dizziness, or palpitations, to be told that they are "neurotic."[31] An explanation to such a patient that there is "a very mild but also very common abnormality of a heart valve, which does sometimes cause ill-understood symptoms of nuisance value only" has in our experience been a more comprehensible explanation from which the patient can receive reassurance.

When an NESC is intermittent or extremely soft, we are not always convinced that primary BML is present. Nevertheless, we consider that primary BML syndrome is often a meaningful diagnosis to make as far as the patient is concerned. We are well aware that such patients diagnosed by us as having primary BML syndrome would be classified by others as examples of neurocirculatory asthenia, Da Costa's syndrome, hyperventilation syndrome, nonspecific T-wave changes, atypical chest pain syndrome, so-called syndrome X, or similar conditions. We seldom make any of those diagnoses in symptomatic patients. There are other patients, however, who are not anxious, have a loud NESC with or without a late systolic murmur, and who complain of the recent onset of a severe fleeting chest pain that is at times incapacitating. Such patients may or may not have electrocardiographic T-wave changes (Fig. 3-27). There are also many patients with the same auscultatory features who have remained asymptomatic for years.

Several studies have provided evidence of abnormal autonomic function in some symptomatic patients with the BML syndrome, in which a hyperadrenergic state or catecholamine sensitivity has been postulated. Symptomatic orthostatic hypotension and ischemic-appearing ST segments in response to forced hyperventilation also suggest autonomic dysfunction. However, the exact relation of these findings to anxiety remains uncertain. We find it difficult to understand how an anomaly of a cardiac valve could correlate with autonomic dysfunction. It would seem more likely to us that the various autonomic disturbances reflect manifestations of anxiety rather than a direct correlation with the valve anomaly. The anxiety, in turn, is often a reaction to the disabling symptoms of chest pain, palpitations, pre-

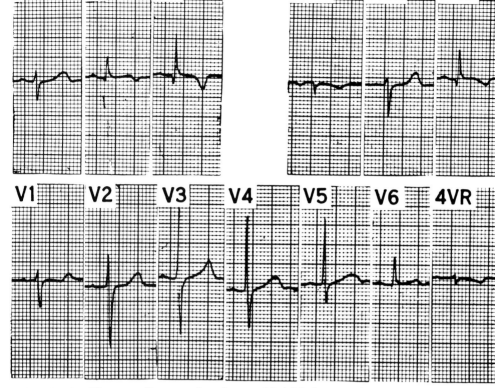

FIGURE 3-27. Electrocardiogram of an 8-year-old child showing Q waves, slightly elevated ST segments, and inverted T waves in leads II, III, and aV_F. This patient died suddenly at the age of 24 years (see text). (From Barlow, JB and Bosman, CK: *Aneurysmal protrusion of the posterior leaflet of the mitral valve. Am Heart J 71:166–178, 1966, with permission.)*

syncope, or even syncope and is not infrequently worsened by unsympathetic medical advisors.

Controversy remains as to whether there is a generalized myocardial disorder in some patients with the primary BML syndrome, especially those complaining of chest pain and those with an abnormal electrocardiogram. Evidence for a diffuse myocardial abnormality has been supported by biopsy studies and histochemical analysis. Malcolm[30] reviewed the data in 1980 and favored that a metabolic or biochemical mechanism was a likely explanation for some symptoms, especially the chest pain. Conclusions drawn from radionuclide studies of left ventricular function in the primary BML syndrome have also been contradictory. To our knowledge, no necropsy evidence supporting "a myocardial factor" has been produced. We do not understand how myocardial function could be significantly affected in the primary BML syndrome, but this possibility requires clarification. Regional abnormalities of left ventricular wall motion have been detected cineangiocardiographically that can probably be attributed to abnormal tension, both in systole and diastole, on chordae and papillary muscles from the billowing mitral leaflets.

ELECTROCARDIOGRAPHIC CHANGES IN THE PRIMARY BML SYNDROME

The prevalence of electrocardiographic abnormalities in patients with the primary BML syndrome varies in different series, depending on the selection of patients, and

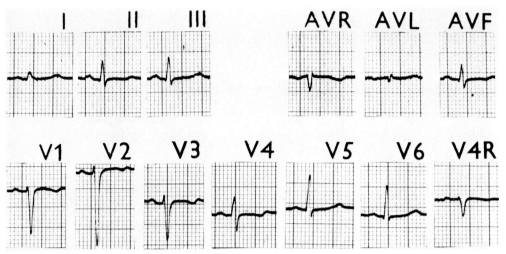

FIGURE 3-28. Electrocardiogram of a 29-year-old woman with an intermittent soft nonejection click. There is inversion of the initial part of the T wave in leads V_2 to V_4. The T waves are flattened in leads II and aV_F. (From Barlow and Pocock,[31] with permission.)

the exact prevalence is unknown. Fifty-three (37 percent) of 144 patients (most of whom were symptomatic) reported by us in 1975[31] had an abnormal electrocardiogram. On the other hand, only 12 (7 percent) of the 168 children detected as having a BML during our survey in 1972[28] had electrocardiographic abnormalities. Furthermore, when electrocardiograms were repeated on 139 of those children four years later,[29] electrocardiographic abnormalities were present in only two children. The most widely recognized pattern is an inverted or partially inverted T wave in leads II, III, and aV_F with resultant abnormally wide mean frontal plane QRS-T angle (Fig. 3-27). Similar T-wave abnormalities may occur in the anterior leads and may or may not be associated with changes in the inferior leads. T-wave inversion may be complete or partial, involving either the initial (Fig. 3-28) or terminal (Fig. 3-29) portion. Deepening of the notch, until the T wave is completely inverted, may develop in the

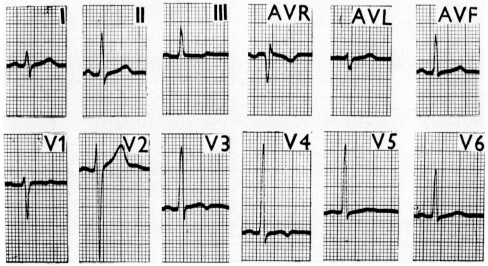

FIGURE 3-29. Electrocardiogram of the 28-year-old man whose soft nonejection click and early, nonpansystolic murmur are demonstrated in Figure 3-14. The terminal portion of the T waves in leads V_3 and V_4 are inverted. (From Barlow and Pocock,[31] with permission.)

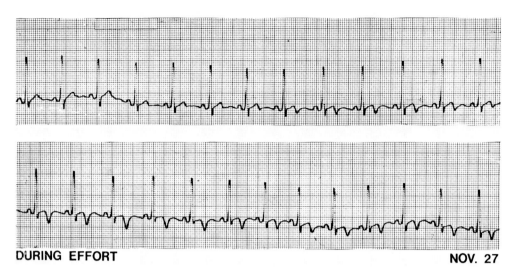

DURING EFFORT   NOV. 27

FIGURE 3-30. Continuous Holter recording of the 28-year-old man whose ECG is shown in Figure 3-29. Progressive T-wave inversion and return to normality within two minutes occurred several times during the period of monitoring, apparently unrelated to emotion, exercise, or change in heart rate. (From Barlow and Pocock,[31] with permission.)

absence of obvious cause or after effort. The ECG may alter spontaneously, and this change may take place within minutes (Fig. 3-30). The adoption of the erect position may also invert T waves. Prominent upright U waves are quite common, especially in the right precordial leads. Prolongation of the QT interval in primary BML syndrome has been reported by several workers but is rare in our experience.

Because chest pain, arrhythmias, and an abnormal ECG are prominent features of both the primary BML syndrome and occlusive coronary artery disease, their differentiation is an important and extremely common problem in clinical practice. The differentiation may be difficult, but after a careful history and stress ECG, the problem can usually be resolved with confidence. In addition, cardiologists are frequently confronted with the assessment of an "abnormal ECG" in asymptomatic subjects, whether or not they have associated evidence of a BML. We are not convinced that there are any essential differences between "nonspecific T-wave changes" and the electrocardiographic abnormalities that we originally ascribed to the primary BML syndrome. Although a comprehensive discussion on the differentiation of "abnormal" ECGs of occlusive coronary artery disease, hypertrophic cardiomyopathy, primary BML syndrome, athlete's heart, or other causes of so-called nonspecific T-wave changes is beyond the scope of this chapter, it is relevant to discuss some guidelines on this very important and common clinical problem. It is not highly relevant whether patients with atypical T-wave changes are diagnosed as primary BML syndrome. The importance lies essentially in differentiating ST segment and T-wave changes at rest or after effort that are due to ischemic heart disease or hypertrophic cardiomyopathy from the relatively or completely "benign" ST segment and T-wave abnormalities of athlete's heart, primary BML syndrome, or nonspecific T-wave changes. It is also important to improve the interpretation of "abnormal" ECGs and hence to reduce considerably the number of so-called false-positive results of stress tests for ischemic heart disease.

ATHLETE'S HEART

With prolonged strenuous exercise, the hearts of physically fit, normal subjects undergo physiological changes, which can result in rhythm changes, conduction

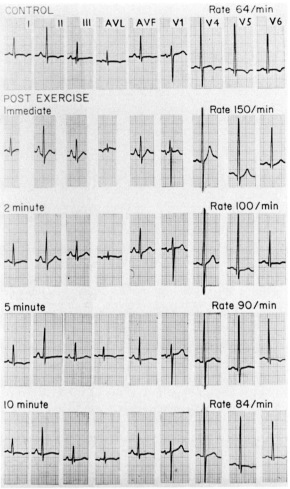

FIGURE 3-31. *Left,* Control and posteffort ECGs of a 22-year-old asymptomatic long-distance runner with an intermittent nonejection systolic click. The large QRS voltages and the inverted T waves, which normalise immediately after effort (see Fig. 3-37, Type III), are typical of an athlete's heart. (From Barlow, JB and Pocock, WA: *Mitral valve prolapse, the athlete's heart, physical activity and sudden death.* Int J Sports Cardiol 1:9–24, 1984, with permission.)

defects, or electrocardiographic alterations. The term "athlete's heart" is suitable to describe these changes in highly trained athletes, but its use must be confined to normal hearts. It is relevant to emphasize that some athletes, albeit physically fit and asymptomatic, might have underlying MVP, a BML, hypertrophic cardiomyopathy, or occlusive coronary artery disease. Although a mild BML may justifiably be regarded as a normal variant, asymptomatic athletes with hypertrophic cardiomyopathy or occlusive coronary artery disease have serious heart disease and are at risk of sudden death, especially during strenuous exercise.

Physiological changes in the hearts of endurance athletes have been shown by echocardiography to comprise an increase in left ventricular wall thickness and left ventricular cavity size, resulting in cardiac enlargement that may reputedly be apparent on chest roentgenogram. Physical force athletes (judo, weight-lifting) simply have an increase in heart size commensurate with their increase in body mass; the ratio of left ventricular cavity radius to wall thickness is decreased as compared with normal controls and endurance athletes. Bar-Shlomo and associates,[32] using radionuclide angiography, showed a response to exercise in endurance athletes that differed from that in normal control subjects. While both had similar increases in ejection fraction, this was achieved in the control subjects by a marked increase in left

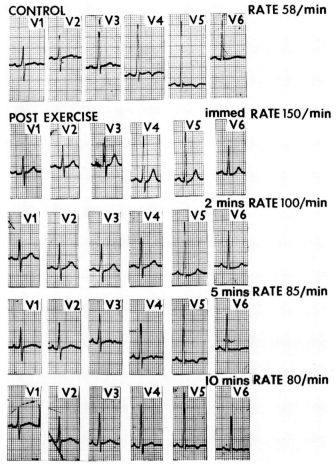

FIGURE 3-31 (*continued*). *Right,* Control and posteffort ECGs of a 30-year-old top-class rugby football player who also has a nonejection click. The electrocardiographic features are again typical of an athlete's heart. (See Fig. 3-37, Type III.)

ventricular end-diastolic volume and lesser degree in end-systolic volume; in the athletes the end-diastolic volume was virtually unchanged, but there was a considerable decrease in the end-systolic volume.

Ventricular hypertrophy is not, in our experience, detectable on physical examination of patients with an athlete's heart. The pulse rate is relatively slow. The physiological vibratory systolic murmur of childhood and young adults may be present in highly trained athletes in their third, fourth, or even fifth, decades. Physiological third heart sounds are common.

The most important clinical features of the athlete's heart can be divided into two main groups: the first relates to the "vagotonia" and the second to the electrocardiographic changes.

Vagotonia

Sinus arrhythmia, often intensified immediately after exercise, and a sinus bradycardia are common. First-, second-, and even third-degree atrioventricular block may occur and have been extensively investigated by Zeppilli and co-workers.[33] These "conduction defects" invariably normalize during strenuous exercise. Rost[34] has suggested that these effects are due more to increased sensitivity of the heart to vagal influences than to a true overaction of the vagus nerve. True abnormalities of the conduction system in young subjects have been reported by Kay and associates,[35] and electrical pacing was reputedly indicated. It should be remembered, however, that highly trained athletes with bradycardia, whether or not accompanied by "heart block," may develop presyncope or even syncope especially after strenuous exercise when the bradycardia returns but systemic peripheral resistance is still low. In such instances, electrical pacing is seldom, if ever, indicated.

Electrocardiographic Changes

The most typical and easily recognized electrocardiographic changes of the athlete's heart comprise increased voltages and T-wave inversion. The T-wave inversion is relatively shallow but may approach 5 mm in the right precordial leads. T-wave inversion returns to normal, or towards normal, immediately after exercise (Fig. 3-31, *left* and *right*). Deep T-wave inversion of more than 5 mm in an asymptomatic or mildly symptomatic athlete is highly suspect of a pathological heart, most notably hypertrophic cardiomyopathy, and has not been encountered by us in lead V_6 in a true athlete's heart. Zeppilli and co-workers[36] have observed normalization of T waves of athletes with isoproterenol infusion and have also emphasized the frequency of the normalization of T waves after effort.

The electrocardiographic T-wave changes of the primary BML syndrome are similar to those of the athlete's heart. Increased voltages are not a recognized feature of the BML syndrome but may occur if the patient is asthenic with a thin chest wall. Because primary BML is common, it is inevitable that a number of athletes will have this condition. The T-wave changes of highly trained sportsmen may indeed be due to associated BML, but this is unlikely to be the only mechanism involved.

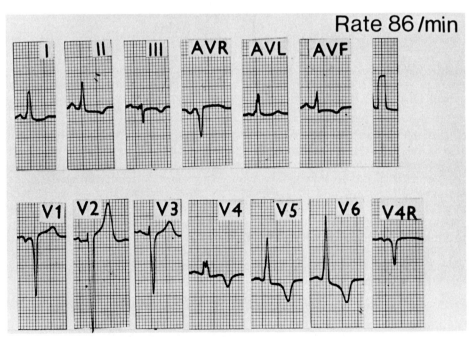

FIGURE 3-32. Resting ECG of a 49-year-old man with severe ischemic heart disease. Selective coronary arteriography confirmed triple vessel disease with considerable left ventricular dysfunction (ejection fraction of 25 percent). Coronary bypass surgery resulted in marked improvement. (See Fig. 3-37, Very Severe 4.) (From Barlow, JB and Pocock, WA: *Mitral valve prolapse, the athlete's heart, physical activity and sudden death.* Int J Sports Cardiol 1:9–24, 1984, with permission.)

OCCLUSIVE CORONARY ARTERY DISEASE

It is often not appreciated that, excluding patients with previous myocardial infarction, so-called unstable angina, and very severe ischemia (Fig. 3-32), the resting ECG of at least 80 percent of patients with occlusive coronary artery disease is normal. Furthermore, subjects known to have had T-wave inversion for years (Fig. 3-33), especially if without significant symptoms or abnormality on clinical examination, are highly unlikely to be suffering from occlusive coronary artery disease. Asymptomatic subjects, but also symptomatic patients complaining of chest pain for months or years, who have abnormal T waves at rest that normalize immediately after effort,

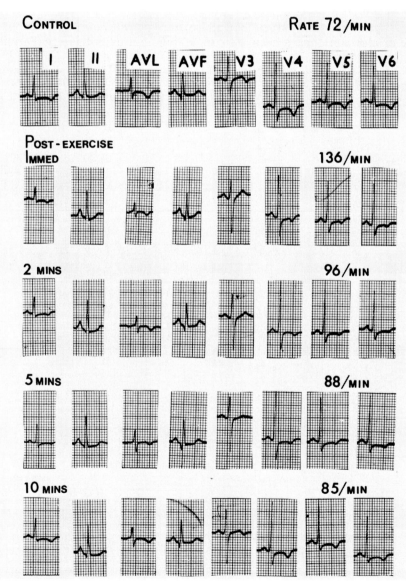

FIGURE 3-33. Control and posteffort ECGs of a 68-year-old woman with a nonejection systolic click and atypical chest pain. The abnormal T waves in the control tracing were known to have been present for at least a year. The T waves are less inverted after effort. (See Fig. 3-37, Type III.) (From Barlow, JB and Pocock, WA: *Mitral valve prolapse, the athlete's heart, physical activity and sudden death.* Int J Sports Cardiol 1:9–24, 1984, with permission.)

are also seldom suffering from occlusive coronary artery disease (Fig. 3-34, *left* and *right;* see also Fig. 3-37).

It is our experience, in fact, that symptomatic or asymptomatic patients who have a normal ECG at rest but who develop ST-segment and T-wave changes after effort (Fig. 3-35, *left* and *right;* see also Fig. 3-37) are more difficult to assess than those who have abnormal T waves at rest.

We have made errors of interpretation in the past and shall probably continue so to do. Nonetheless, we are convinced that discernible differences are usually apparent; an awareness of these should decrease the number of so-called false-positive stress ECGs and therefore improve the clinical contribution of this most important method of examination. Many papers that discuss the prevalence of false-positive stress tests do not illustrate the ECGs. When ECGs are shown, the configuration of the ST segments often has features unusual for ischemia. The situation is analogous to the assessment of a patient with an isolated systolic murmur. A systolic murmur may or may not denote heart disease; systolic murmurs have similarities but

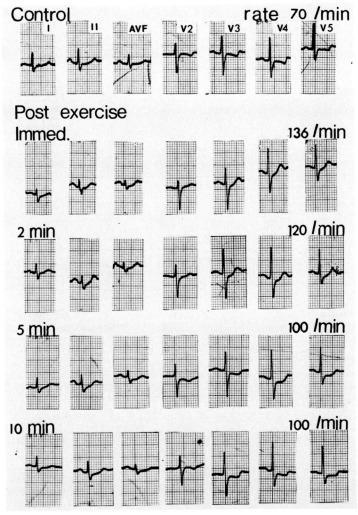

FIGURE 3-34. *Left,* Control and posteffort ECGs of a 59-year-old man who had complained of severe chest pain for two years and had been diagnosed elsewhere as "severe coronary artery disease." The T waves normalise after effort. Selective coronary arteriography was normal, and a left ventriculogram confirmed primary BML with minimal mitral regurgitation. (See Fig. 3-37, Type III.) (From Barlow, JB and Pocock, WA: *Mitral valve prolapse, the athlete's heart, physical activity and sudden death.* Int J Sports Cardiol 1:9–24, 1984, with permission.)

also detectable differences. We consider that there are probably always detectable differences in the timing or configuration, or both, of ST-segment and/or T-wave changes that develop during and after exercise, that are caused by myocardial ischemia as opposed to "benign" conditions such as the primary BML syndrome, anxiety, or nonspecific T-wave changes (Fig. 3-36).

Whether or not the ECG is monitored during exercise, it is important for the patient to try to complete submaximal effort. We record 12-lead tracings immediately, and at 2, 5, and 10 minutes after cessation of exercise. ST-segment and T-wave changes that occur during and after exercise have to be assessed for time of onset and duration (Fig. 3-37) as well as their configuration.

Time of Onset and Duration of ST-Segment and T-Wave Changes

On configuration alone, the nonischemic ST-T may be difficult or impossible to distinguish from those of ischemia, but they have different time-course patterns after

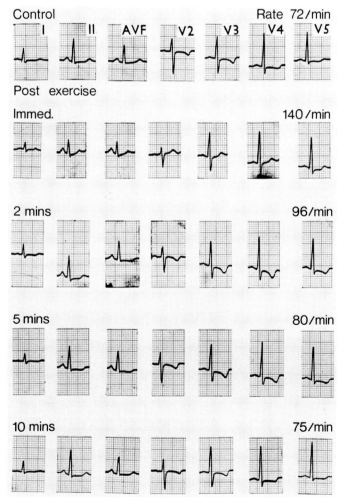

FIGURE 3-34 (continued). Right, Control and posteffort ECGs of a 52-year-old woman with an isolated nonejection systolic click and disabling chest pain, who had previously been diagnosed by several physicians as suffering from "severe coronary artery disease." The T waves normalise immediately after exercise. Selective coronary arteriography was normal. (See Fig. 3-37, Type III.) (From Barlow, JB, Pocock, WA, and Obel, IWP: Mitral valve prolapse—primary, secondary, both, or neither? Am Heart J 102:140–143, 1981, with permission.)

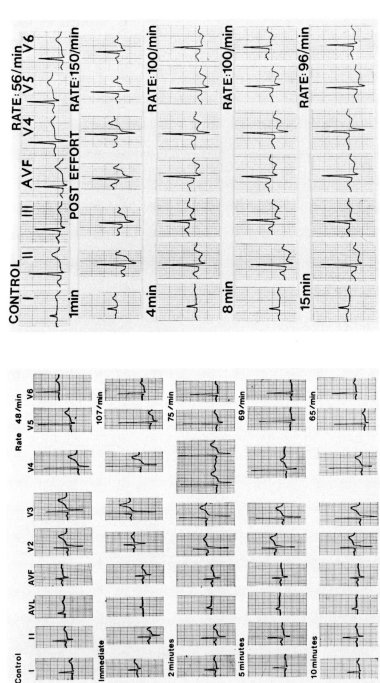

FIGURE 3-35. *Left,* Control and posteffort ECGs of an asymptomatic 53-year-old jogger. We interpreted the control tracing as normal but originally and correctly favored that the ST-segment depression immediately and two minutes after effort—most apparent in standard leads 2, V_4, V_5, and V_6—was suggestive of mild myocardial ischemia. Selective coronary arteriography was completely normal. This man also had a nonejection click on auscultation. (See Fig. 3-37, Type II). (From Barlow, JB and Pocock, WA: *Mitral valve prolapse, the athlete's heart, physical activity and sudden death.* Int J Sports Cardiol 1:9–24, 1984, with permission.)

Right, Control and posteffort ECGs of a 50-year-old woman complaining of chest pain. The ST segments are apparently depressed but upsloping one minute after effort. Thereafter, some ST-segment depression with a downsloping ST segment remains for at least 15 minutes after the exercise. Because of her good exercise performance, the relatively late onset of apparent ischemic ST segments (four minutes) and the sustained ST segment abnormalities (at least 15 minutes), an ischemic cause of these ST segment changes was not favored. Coronary arteriography was, in fact, later shown to be completely normal. (See Fig. 3-37, Type I.) (From Barlow,[37] with permission.)

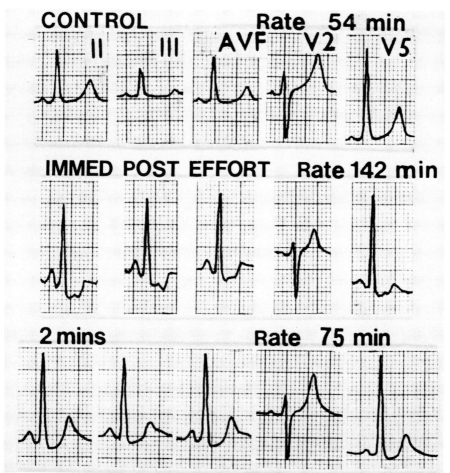

FIGURE 3-36. Control and posteffort ECGs of a 33-year-old highly trained athlete who complained of atypical chest pain. The ST segments are abnormal immediately posteffort but normalise two minutes after effort with a rate of 75 per minute. These changes are incompatible with myocardial ischemia. Selective coronary arteriography was normal. (See Fig. 3-37, Type II.) (From Barlow,[37] with permission.)

cessation of exercise. The time-course patterns of ischemic and nonischemic ST depression or T inversion are outlined in Figure 3-37. It must again be emphasized that in the absence of previous myocardial infarction, very severe ischemia, "unstable angina," or discernible factors such as left ventricular hypertrophy, conduction defects, drug therapy, or electrolyte imbalance, the ECG of patients with uncomplicated occlusive coronary artery disease is usually normal, or near normal, at rest. Thus, patients with mild ischemia have a normal ECG at rest (Fig. 3-37, Mild 1) and develop ST-T changes 2 to 3 minutes postexercise. The ST-T alterations are maximal 4 to 5 minutes postexercise, and these return to normal relatively early, at about 6 minutes. Patients with moderate ischemia (Fig. 3-37, Moderate 2) show earlier onset and later offset of ST-T abnormalities. Most patients with severe (Fig. 3-37, Severe 3) ischemia also have normal ST segments and T waves at rest, but some are slightly abnormal (Fig. 3-37, Severe 3a). In both instances, conclusively abnormal ST-T develops during exercise, maximal changes are seen 3 to 6 minutes postexercise, and the abnormal ST-T persists at 10 minutes. Ischemic ST-T at rest denotes very severe ischemia (Fig. 3-37, Very Severe 4), and it increases immediately with exercise and remains more marked at 10 minutes than in the resting tracing.

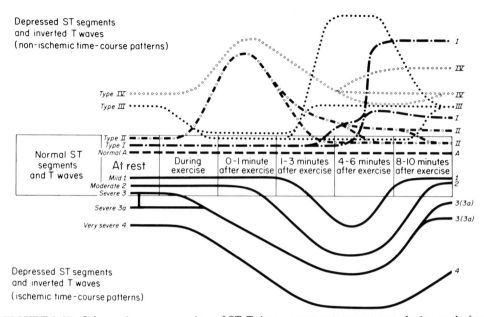

FIGURE 3-37. Schematic representation of ST-T time-course patterns at rest, during and after exercise. Lines within the rectangular panel reflect normal appearances at the relevant times. Thus, the line "Normal" illustrates the ST-segment and T-wave appearances of completely normal subjects at rest, during exercise, and throughout the 10-minute interval after exercise. The time-course patterns of nonischemic ST-depression and T-wave inversion are drawn above the rectangular panel, whereas those of ischemia appear below the panel. The extent of ST depression or T-wave inversion is represented by the vertical distance above (nonischemic) or below (ischemic) the panel. For example, the ST segments and T waves of the nonischemic Type II time-course pattern are normal at rest, maximal ST depression and T inversion occur during or approximately one minute after exercise, and rapid improvement is demonstrated by the line "Type II" returning towards, or entering, the panel within three minutes after exercise. Deviations of abnormality at rest for nonischemic (Types III and IV above the panel) and ischemic (Severe 3a and Very Severe 4 below the panel) ST-T are somewhat arbitrary for an individual patient, but the amount of change during and after exercise should be compared with the resting level.

Whereas ischemic ST depression and T-wave inversion consistently follow a general behavior of early onset/late offset and late onset/early offset, the time-course responses to exercise of nonischemic cases are more variable. Four types of time-course behavior for the nonischemic ST-T have been delineated.[37] In Type I, the ST segments and T waves are normal at rest (Fig. 3-37, Type I) and are still normal or become only disputably abnormal until 2 to 6 minutes postexercise, when definite ST-T changes supervene (Fig. 3-38), which may persist for at least 10 minutes into the recovery phase (see Fig. 3-35, *right*). The Type I nonischemic time-course behavior was encountered by Malcolm and Ahuja[38] who commented that it "distinctly differed" from that of coronary artery disease. The inappropriately late development of the marked ST-T abnormalities distinguishes Type I from those cases with ischemic time-course behavior (see Fig. 3-37, Severe 3) in which abnormal ST-T also remain for 10 minutes, or longer, after cessation of exercise (Fig. 3-39). Type II is the other non-ischemic pattern in which the resting electrocardiogram is normal (see Fig. 3-37, Type II). The essential time-course features of Type II were suggested in 1977 by Lozner and Morganroth[39] to be of value in identifying subjects without coronary artery disease in whom ST-T changes occur during exercise. Ellestad[40] has observed that the ST segment depression in Type II may be considerable either during or immediately after exercise (see Fig. 3-36). Although the ST segments and T waves usually normalize at 2 minutes, in a minority they improve at

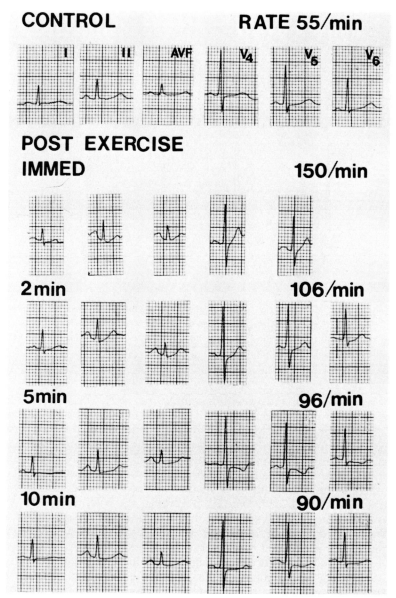

FIGURE 3-38. Late-onset (five minutes) ST segment changes in a 45-year-old man. The ST segments remain abnormal at 10 minutes. This pattern of change is not that of myocardial ischemia. (See Fig. 3-37, Type I.)

that time but remain abnormal for several minutes. Whether or not they persist for 5, 10, or more minutes, the very early onset of the ST-T alterations followed by improvement or normalization within 3 minutes is not in accord with ischemic time-course behavior.[38] Type IV (see Fig. 3-37, Type IV) has virtually the same time-course pattern as Type II except that ST-T are present at rest and throughout the post exercise observation period (Fig. 3-40). As with Type II, the Type IV time-course pattern of an immediate increase in the ST-T abnormalities followed by improvement within 3 or 4 minutes after cessation of exercise should make differentiation from an ischemic response apparent. Some patients can be interchanged between Types II and IV depending on the resting status of the ST segments and T waves at the time of the stress test. It is known that ST-T may be affected by posture and hyperventila-

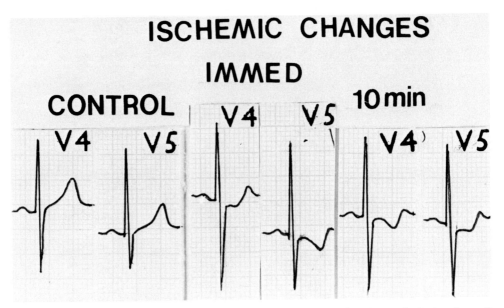

FIGURE 3-39. Electrocardiographic leads V_4 and V_5 recorded before *(control)*, during *(immed)*, and 10 minutes after effort in a 56-year-old man with severe coronary artery disease. The early onset and prolonged duration of the abnormal ST-segment changes are typical of severe myocardial ischemia. (See Fig. 3-37, Severe 3.)

tion, or may vary spontaneously within minutes or days.[31] Type III (see Fig. 3-37, Type III) is an important nonischemic pattern, and many cases of mitral valve prolapse and athlete's heart (see Fig. 3-31) demonstrate the Type III time-course behavior. The ECG is abnormal at rest, thereby simulating very severe ischemia, but the ST-T changes partially or completely normalize during or shortly after exercise, and later either return to the resting pattern or become more abnormal (see Fig. 3-34). There is thus an important difference in the time-course patterns of Type III and marked ischemia (see Fig. 3-37, Type III, Severe 3a, and Very Severe 4).

It is our ongoing clinical experience that estimation of ST-segment and T-wave time-course behavior during and after exercise, combined with the generally accepted practice of evaluating the history, clinical examination, exercise variables, and ST-T configuration, enhances the diagnostic value of an exercise test. In many instances, depending on the clinical setting, these practices also avoid the necessity for expensive additional investigations, such as radionucleotide studies or coronary arteriography. Irrespective of the age, sex, symptoms, or risk factors of a patient, stress testing remains a most practicable and cost-effective method for detecting ischemic heart disease. This useful investigation should not be judged unreliable because of the reputedly high prevalence of false-positive results. It is we, the observers, whose reliability has been suspect.

ST-Segment Configuration

As has been emphasized by Schamroth,[41] true ST-segment depression occurs only if the J point is below the continuation of the PQ segment. ST-segment depression of at least 1 mm that is downsloping (Fig. 3-39) or horizontal for 0.08 second (Fig. 3-41) is accepted by most investigators as indicative of ischemia. The magnitude of the ST-segment depression should also be correlated with the R-wave amplitude. Although an increase of the R-wave amplitude after exercise is itself a sign of ischemia, ST-segment depression of 1 mm with an R wave of 6 mm is surely more

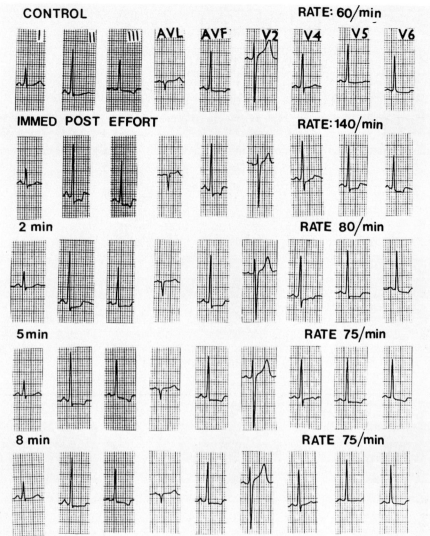

CONTROL   **RATE: 60/min**

IMMED POST EFFORT   **RATE: 140/min**

2 min   **RATE 80/min**

5 min   **RATE 75/min**

8 min   **RATE 75/min**

FIGURE 3-40. A more gradual upward coving of the depressed ST segment compared with Figure 3-42. The ST segments are abnormal at rest, but ST changes are most marked immediately after effort. Coronary arteriography was normal. (See Fig. 3-37, Type IV.) (From Barlow,[37] with permission.)

significant than similar ST-segment depression with an R wave of 20 mm. ST-segment depression that remains upsloping in all tracings after effort, despite a fairly distinct demarcation between the ST segment and the T wave (see Fig. 3-35, *left*), is probably seldom ischemic.

We have observed, both in published reports and in our own experience, ST-segment depression after effort but with an upward coving of the ST segment *after* the J wave. The upward cove may be sharp and narrow (Fig. 3-42) or more gradual (Fig. 3-40). Some patients with this pattern have had an NESC on auscultation; others have been physically very fit. Although we have observed similar upward coving in a few cases of occlusive coronary artery disease, this ST configuration may then reflect secondary BML or coincidentally associated primary BML. In most instances, this ST configuration does not occur in ischemic patients and is different from the usual flat or downward-sloping ST-segment depression. When this upward cove is

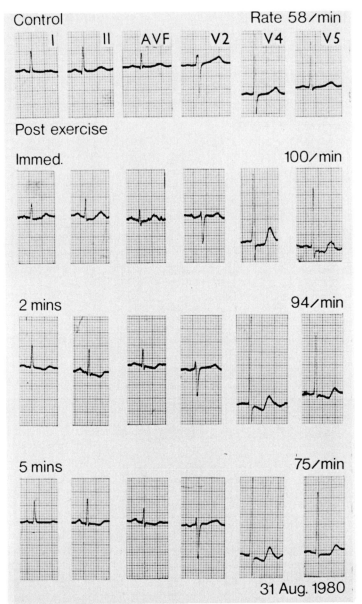

FIGURE 3-41. Normal control with typical ischemic ST-segment changes occurring immediately after exercise in the 40-year-old man whose cineangiocardiogram is shown in Figure 3-18. This man has primary billowing mitral leaflets and severe triple-vessel coronary artery disease.

associated with a time of onset and offset incompatible with ischemia (see Figs. 3-36, 3-40, 3-42), the differentiation is easier (see Fig. 3-37).

CONCURRENT PRIMARY BML (OR NONSPECIFIC T-WAVE CHANGES) AND MYOCARDIAL ISCHEMIA OR INFARCTION

As has been discussed, it is now widely accepted that MVP or BML may result from ischemic heart disease on the basis of papillary muscle dysfunction or fibrosis; but occlusive coronary artery disease and primary BML are common conditions, and

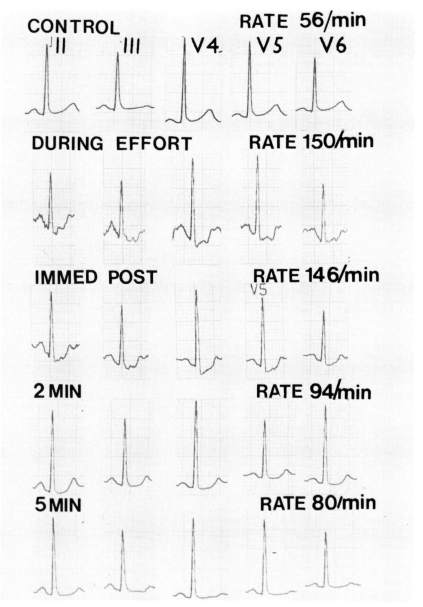

FIGURE 3-42. Upward coving of the ST segment after the J wave occurring during and immediately after exercise, in a 53-year-old man with atypical chest pain and a nonejection systolic click. This configuration should be differentiated from depressed ST segments of myocardial ischemia. The early onset and short duration of the ST changes are also not ischemic. (See Fig. 3-37, Type II.) (From Barlow,[37] with permission.)

there has to be a number of patients with both of these. Whenever selective coronary arteriography confirms occlusive coronary artery disease and left ventriculography shows a relatively mild BML, it is impossible to be certain whether the BML is primary or a result of myocardial ischemia. When the BML is marked, we favor the conclusion that the two conditions are occurring coincidentally (see Fig. 3-18).

The ECG, at rest or after effort, may show abnormalities in which changes of myocardial ischemia or of a primary BML may predominate (Fig. 3-43). The inevitability of these two conditions occurring together, and therefore of having electro-

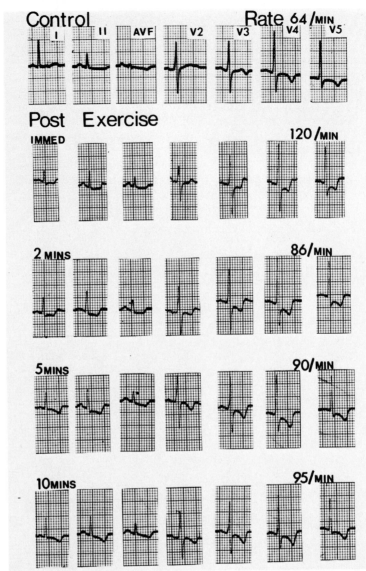

FIGURE 3-43. Control and posteffort ECGs of a 55-year-old man complaining of intractable, but very atypical, chest pain. A nonejection click was present and the control ECG is compatible with primary BML. Immediately two and five minutes after effort, there is at least 2 mm ST-segment depression in the left precordial leads. Cardiac catheterization confirmed BML, and selective coronary arteriography showed complete occlusion of the right coronary artery. We believe that this man has asymptomatic myocardial ischemia but that his chest pain is due to his BML. (From Barlow, JB and Pocock, WA: *Mitral valve prolapse, the athlete's heart, physical activity and sudden death.* Int J Sports Cardiol 1:9–24, 1984, with permission.)

cardiographic changes reflecting both conditions, has received little attention in the scientific literature. Recognition of this is important, because the explanation for chest pain in an individual patient is not necessarily resolved by confirmation of a BML or of anatomical occlusive coronary artery disease. Severe occlusive coronary artery disease with myocardial ischemia may not produce angina. Conversely, patients with the primary BML syndrome with normal coronary arteries and no demonstrable myocardial ischemia may suffer severe chest pain which occasionally is impossible to differentiate from true angina. There must, therefore, be a number of patients with angiographically proven coronary artery disease in whom the severe chest pain does not necessarily reflect myocardial ischemia. Furthermore, the primary BML syndrome is not the only condition that may be considered as an alternative diagnosis to coronary artery disease. So-called atypical chest pain syndrome, nonspecific T-wave changes, Da Costa's syndrome, neurocirculatory asthenia, hyperventilation syndrome, or "athlete's heart" must also be distinguished from ischemic heart disease, because of the patient's symptoms or electrocardiographic changes, or both. Regardless of whether most patients with these "Diseases of Yesteryear" are examples of the primary BML syndrome, as convincingly argued by Wooley,[42] their "cardiac disorder" is no prophylaxis against the future development of occlusive coronary artery disease! What then is the character of the chest pain of a patient with Da Costa's syndrome who develops myocardial ischemia from occlusive coronary artery disease? What are the electrocardiographic patterns of an athlete, or of an individual with nonspecific T-wave changes, or of a symptomatic patient with a primary BML, when the manifestations of occlusive coronary artery disease supervene? We should not forget that, just as not all chest pain is angina, not all chest pain in patients with severe occlusive coronary artery disease is due to myocardial ischemia. We should also not forget that every patient with the primary BML syndrome, Da Costa's syndrome, nonspecific T-wave changes, "athlete's heart," or atypical chest pain syndrome will eventually die and that the cause of death will often be occlusive coronary artery disease!

Another problem relates to the possible causal relationship between a primary BML and myocardial ischemia or infarction in the presence of anatomically normal or near-normal coronary arteries. The entity of myocardial ischemia or infarction with anatomically normal or near-normal coronary arteries is generally accepted. Many investigators favor that coronary artery spasm is the cause, but the reason for such spasm is unknown. In 1976, we reported four patients with the primary BML syndrome, myocardial infarction, and anatomically normal coronary arteries and postulated that coronary artery spasm or coronary artery emboli may be causally related to the BML syndrome.[43] One of those four patients, a 23-year-old man, had a small parietal lobe infarct, presumably embolic, about 22 months after his myocardial infarction. Since our original study, we have had similar patients. One was a 39-year-old man with an NESC who had had several systemic emboli over a two-year period and a clinically silent large apical myocardial infarction (Figs. 3-44, 3-

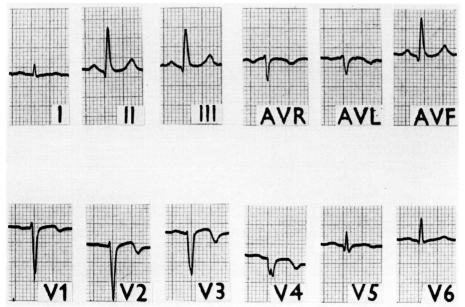

FIGURE 3-44. Electrocardiogram of a 39-year-old man with mild BML and a large "silent" apical myocardial infarction.

45). Coronary arteriography showed normal coronary arteries. Although a few observers, including Wigle's group in Toronto,[44,45] have now reported an association between coronary artery spasm and BML, the possibility of a causal relationship between the primary BML syndrome and myocardial ischemia or infarction has not to date aroused much interest. Vincent and colleagues[46] recently reported a 29-year-old woman with angiographically normal coronary arteries who sustained an acute myocardial infarction during selective coronary angiography. Coronary artery spasm and thrombosis were both demonstrated. The patient also had the primary BML syndrome on a familial basis, but neither Vincent and colleagues[46] nor Conti,[47] in a related editorial, mentioned the possible relationship between the two conditions.

We continue to question whether there is a causal relationship between the BML syndrome and myocardial ischemia or infarction, possibly induced by coronary artery spasm, which in turn may be provoked by coronary emboli. The chest pain of the primary BML syndrome can be differentiated in most instances from angina due to coronary artery disease. However, true angina may be atypical and have "widely variable expression," whereas the chest pain of some patients with the BML syndrome may closely simulate angina. We have encountered a relatively small group of patients in whom stress electrocardiography, selective coronary arteriography, and, most importantly, the recording of an ECG during the pain, have singly or in combination been essential in order to clarify the assessment.

Cerebral emboli, usually small, are a rare but generally recognized complication of a BML. We are well aware of the high prevalence of BML in both asymptomatic and symptomatic subjects and therefore of the possible fallacy in attributing systemic emboli to a relatively minor valve abnormality that is so common. Nevertheless, deposits of fibrin and platelet thrombi on the atrial surface of the posterior leaflet have been detected,[48] and these are a potential source of bland emboli.

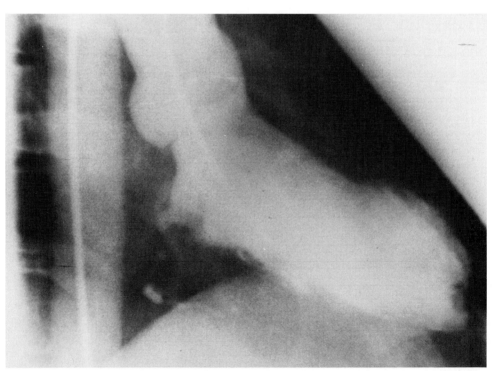

FIGURE 3-45. Left ventricular cineangiocardiogram of the 39-year-old man whose ECG is shown in Figure 3-44. Apical dyskinesia and thrombus are demonstrated. In addition, mild billowing of the mitral valve can be observed.

Furthermore, an association between the BML syndrome and migraine has been reported,[49] and increased platelet aggregability may be the pathophysiological mechanism. Patients of ours with BML and transient cerebral ischemic episodes have responded well to aspirin and dipyridamole. Patients with primary BML who have had myocardial infarction despite normal or near-normal coronary arteries have also done well on this therapy, but we give them coronary vasodilator therapy, usually nifedipine, as well.

HYPERTROPHIC CARDIOMYOPATHY

Most patients with hypertrophic cardiomyopathy encountered by cardiologists are symptomatic and have characteristic clinical and electrocardiographic features of that condition, although the resting ECG is occasionally normal. The systolic murmur of hypertrophic cardiomyopathy may be of relatively late onset but has a different cadence and starts earlier than the late systolic murmur of MVP (Fig. 3-46). Some subjects, including highly trained athletes with undoubted hypertrophic cardiomyopathy, are asymptomatic. We have reported a 32-year-old asymptomatic jogger in whom no abnormality was detected on physical examination.[50] His resting ECG indicated considerable left ventricular hypertrophy with deeply inverted T waves, including lead V_6, highly suggestive of the so-called apical hypertrophic cardiomyopathy, which has hitherto received most attention in the Japanese literature.[51] The T waves became deeper after exercise (Fig. 3-47). Angiocardiography and echocardiography confirmed the apical myocardial hypertrophy. Recently, we encountered a similar example of this condition in a 47-year-old man who was referred to us with the provisional diagnosis of "athlete's heart." He was symptomatic in that he com-

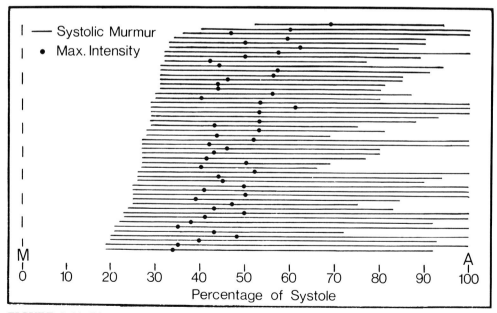

FIGURE 3-46. Diagrammatic representation of the delayed onset systolic murmurs of 50 patients with hypertrophic cardiomyopathy. The time of onset, maximal intensity, and end of each murmur are expressed as a percentage of the MA interval and can be compared with the late systolic murmurs of MVP in Figure 3-4. (From Tucker, RBK, Zion, MM, Pocock, WA, and Barlow, JB: *Auscultatory features of hypertrophic obstructive cardiomyopathy: A study of 90 patients.* S Afr Med J 49:179–186, 1975, with permission.)

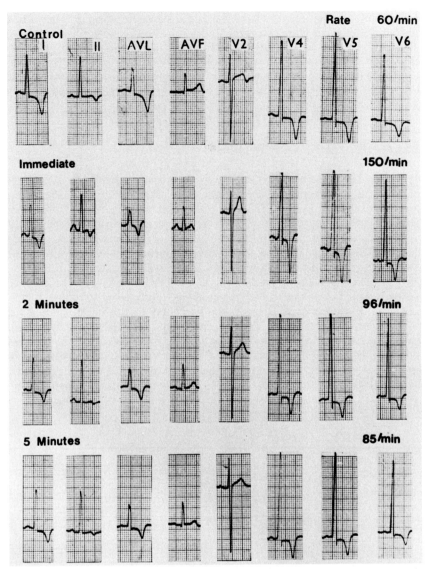

FIGURE 3-47. Control and posteffort ECGs of a 32-year-old asymptomatic jogger with apical hypertrophic cardiomyopathy. (From Barlow, JB and Pocock, WA: *Mitral valve prolapse, the athlete's heart, physical activity and sudden death.* Int J Sports Cardiol 1:9–24, 1984, with permission.)

plained of palpitations and a mild central chest pain on effort. On examination, his apex beat was abnormally forceful and compatible with left ventricular hypertrophy. An ECG recorded seven years previously was unusual but showed upright T waves (Fig. 3-48), whereas his current ECG (Fig. 3-49) showed large QRS voltages and deeply inverted T waves. The T-wave inversion did not change after exercise, but the ST-segment depression increased (Fig. 3-50). Echocardiography confirmed left ventricular hypertrophy, and coronary arteriography was normal. This patient also had a clearly audible atrial sound, which, despite some literature to the contrary, we consider as always indicative of an abnormal heart.

It is relevant to emphasize again that various combinations of athlete's heart, the primary BML syndrome, hypertrophic cardiomyopathy, and occlusive coronary artery disease may occur in the same subject.

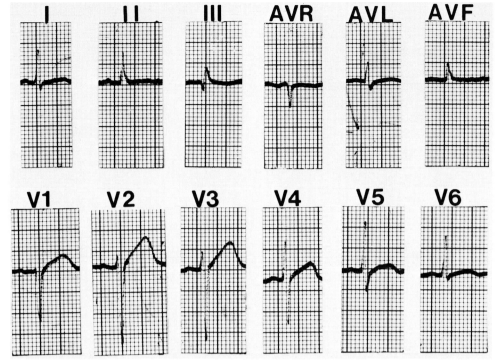

FIGURE 3-48. ECG of a man, then aged 40 years, who seven years later developed electro-cardiographic and clinical evidence of hypertrophic cardiomyopathy (see Fig. 3-49). The T waves are unusual but are upright in most leads. (From Barlow, JB and Pocock, WA: *Mitral valve prolapse, the athlete's heart, physical activity and sudden death.* Int J Sports Cardiol 1:9–24, 1984, with permission.)

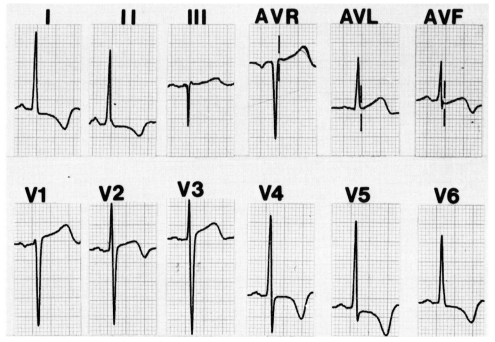

FIGURE 3-49. Large QRS voltages and deeply inverted T waves of the man of Figure 3-48, now aged 47 years (see Fig. 3-48). (From Barlow, JB and Pocock, WA: *Mitral valve prolapse, the athlete's heart, physical activity and sudden death.* Int J Sports Cardiol 1:9–24, 1984, with permission.)

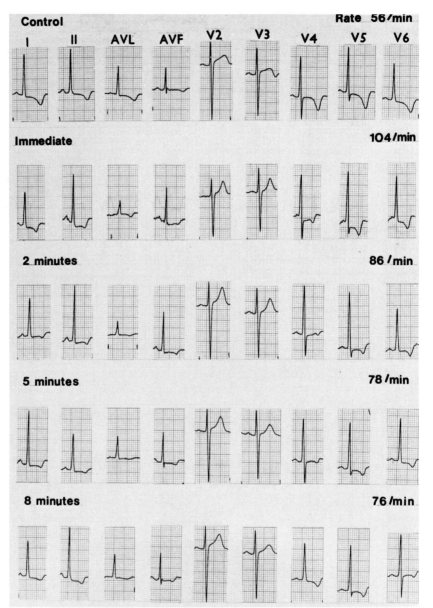

FIGURE 3-50. Control and posteffort ECGs of the man whose resting ECGs are shown in Figures 3-48 and 3-49. The post-effort tracings show marked ST segment depression, although the T-wave inversion does not alter significantly. (From Barlow, JB and Pocock, WA: *Mitral valve prolapse, the athlete's heart, physical activity and sudden death.* Int J Sports Cardiol 1:9–24, 1984, with permission.)

COURSE, PROGNOSIS, AND GENERAL MANAGEMENT OF PRIMARY MITRAL LEAFLET BILLOWING AND PROLAPSE

ASYMPTOMATIC PRIMARY BML AND MVP

Primary BML or MVP in asymptomatic individuals may be recognized during routine examinations, including those for employment or life insurance, or in surveys of schools and other institutions. The condition is sometimes detected because of an abnormal ECG, which may have been performed under similar circumstances. The asymptomatic subject may have been informed of the abnormality and must then be regarded as a "patient." Irrespective of whether the BML or the MVP is in a subject, a patient, or a trained athlete, a reasonable practical approach to management may be found in the following sections.

Isolated Nonejection Systolic Click on Auscultation (With or Without T-Wave Changes on ECG)

The asymptomatic subject, patient, or athlete either should not be informed about the click or, if he or she knows about it already, should be strongly reassured that it is virtually a "normal variant" that occurs in a large number of healthy people. A similar approach should be applied to subjects in whom a BML is detected on echocardiography, whether "silent" to auscultation or associated with an isolated NESC. We do not consider that there are always valid reasons to perform a stress electrocardiograph or Holter monitoring in such subjects. An effort electrocardiograph is indicated if the individual is employed in an important public service capacity, such as an airline pilot. A stress electrocardiograph is probably indicated if a BML is detected during examination for a life insurance policy or even during a routine check-up. Although asymptomatic subjects may occasionally develop arrhythmias after effort, the prognostic significance of this observation remains to be clarified. We have seldom observed any "important" arrhythmia in such asymptomatic subjects with a primary BML. By "important" arrhythmia, we refer to supraventricular tachycardia or ventricular ectopic beats falling into Lown's Grade 3, 4A, 4B, or 5 classification (Table 3-2). Using Holter monitoring during exercise, Pantano and Oriel[52] detected Grade 3 and 4A ventricular ectopy in "apparently normal" well-trained runners. They did not observe Grade 4B or 5. It is debatable whether athletes who develop Grade 3 or 4A ventricular premature beats are indeed normal. It remains important, however, that those runners were asymptomatic and, on currently available information, it is surely correct that they be permitted to continue their sport. The situation is somewhat hypothetical, but should athletes who are subjected to a stress electrocardiograph or Holter monitoring during their particular form of exercise develop Lown's Grade 4B or 5 ventricular ectopy, sport should presumably be stopped. It does not seem to be either practicable or helpful for these patients to receive antiarrhythmic therapy while they remain asymptomatic.

It is not justifiable for most other subjects with an isolated NESC detected during routine surveys to be subjected to a stress electrocardiograph. This applies, for example, to schoolchildren, students, employees in a factory, and so forth. We have encountered an analogous situation on routine screening of the ECGs of healthy young women who are prospective employees, as air hostesses, of South African Airways. A number of these women have had ST-segment and T-wave changes,

TABLE 3-2. Grading System for Ventricular Ectopy

GRADE	CHARACTERISTIC
1	Uniform ventricular premature beats (fewer than 30/hour)
2	Uniform ventricular premature beats (more than 30/hour)
3	Multiform ventricular premature beats
4A	Couplets (two consecutive ventricular premature beats
4B	Triplets (three or more consecutive ventricular premature beats)
5	R on T phenomenon

Adapted from Lown, B, and Wolf, M: Circulation 44:130–142, 1971.

compatible with a BML, and have then been examined by one of us (JBB). An isolated NESC is often present. We have not thought it meaningful to subject those young women to a stress test. An air hostess singled out from her peers for an effort electrocardiograph would require an explanation, would become anxious, and may even develop a cardiac neurosis. Should, in fact, a posteffort electrocardiogram reveal ventricular ectopy, we see little reason to believe that the woman should be informed, then reassurance attempted, and an antiarrhythmic agent prescribed.

The management of asymptomatic subjects with an isolated NESC with regard to prophylaxis against infective endocarditis is also controversial. Although there have been occasional cases of infective endocarditis, not only is prophylaxis in the majority of subjects involved impracticable but the overall benefit derived from it is highly questionable. We do not recommend antibiotic prophylaxis against infective endocarditis in patients or subjects with an isolated NESC. Similarly, we see no justification for recommending such prophylaxis in cases with echocardiographic evidence of BML unless there is auscultatory confirmation of associated MVP.

Nonpansystolic Mitral Murmur (With or Without an "Abnormal" ECG)

If a late systolic murmur, albeit intermittent, is detected, this denotes mitral regurgitation and the risk of infective endocarditis is almost certainly greater. The patient should be informed of the MVP and advised to take prophylactic antibiotics before dental treatment or other procedure of "risk," Our policy regarding the detection and management of arrhythmias is the same as that described above for asymptomatic subjects with an isolated NESC.

Most subjects with a constant late systolic murmur on auscultation can be shown to have BML on echocardiography. The BML is confined to late systole on M-mode echocardiography (see Fig. 3-20), and this timing can be confirmed on 2-D echocardiography (Fig. 3-51). An asymptomatic subject with a late systolic murmur should be assessed annually for evidence of progression of MVP on auscultation and of increase in extent of BML on echocardiography. In our experience, most late systolic murmurs do not change over many years.

It is more difficult to define a definite policy in subjects who have an early nonpansystolic apical murmur. These murmurs have received little attention in the literature, but we believe, particularly when they are confined to the apex and associated with an NESC, that they denote mild mitral regurgitation and therefore MVP. Whereas the typical cadence of a late systolic murmur makes it easy to identify, the differentiation of an early mitral systolic murmur from an ejection systolic murmur heard at the apex may be difficult. Nonetheless, despite our frequent inability to confirm the BML on echocardiography, we manage subjects with a mitral early systolic murmur on the same lines as those with a late systolic murmur.

Pansystolic Mitral Murmur (With or Without an "Abnormal" ECG)

We are considering now asymptomatic subjects with BML and MVP who have a pansystolic murmur of *mild* mitral regurgitation. There should be no clinical, electrocardiographic, or radiological evidence of left ventricular or left atrial enlargement; splitting of the second sound should be normal; and the presence of a third heart sound must be judged "physiological." Physiological third heart sounds are extremely common in children and young adults, but also in physically fit older individuals. Echocardiography will now invariably confirm the BML that is pansystolic (the so-called hammock pattern) and relatively severe (see Fig. 3-21).

Of course, prophylaxis against infective endocarditis is indicated, as is regular evaluation of the severity of the mitral regurgitation. If the patient is involved in a sport requiring strenuous exercise, some cardiologists may prefer to subject him or

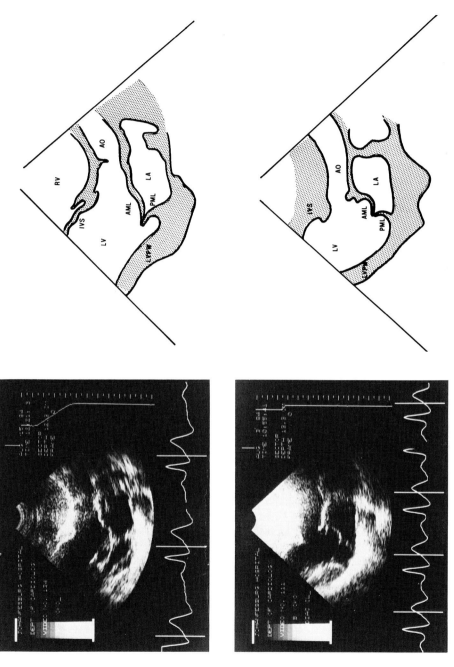

FIGURE 3-51. Parasternal long-axis views and labelled drawings of 2-D echocardiograms recorded in early *(top left, right)* and late *(bottom left, right)* systole. Billowing of the mitral leaflets towards the left atrium is demonstrated during late systole. This is the same patient as in Figure 3-20.

her to a submaximal stress electrocardiograph or to Holter monitoring during the sport activity itself. Based on data currently available, and we emphasize that the patient must be truly asymptomatic, we consider that the development of an arrhythmia (provided it is not Lown's Grade 4B or 5) should be managed as previously described in a manner similar to that of subjects with a BML with or without nonpansystolic MVP. Thus, the sport participation should be allowed to continue, and antiarrhythmic therapy is not warranted.

There are cardiologists who would advise against very strenuous sport in an athlete with a pansystolic murmur of MVP and holosystolic BML on echocardiography, because of the possibility of the exercise causing deterioration of the valve lesion. We find it impossible to generalize in this regard.

SYMPTOMATIC PRIMARY BML AND MVP

Because the patient is symptomatic, the symptoms are of concern to the patient, and he or she is seeking assistance. Whether or not the clinician believes that some or none of the symptoms can be attributed to the primary BML, a compassionate attitude to the patient is essential. The more prominent features of the syndrome will be considered in relation to management.

Anxiety

Numerous patients with the primary BML syndrome are anxious, but they also have other cardiovascular symptoms, such as chest pain, palpitations, or dizziness, which are not necessarily features of anxiety states caused by domestic problems, inability to cope at work, or other stressful situations prevalent in modern society. In other words, the anxiety associated with the BML syndrome invariably has a cardiac connotation, and there is a fear of serious heart disease or sudden death. The symptomatic presentation is therefore very similar to, if not identical with, so-called irritable heart, neurocirculatory asthenia, soldier's heart, Da Costa's syndrome, atypical chest pain syndrome, and similar disorders. As previously mentioned, the anxiety of these patients has often been exacerbated, and not alleviated, by the insistence of medical attendants that there is no organic heart disease present or that the symptoms are not of cardiac origin. It is not reassuring to patients with disturbing symptoms, particularly chest pain and palpitations, to be told that they are "neurotic," that the symptoms are "all in the mind," or that they should "forget about it and pull themselves together." We have found it more reassuring and consoling to the patient to be told that "the valve anomaly is extremely common, valve function normal (BML) or very mildly abnormal (MVP), and that the associated symptoms are genuine, albeit ill understood, but are of nuisance value only."

A beta-receptor blocking agent invariably alleviates the systemic effects of the anxiety whether or not it also directly affects the underlying causes of the symptoms, such as by suppressing an arrhythmia predisposing to palpitations or by decreasing the force of myocardial contractility (which thus relieves chest pain).

Chest Pain

Despite the large number of anxious patients with the BML syndrome and chest pain, we have also been impressed by the presentation of chest pain, sometimes severe and disabling, in somewhat stoical subjects who were previously unaware of having a BML, MVP, or any other cardiac abnormality. Although so-called atypical chest pain is a symptom that may have many causes, we believe that a BML is one of them. We readily concede that there are some patients with similar chest pain who have no conclusive evidence of a BML. When a primary BML is detected or even suspected, and provided that ominous or other treatable causes of chest pain have been excluded, we find it meaningful to attribute the chest pain to the BML and to inform the patient of that opinion.

Although chest pain may be more frequent in patients with the BML syndrome who have an abnormal ECG, there are others in whom the ECG, both at rest and after effort, remains normal. The mechanism of production of the chest pain is ill understood. Cobbs,[53] Jeresaty,[54] as well as ourselves,[55] independently suggested that increased tension from chordae tendineae may tug on a papillary muscle and produce pain. Increased tension on papillary muscles would be compatible with the observation that T-wave inversion develops or becomes more marked with standing or amyl nitrite inhalation, both of which result in greater billowing of leaflets. Following their angiocardiographic observations on regional left ventricular wall movement abnormalities in patients with the BML syndrome, Gibson and Brown[56] more recently also considered the possibility that regional subendocardial ischemia may be a factor in causing chest pain and arrhythmias.

The pain is most commonly sharp, fleeting, left-sided, and localised to the apical region. There is seldom a relation to exercise or emotion. Some patients insist that they have to sit or even lie down. The pain may be sufficiently severe to cause considerable anxiety or a feeling of "impending doom." It may occur in bed at night but seldom wakes the patient. Holter monitoring has not demonstrated a correlation between transient T-wave changes and chest pain. These characteristics have left some clinicians unconvinced that the chest pain is cardiac, or indeed organic, in origin. Other patients, invariably with associated anxiety, complain of a constant localised chest pain lasting for hours or even days. We do not dispute the concept that anxiety is an aggravating factor, and in some instances probably the principal factor, that contributes to chest pain in symptomatic patients with the primary BML syndrome.

A few patients complain of chest pain indistinguishable from angina. It is possible that some have learnt of the nature of true angina pectoris from other patients or medical attendants. In our experience, a stress electrocardiogram is highly contributory in excluding occlusive coronary artery disease, but, depending on the context of the situation, selective coronary arteriography or radionucleotide studies may be necessary for confirmation. The problem is obviously easier to resolve in, for example, a 20-year-old female as opposed to a middle-aged man. It is amongst this group of patients with "typical angina," albeit usually at rest, that the possibility of coronary artery spasm arises. There is support in the literature for the diagnostic role of ergonovine injection in provoking coronary artery spasm in such patients. We consider that the most contributory method of excluding the possibility of coronary artery spasm is to record an electrocardiogram during an attack of the "typical angina pectoris." It must be emphasized, however, that this possibility of coronary artery spasm arises in only a very small minority of patients with the primary BML syndrome who complain of chest pain.

Reassurance is important in the management of patients with the BML syndrome who complain of chest pain. We consider that beta-receptor blocking agents are also contributory, irrespective of their effect on anxiety. As stated previously, our patients with definite primary BML, normal or near-normal coronary arteries, and myocardial ischemia or infarction, have responded well to aspirin, dipyridamole, and nifedipine therapy.

Systemic Emboli

Irrespective of whether the condition is detected by auscultation or by echocardiography, BML is common in "normal" populations. Some clinicians thus remain unconvinced that transient cerebral ischemic attacks, hemiplegia, or other cases of systemic embolization of unknown or uncertain origin, have a causal relationship with the BML. We have observed, or been informed of, approximately 40 patients in our institution who have had bland systemic emboli with no source of origin other than a BML. Almost all of these patients had previously been asymptomatic, and it is rare, in our experience, for a patient with primary BML syndrome and symptoms to suffer subsequently a bland systemic embolus. It is therefore not our policy to prescribe antithrombotic therapy routinely to patients with a BML. As previously stated, patients who have had embolic events have responded well to antithrombotic (usually aspirin and dipyridamole) therapy as well as, in a few instances when indicated, the coronary vasodilator drug nifedipine.

Progressive Mitral Regurgitation

It is impossible to predict with certainty the future course of an individual patient with a primary BML as regards the progression to significant mitral regurgitation. Jeresaty[57] summarized the data (much of which is incomplete or influenced by selection of cases) that were available prior to 1979. Our four-year follow-up of young subjects with an isolated NESC confirmed our general clinical impression that progression to mitral regurgitation is rare and that rapid progression to significant mitral regurgitation is extremely rare. We have observed patients with MVP reflected by a late systolic murmur advance to a pansystolic murmur during a 10- to 20-year period, but rapid progression is very unusual in the absence of infective endocarditis or Marfan's syndrome. A few patients with a late systolic murmur are presumably suffering from the "floppy valve syndrome" without skeletal manifestations of Marfan's syndrome, but we find it difficult or impossible to identify these with certainty. Obvious BML on echocardiography does not mean that marked MVP will inevitably ensue. It is probable that some, especially middle-aged or elderly men, will develop severe mitral regurgitation associated with rupture of chordae to the posterior leaflet. We have observed this progression but seldom. Middle-aged or elderly Caucasian patients with floppy valves or the syndrome of "idiopathic rupture of chordae" requiring mitral valve surgery are not uncommon, and we operate on approximately seven such patients annually. It is a minority of these who have reliable evidence of having previously had a late systolic murmur or echocardiographic signs of a BML. Four such patients in whom MVP had been documented 4 to 11 years earlier have recently been discussed by Jeresaty and co-workers.[58] Some patients presenting with acute severe mitral regurgitation would presumably have had auscultatory and echocardiographic evidence of primary BML many years previously, but the reason for the sudden onset of severe mitral regurgitation remains unknown in the majority.

We conclude that most patients, regardless of age or sex, who have a late or early nonpansystolic murmur of MVP associated with BML on echocardiography will run a favorable course and will not progress to severe mitral regurgitation. Yearly observation is, however, mandatory. The outcome of mild mitral regurgitation in a patient with a pansystolic murmur and pansystolic billowing on echocardiography is less certain, but progression to severe mitral regurgitation, in the absence of Marfan's syndrome or infective endocarditis, has seldom been observed.

Infective Endocarditis

We have discussed the prophylaxis against infective endocarditis, and it is our policy not to recommend antibiotic prophylaxis in patients with a BML unless definite MVP, detected by a mitral systolic murmur, is present.

We have encountered several cases of infective endocarditis in patients with BML and without MVP, but this is probably very rare. The prevalence of infective endocarditis on a BML, with or without MVP, is not known. It is probable that some patients with infective endocarditis on a "normal valve" originally had an underlying BML.

Arrhythmias and Conduction Defects

Symptoms such as palpitations, lightheadedness, dizziness, or syncope suggest the presence of arrhythmias or conduction defects, but exercise electrocardiography or ambulatory monitoring may be necessary for confirmation. Arrhythmias may occasionally occur without symptoms and, conversely, dizziness and palpitations have been prominent complaints at times when electrocardiographic monitoring or clinical examination provided no objective explanation. Orthostatic hypotension should be excluded in all patients with these symptoms, particularly if 24-hour ambulatory monitoring is negative.

A wide variety of arrhythmias has been encountered in association with the primary BML syndrome and includes supraventricular tachycardia, atrial fibrillation, atrial flutter, atrial ectopic beats, ventricular tachycardia, and ventricular fibrillation. Ventricular extrasystoles (Figs. 3-52, 3-53) are the most common rhythm disturbance, may be unifocal or multifocal, and may display the R on T phenomenon. They are often precipitated or aggravated by emotion and exercise. Ventricular extrasystoles may occur with an otherwise normal ECG, irrespective of whether they are unifocal or multifocal or whether they are present at rest or only after exercise. The cause of the arrhythmias is speculative. Ventricular arrhythmias may result from abnormal tension on papillary muscles, with secondary papillary muscle and adjacent myocardial ischemia. This theory would be compatible with the cineangiocardiographic observations of Gibson and Brown[56] of regional wall abnormalities in systole and diastole. Endocardial friction lesions, produced by contact between the chordae and left ventricular endocardium, have been emphasized by Chesler and co-workers[48] to be associated with myxomatous mitral valves, and the friction responsible for the lesions may be a cause of the ventricular dysrhythmias. Deposits of fibrin and platelets found in the angle between the posterior mitral leaflet and the left atrial wall could be a cause of coronary embolism, again possibly leading to ventricular arrhythmias. It would be difficult to explain atrial arrhythmias on these

I MIN POST EXERCISE

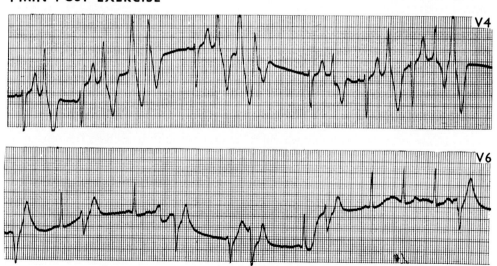

FIGURE 3-52. Numerous multifocal ventricular extrasystoles recorded in leads V_4 and V_6 approximately one minute after exercise in a 38-year-old woman.

Immed. Post Exercise

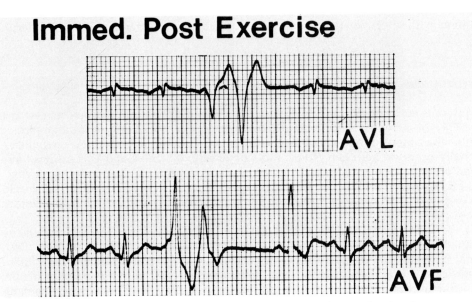

FIGURE 3-53. Multifocal ventricular ectopic beats that occurred immediately after strenuous exercise in the young woman whose ECG is shown in Figure 3-28. (From Barlow and Pocock,[31] with permission.)

mechanisms. Wit and associates[59] demonstrated spontaneous diastolic depolarization of muscle fibres in the anterior mitral leaflet of the dog when these were stretched or exposed to catecholamines, and they suggested that the mitral valve could act as a site of ectopic impulse initiation. A similar mechanism in humans may explain some of the atrial arrhythmias with the primary BML syndrome, in which there may be considerable stretching of the leaflets.

Conduction disturbances have been observed and include sinoatrial block, left and right bundle branch block, and left anterior hemiblock. Prolongation of the PR interval has also been encountered. An association of a primary BML with the Wolff-Parkinson-White syndrome has been reported, but it remains uncertain whether this conduction defect is a consequence of the primary BML, whether it is a chance association, or whether the abnormal activation of ventricular contraction results in the BML.

The mechanism of the conduction disturbances has not been clarified. Trent and co-workers[60] described interruption of the conduction system as a result of fibrosis in the myocardium in one patient. In 1981, Bharati and associates[61] made a detailed study of the conduction system in three cases of BML and observed premature aging and sclerosis of the atrioventricular node and trifascicular conduction system, thrombosis of the sinoatrial nodal artery, and fatty infiltration in the approach to the sinoatrial and atrioventricular nodes. In 1967, James[62] had described in Marfan's syndrome a degenerative process of small coronary vessels supplying the sinus and atrioventricular nodes, the His bundle, and its branches. The relevance of these histological findings in the pathogenesis of conduction defects or tachyarrhythmias needs elucidation. Whatever the mechanism of conduction disturbances, a conduction disturbance as the possible cause of palpitations or syncope should be excluded before starting treatment with antiarrhythmic drugs, especially beta-receptor blocking agents.

The management of conduction defects or supraventricular arrhythmias in patients with the primary BML syndrome does not differ from that of patients without a BML and will not be further discussed.

The detection and management of ventricular arrhythmias is probably the most important challenge for the clinician confronted with symptomatic patients, including athletes, with the BML syndrome. The symptoms suggestive of episodes of arrhythmia are palpitations, lightheadedness or dizziness, and syncope. All patients with such symptoms should be subjected to 24-hour Holter monitoring or to a stress electrocardiograph. If the rhythm remains normal or if unifocal ventricular ectopic beats develop, our policy is to treat symptoms with firm reassurance and sometimes a beta-receptor blocking agent. A good response can be anticipated. If Grade 3, 4A, 4B, or 5 ventricular ectopy is detected, then the arrhythmia should be treated until control is achieved or symptoms are considerably improved. Beta-receptor blocking agents are again the standby of drug therapy. The beta-receptor blocking agent, sotalol, is unique as a beta-receptor blocking agent in that it also has Class III antiarrhythmic activity.[63] We have had favorable results over several years using this beta-receptor blocking agent for the treatment of supraventricular and ventricular arrhythmias due to any underlying pathology. In recent months, we have also had a favorable, albeit relatively small, experience using sotalol in symptomatic patients with the BML syndrome and ventricular ectopy. Because of the possible occurrence of torsade de pointes if hypokalemia supervenes, sotalol therapy should be avoided in any patient concurrently receiving diuretic therapy. Sotalol should also be used cautiously in conjunction with other drugs known to prolong the QT interval, such as Class I antiarrhythmic agents, phenothiazines, and tricyclic antidepressants.

All effective antiarrhythmic drugs may have serious or dangerous side effects. Side effects of disopyramide and quinidine have led us almost to abandon their use. Amiodarone is the most effective antiarrhythmic agent that we have used to date in the treatment of refractory ventricular tachyarrhythmias. The potentially serious side effects of that drug mitigate against its use, except in severe cases intractable to other therapy.

Sudden Death

In 1970, we subjected 12 patients with the primary BML syndrome to a submaximal effort test and detected multifocal ventricular extrasystoles in three.[55] We therefore emphasized the importance of exercise in precipitating premature ventricular contractions and warned of a risk of sudden death, should multifocal ventricular ectopy develop. At that time, sudden death was not a recognized complication of the BML syndrome, although one such patient had been reported by Hancock and Cohn[64] in 1966 and another by us[25] in 1968. Following that original warning, however, numerous studies on BML and MVP, as well as our own increased experience, revealed that the BML syndrome was highly prevalent. Furthermore, despite detection of potentially lethal ventricular ectopy after exercise or on 24-hour Holter monitoring, reports of sudden death were scanty and clinical details or necropsy findings were usually absent or incomplete. It therefore became widely accepted that a primary BML is a benign condition with a generally excellent prognosis. The problem of sudden death has been compounded by the probability in some instances that the BML was a secondary or associated feature. The arrhythmogenic effect of drugs, notably quinidine, may well have been responsible for sudden demise in other cases. In addition, sudden unexpected death, with or without preceding observation of potentially fatal ventricular arrhythmias, has occasionally been encountered in young adults in whom necropsy neither showed evidence of a BML nor provided a satisfactory explanation for the cause of death.

The demonstration of multifocal ventricular extrasystoles, especially when showing the R on T phenomenon or causing appropriate symptoms, cannot be ignored regardless of whether an underlying or associated cardiac condition, including BML or MVP, is present. The nature of the cardiac condition, the presence of relevant symptoms, and the context of the situation in which the ventricular ectopy is detected are crucial factors in assessing an individual patient. It is difficult to generalize. Few cardiologists would dispute that patients with multifocal ventricular extrasystoles and coronary artery disease or hypertrophic cardiomyopathy are at significant risk of sudden death. On the other hand, the prognosis of patients with multiform ventricular ectopy, occurring with BML or without detectable underlying cardiac pathology, is generally good. Because of our known interest in the BML syndrome, we have received information from other centers on unpublished cases of unexpected sudden death in which BML or floppy leaflets were detected at necropsy. Chesler and co-workers[48] have recently reported the necropsy findings of similar cases. Comprehensive clinical data was seldom available, and it remains impossible to estimate the incidence of this unfortunate outcome. The overall prevalence has to be very low and the risk small. Motulsky's[65] comment in 1978 that "for every patient with symptomatic mitral valve prolapse there are hundreds of asymptomatic persons" remains pertinent. It is also pertinent to re-emphasize that the majority of symptomatic patients have complaints largely attributable to anxiety with no confirmation, including by Holter monitoring and stress electrocardiography, of potentially fatal ventricular ectopy. These facts are no consolation to the relatives of the few subjects who do die suddenly. Doctors, especially pathologists, must become aware that a primary BML should be actively sought in cases of unexpected sudden death, in addition to the hitherto better-recognized and more obvious causes, such as occlusive coronary artery disease, congenital anomalies of coronary arteries, hypertrophic cardiomyopathy, aortic stenosis, acute viral myopericarditis, the congenital prolonged QT syndrome, conduction system abnormalities, cardiac neoplasm, and acute pulmonary embolism.

Despite our long experience of asymptomatic and symptomatic subjects or patients in whom we have diagnosed BML, we are aware of unexpected death in only one of our own patients. We do not claim to have conducted a thorough follow-up of our large series of patients, but "bad news travels fast" and we think that we would have been informed of unexpected deaths. In addition to our own patient, we have documented unexpected deaths in two subjects with BML in whom relevant information strongly suggests that the mitral valve anomaly was a relevant factor.[66] The first was a 39-year-old man who died while mowing a lawn. He had marked BML at necropsy (Fig. 3-54) and reputedly no coronary artery disease. The other was a 43-year-old woman who had complained of palpitations and who had been rec-

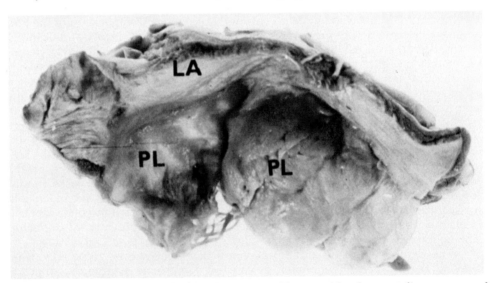

FIGURE 3-54. Posterior mitral leaflet of a 39-year-old man with a late systolic murmur and click who died suddenly during mild exercise. The valve is viewed from the atrial aspect. At necropsy the voluminous leaflet was inadvertently cut, and this has been sutured. The chordae are thin and elongated. PL = posterior leaflet; LA = left atrial wall. (From Barlow et al,[25] with permission.)

ognized by Kleynhans and his colleagues in Bloemfontein[66] as an example of primary BML syndrome on the basis of an apical late systolic murmur and NESC, intermittent transient T-wave inversion in the inferior leads of the electrocardiograph, and late systolic billowing on M-mode echocardiography. She had developed multifocal ventricular extrasystoles and a short run of ventricular tachycardia after a stress test. That woman's electrocardiograms have been examined by us, and although we have no information concerning a necropsy, we accept her as a typical case of the primary BML syndrome.

Because well-documented cases with clinical details and necropsy findings are rare, it is relevant to provide details of our 24-year-old female patient whom we have recently reported.[66] She was referred to us as an asymptomatic child, aged 8 years, for assessment of a loud late systolic murmur and NESC (see Fig. 3-5). The ECG showed slightly elevated ST segments with T-wave inversion in leads 2, 3, and aV$_F$ (see Fig. 3-27). Left ventricular cineangiography demonstrated mild mitral regurgitation and considerable billowing of the posterior mitral leaflet (Fig. 3-55). She was not subjected to stress electrocardiography at that time. Relatives were examined, and her father had an isolated NESC. She attended our clinic at six-month intervals and remained asymptomatic. At 13 years of age, numerous multifocal ventricular extrasystoles were recorded after a strenuous exercise test (Fig. 3-56). On propranolol, 80 mg daily, and diphenylhydantoin, 300 mg daily, the arrhythmia was sup-

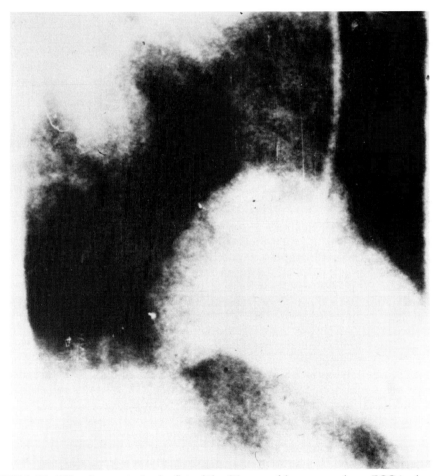

FIGURE 3-55. Billowing posterior leaflet of the 24-year-old woman whose ECG is shown in Figure 3-27. (From Barlow, JB and Bosman, CK: *Aneurysmal protrusion of the posterior leaflet of the mitral valve.* Am Heart J 71:166–178, 1966, with permission.)

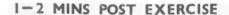

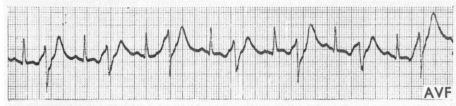

NO TREATMENT

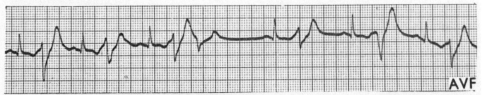

PROPRANOLOL 80 mg. DAILY

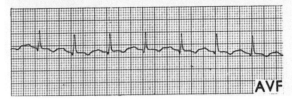

FIGURE 3-56. Postexercise ECGs before and after treatment in a 13-year-old girl. This is the same patient who was originally seen at age 8 (see Figs. 3-27, 3-55). *Top,* Multifocal ventricular extrasystoles in bigeminal rhythm. *Middle,* Extrasystoles persist after one month on propranolol, 80 mg daily. *Bottom,* No ectopic beats appear after one month on propranolol, 80 mg daily, and phenytoin (diphenylhydantoin), 300 mg daily. It is noteworthy that several of the ectopic beats occur early and are of the R on T variety. (From Pocock and Barlow,[55] with permission.)

pressed (Fig. 3-56). She was thereafter assessed at yearly intervals by our colleague (CK Bosman), who was in practice near her residence, and she remained well with no change in electrocardiographic or auscultatory features. At 22 years of age, she admitted to occasional palpitations when she was tired or excited. At no time was there syncope or presyncope. Suppression of the arrhythmia varied with patient compliance and alteration in drug regimen, but premature ventricular contractions could usually be provoked by effort. In May 1980, frequent multifocal ventricular extrasystoles (Fig. 3-57) were noted on a routine electrocardiogram. Treatment was altered to disopyramide, 100 mg twice daily, and acebutolol, 100 mg twice daily; and when she was seen again after six months, no arrhythmia was detected. Six months after that, while talking to her sister and without any emotional disturbance, she collapsed and could not be resuscitated.

Pathological findings were confined to the heart. The posterior leaflet of the mitral valve showed extensive interchordal hooding and billowing towards the left atrium. The leaflet was opaque and thickened, and its related chordae tendineae were elongated and thickened (see Fig. 3-25). The anterior leaflet was also thickened but not redundant. A discrete, 1 cm × 1 cm area of endocardial thickening was present above the posteromedial commissure of the mitral valve and was interpreted as a "jet lesion" resulting from mitral regurgitation. The left ventricle was of normal size and thickness. Adjacent to the posterior mitral leaflet the mural endocardium

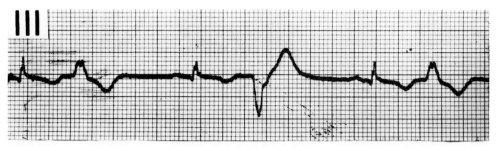

FIGURE 3-57. ECG (standard lead III) recorded one year prior to patient's death, showing multifocal premature contractions. See text. (From Pocock et al,[66] with permission.)

showed fibrous thickening, which was confluent in one area. In the angle between the left atrial wall and the posterior leaflet, there was a linear array of hemorrhagic lesions that microscopically consisted of aggregates of connective tissue, fibrin, platelets, leukocytes, and red cells. The coronary arteries were normal. Microscopic examination of the posterior leaflet showed marked thickening of the spongiosa, which encroached upon and disrupted the fibrosa (Fig. 3-58). The spongiosa of the anterior mitral leaflet was also increased but less extensively. No microscopic abnormalities were detected in the myocardium.

The circumstances of this patient's death suggest that she had ventricular fibrillation, probably related to the multifocal premature ventricular contractions that had been present intermittently for at least 11 years. Drug-induced fibrillation is unlikely, since the dose of disopyramide was very low and there had been no recent change in her drug regimen nor on the ECG. A disturbing feature of this case was that the young woman had originally been asymptomatic and later had mild symptoms only. She had therefore not always been compliant in adhering to the drug regimen. The fact that marked BML with MVP were detected at the age of 8 years, reflected clinically by the loud, constant, late systolic murmur and confirmed cineangiocardiographically, also places her in a small minority group.

Based on the 25 documented cases of sudden unexpected deaths collected by Jeresaty in 1979,[57] the necropsy and other material reported by Chesler and co-workers,[48] our own recent review[66] of a further 17 cases, and the information available to us from conversation or correspondence, we have attempted to identify the small number of patients at higher risk. A prominent BML, readily demonstrated on M-mode or 2-D echocardiography, and indisputable MVP, evaluated clinically by a constant apical late systolic murmur that becomes louder and longer on standing, are pertinent features especially if detected at an early age. Abnormal T waves and ventricular ectopy on the resting ECG are other probable risk factors. Sudden unexpected deaths have a preponderance of women. Regrettably, there are exceptions to all those "higher risk" features. Nonetheless, and until more data allow a more accurate profile of the patient at risk to be obtained, a policy has to be formulated that will not create anxiety or even cardiac neurosis in a large number of asymptomatic or symptomatic patients. On current evidence we suggest that symptomatic patients with ventricular ectopy at rest, especially when there is a convincing history of palpitations, syncope, or even presyncope, be subjected to 24-hour ambulatory monitoring or, if facilities are not readily available, to a strenuous stress test. Those who develop multiform ventricular extrasystoles or other potentially dangerous arrhythmias should be maintained on antiarrhythmic drugs with regular monitoring to ensure that control is adequate. Any beta-receptor blocking agent may contribute to therapy, but we have already suggested the advantages of giving sotalol, which has Class III antiarrhythmic activity, in some cases. Amiodarone, because of significant side effects, should be used only for intractable and serious ventricular arrhythmias. If patients continue to exhibit dangerous arrhythmias despite sotalol, amiodarone, or

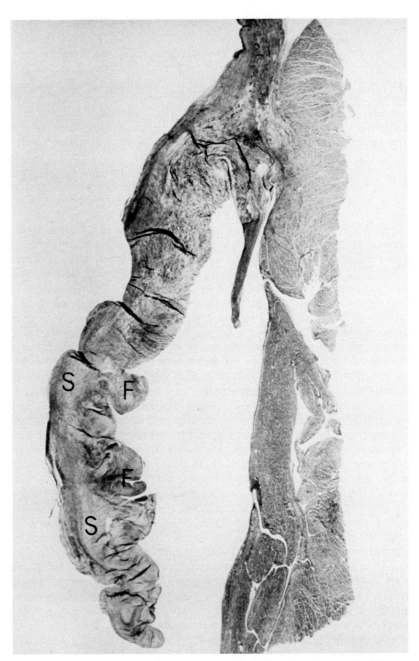

FIGURE 3-58. Photomicrograph of posterior mitral leaflet showing marked increase in the spongiosa layer (*S*), which encroaches upon the fibrosa (*F*). See text. (From Pocock et al,[66] with permission.)

other antiarrhythmic agents, the question of mitral valve surgery arises. Cobbs and King[67] referred a patient with recurrent ventricular fibrillation for mitral valve replacement in 1973 and observed improvement following surgery. In 1979, Jerome Kay and co-workers[68] reported improvement after mitral valve repair in six very symptomatic patients with severe billowing but mild mitral regurgitation. It must be emphasized that the indication for mitral valve surgery related to the symptoms and the arrhythmias and not to the hemodynamically mild mitral regurgitation. Kay[69] has extended this experience and remains satisfied with the long-term results. In 1985, Denton Cooley's group[70] in Houston published favorable results following mitral valve repair in 37 symptomatic patients with the primary BML syndrome. A policy of surgical treatment for ventricular arrhythmias or disabling symptoms in patients with the primary BML syndrome without significant mitral regurgitation may seem unduly aggressive. On the other hand, we will never know whether the young woman reported by us would be alive today if she had been subjected to a mitral valve repair procedure. Fortunately, we have no such patient at present, but we would now regard the combination of advanced billowing demonstrated echocardiographically and confirmed angiocardiographically, some mitral regurgitation, important symptoms such as presyncope or syncope, and dangerous ventricular arrhythmias unresponsive to treatment with antiarrhythmic agents as an indication for mitral valve repair even in the absence of hemodynamically significant regurgitation.

CONCLUDING REMARKS

Although we have not reviewed the literature in this chapter, we claim to have read during the last two decades nearly all of the vast number of English language publications relating to so-called mitral valve prolapse. We have attempted to correlate this literature with our own experience, to clarify some features, and to emphasize others.

In our view, current confusion would be considerably reduced if Carpentier's concept[15] of "billowing" and "prolapse," which is based on functional anatomical factors, was generally recognized and accepted. We have expanded that concept[16] in an attempt to clarify terminology. The normal mitral leaflets billow slightly after closure but an exaggeration of that should be termed "billowing" mitral leaflets (BML). This can often be detected on auscultation by a nonejection systolic click and may be confirmed on echocardiography or cineangiocardiography depending on the extent of the billowing of the scallops or leaflets. A "floppy valve" is thus an extremely severe form of BML whereas very mild BML, sometimes involving part of one scallop, could justifiably be regarded as a variant of normal. Prolapse (MVP) occurs when part of the leaflet edges no longer appose, mitral regurgitation is an inevitable consequence, and this is most reliably and practicably detected by the presence of a mitral systolic murmur on auscultation. Although there are causes of MVP without BML, this chapter is concerned mainly with the MVP that supervenes on more advanced BML. "Flail" is an exaggeration of MVP and occurs when chordae rupture or are very elongated; the flail leaflet edge can be observed on echocardiography, and the associated mitral regurgitation is usually hemodynamically significant.

The eponym, Barlow's syndrome, has not infrequently been used as synonymous with BML or MVP. If an eponym is used at all, this should surely be confined to the syndrome relating to *primary* BML with or without supervening MVP. We consider it important to recognize that primary BML is a degenerative, albeit usually mild, condition of the leaflets and chordae, which is highly prevalent, seldom significantly progressive, and usually benign. It is frequently asymptomatic but may be associated with symptoms dominated mainly by anxiety. Policies of management relating to symptoms, the occurrence of systemic emboli, the detection of arrhythmias, and prophylaxis against infective endocarditis have to be formulated. We cannot claim to have provided answers to many questions, some of which are of academic interest but others of great clinical importance. Clarification of the roles of autonomic dysfunction, myocardial disorder or dysfunction, and an explanation for the electrocardiographic ST-segment and T-wave changes may be of much academic interest, but are unlikely to influence clinical management in the near future.

We have also attempted to emphasize the importance in recognizing BML and MVP that are secondary to underlying myocardial pathology such as ischemic heart disease or cardiomyopathy. The coincidental association of primary BML with numerous conditions, whether they are uncommon or not, is also emphasized. In our experience, either because of electrocardiographic changes or symptoms including chest pain and palpitations, benign syndromes such as the primary BML syndrome, Da Costa's syndrome, atypical chest pain syndrome, nonspecific T-wave changes, hyperventilation syndrome, or so-called athlete's heart must be differentiated from more serious heart disease notably occlusive coronary artery disease and hypertrophic cardiomyopathy. It is our contention that exercise electrocardiographic testing remains a most practicable and cost-effective investigation for identifying occlusive coronary artery disease and that the high prevalence of false-positive results could be considerably reduced by improved assessment of ST-segment and T-wave time-course behavior. We may overdiagnose the primary BML syndrome but give reasons why we consider that that policy is beneficial to an individual patient.

The management of intractable and dangerous arrhythmias as well as the prevalence and prevention of sudden death in the primary BML syndrome remain problems that will not be resolved until additional information is forthcoming. It is not appropriate for this important entity to be regarded as "a fiasco," as described by Leatham and Brigden,[71] to range from a "harbinger of death" to a "variant of normal" as discussed recently by Oakley,[72] or for some aspects to remain "an enigma," which seems to us to be the current status.[15]

REFERENCES

1. GRIFFITH, JPC: *Midsystolic and late systolic mitral murmurs.* Am J Med Sci 104:285, 1892.

2. HALL, JN: *Late systolic mitral murmurs.* Am J Med Sci 125:663–666, 1903.

3. LEWIS, T: *Diseases of the Heart,* ed 4. McMillan & Co, Ltd, London, p 154, 1949.

4. MACKENZIE, J: *Diseases of the Heart,* ed 4. Oxford University Press, London, p 357, 1925.

5. EVANS, W: *Mitral systolic murmurs.* Br Med J 1:8–9, 1943.

6. GALLAVARDIN, L: *Pseudo dédoublement du deuxième bruit du coeur simulant le dédoublement mitral par bruit extra-cardiac télésystolique surajouté.* Lyon Méd 121:409–477, 1913.

7. McKUSICK, VA: *Symposium on cardiovascular sound.* Circulation 16:412–414, 1957.

8. WHITE, PD: *Heart Disease,* ed 2. Macmillan, New York, p 211, 1937.

9. REID, JVO: *Mid-systolic clicks.* S Afr Med J 35:353–355, 1961.

10. BARLOW, JB, POCOCK, WA, MARCHAND, P, AND DENNY, M: *The significance of late systolic murmurs.* Am Heart J 66:443–452, 1963.

11. BARLOW, JB: *Conjoint clinic on the clinical significance of late systolic murmurs and nonejection systolic clicks.* J Chron Dis 18:665–673, 1965.

12. HUMPHRIES, JO AND McKUSICK, VA: *The differentiation of organic and "innocent" systolic murmurs.* Progr Cardiovasc Dis 5:152–171, 1962.

13. POCOCK, WA AND BARLOW, JB: *Etiology and electrocardiographic features of the billowing posterior mitral leaflet syndrome.* Am J Med 51:731–739, 1971.

14. CRILEY, JM, LEWIS, KB, HUMPHRIES, JO, AND ROSS, RS: *Prolapse of the mitral valve: Clinical and cine-angiocardiographic findings.* Br Heart J 28:488–496, 1966.

15. BARLOW, JB AND POCOCK, WA: *The mitral valve prolapse enigma—two decades later.* Mod Concepts Cardiovasc Dis 3:13–17, 1984.

16. BARLOW, JB AND POCOCK, WA: *Billowing, floppy, prolapsed or flail mitral valves?* Am J Cardiol 55:501–502, 1985.

17. ROBERTS, WC: *Congenital cardiovascular abnormalities usually "silent" until adulthood: Morphologic features of the floppy mitral valve, valvular aortic stenosis, discrete subvalvar aortic stenosis, hypertrophic cardiomyopathy, sinus of Valsalva aneurysm, and the Marfan syndrome.* In ROBERTS, WC (ED): *Congenital Heart Disease in Adults.* FA Davis, Philadelphia, 1979, pp 407–453.

18. DOCK, W: *The mode of production of the systolic clicks due to the prolapse of the mitral cusps.* Arch Intern Med 132:118–125, 1973.

19. HAIKAL, M, ALPERT, MA, WHITING, RB, AHMAD, M, AND KELLY, D: *Sensitivity and specificity of M-mode echocardiographic signs of mitral valve prolapse.* Am J Cardiol 50:185–190, 1982.

20. SHAH, PM: *Update of mitral valve prolapse syndrome: When is echo prolapse a pathological prolapse?* Echocardiography: A Review of Cardiovascular Ultrasound 1:87–95, 1984.

21. ALPERT, MA, CARNEY, RJ, FLAKER, GC, SANFELIPPO, JF, WEBEL, RR, AND KELLY, DL: *Sensitivity and specificity of two-dimensional echocardiographic signs of mitral valve prolapse.* Am J Cardiol 54:792–796, 1984.

22. COBBS, BW: *Rheumatic heart disease and other acquired valvular diseases.* In HURST, JW, LOGUE, RB, SCHLANT, RC AND WENGER, NK (EDS): *The Heart: Arteries and Veins.* McGraw-Hill, New York, 1974, p 882.

23. KALBIAN, VV: *The mechanism of mitral regurgitation in carditis of acute rheumatic fever.* Am Heart J 85:139–140, 1973.

24. PHILLIPS, JH, BURCH, GE, AND DE PASQUALE, NP: *The syndrome of papillary muscle dysfunction. Its clinical recognition.* Ann Intern Med 59:508–520, 1963.

25. BARLOW, JB, BOSMAN, CK, POCOCK, WA, AND MARCHAND, P: *Late systolic murmurs and non ejection ("mid-late") systolic clicks. An analysis of 90 patients.* Br Heart J 30:203–218, 1968.

26. SOMERVILLE, J, KAKU, S, AND SARAVALLI, O: *Prolapsed mitral cusps in atrial septal defect. An erroneous radiological interpretation.* Br Heart J 40:58–63, 1978.

27. POMERANCE, A: *Ballooning deformity (mucoid degeneration) of atrio-ventricular valves.* Br Heart J 31:343–351, 1969.

28. McLAREN, MJ, HAWKINS, DM, LACHMAN, AS, LAKIER, JB, POCOCK, WA, AND BARLOW, JB: *Nonejection systolic clicks and mitral systolic murmurs in black schoolchildren of Soweto, Johannesburg.* Br Heart J 38:718–724, 1976.

29. COHEN, M, POCOCK, WA, LAKIER, JB, McLAREN, MJ, LACHMAN, AS, AND BARLOW, JB: *Four year follow-up of Black schoolchildren with nonejection systolic clicks and mitral systolic murmurs.* Am Heart J 95:697–701, 1978.

30. MALCOLM, AD: *Myocardial mysteries surrounding mitral leaflet prolapse.* Am Heart J 100:265–267, 1980.

31. BARLOW, JB AND POCOCK, WA: *The problem of nonejection systolic clicks and associated mitral systolic murmurs: Emphasis on the billowing mitral leaflet syndrome.* Am Heart J 90:636–655, 1975.

32. BAR-SHLOMO, BZ, DRUK, MN, MORCH, JE, JABLONSKY, G, HILTON, JD, FEIGLIN, DHI, AND McLAUCHLIN, PR: *Left ventricular function in trained and untrained healthy subjects.* Circulation 65:484–488, 1982.

33. ZEPPILLI, P, FENICI, R, SASSARA, M, PIRRAMI, MN, AND CASELLI, G: *Wenckebach 2nd degree AV block in top ranking athletes: An old problem revisited.* Am Heart J 100:281–294, 1980.

34. ROST, R: *The athletes heart.* Eur Heart J 3:193–198, 1982.

35. KAY, R, ESTIOKO, M, AND WEINER, I: *Primary sick sinus syndrome as an indication for chronic pacemaker therapy in young adults. Incidence, clinical features, and long-term evaluation.* Am Heart J 103:338–342, 1982.

36. ZEPPILLI, P, PIRRAMI, MM, SASARA, M, AND FENICI, R: *T wave abnormalities in top ranking athletes: Effects of isoproterenol, atropine and physical exercise.* Am Heart J 100:213–222, 1980.

37. BARLOW, JB: *The "false-positive" exercise electrocardiogram. Value of time-course patterns in assessment of depressed ST segments and inverted waves.* Am Heart J 110:1328–1336, 1985.

38. MALCOLM, AD AND AHUJA, SP: *The electrocardiographic response to exercise in 44 patients with mitral leaflet prolapse.* Eur J Cardiol 8:359–370, 1978.

39. LOZNER, EC AND MORGANROTH, J: *New criteria to enhance the predictability of coronary artery disease by exercise testing in asymptomatic subjects.* Circulation 56:799–802, 1977.

40. ELLESTAD, MH: *Stress Testing. Principles and Practice,* ed 2. FA Davis, Philadelphia, 1980, pp 203–218.

41. SCHAMROTH, L: *The Electrocardiology of CAD,* ed 2. Blackwell Scientific Publications, Oxford, London, Edinburgh, Boston, Melbourne, 1984, pp 175–177.

42. WOOLEY, CF: *Where are the diseases of yesteryear? Da Costa Syndrome, soldiers heart, the effort syndrome, neurocirculatory asthenia and the mitral valve prolapse syndrome.* Circulation 153:749–751, 1976.

43. CHESLER, E, MATISONN, RE, LAKIER, JB, POCOCK, WA, OBEL, IWP, AND BARLOW, JB: *Acute myocardial infarction with normal coronary arteries. A possible manifestation of the billowing mitral leaflet syndrome.* Circulation 54:203–209, 1976.

44. BUDA, AJ, LEVENE, DL, MYERS, MG, CHISHOLM, AW, AND SHANE, SJ: *Coronary artery spasm and mitral valve prolapse.* Am Heart J 95:457–462, 1978.

45. HUCKELL, VF, MCLAUGHLIN, PR, MORCH, JE, WIGLE, ED, AND ADELMAN, AG: *Printzmetal's angina with documented coronary artery spasm. Treatment and follow-up.* Br Heart J 45:649–655, 1981.

46. VINCENT, GM, ANDERSON, JL, MARSHALL, HW: *Coronary spasm producing coronary thrombosis and myocardial infarction.* N Engl J Med 309:238–239, 1983.

47. CONTI, CR: *Coronary artery spasm and myocardial infarction.* N Engl J Med 309:238–239, 1983.

48. CHESLER, E, KING, RA, AND EDWARDS, JE: *The myxomatous mitral valve and sudden death.* Circulation 67:632–639, 1983.

49. LITMAN, GI AND FRIEDMAN, HM: *Migraine and the mitral valve prolapse syndrome.* Am Heart J 96:610–614, 1978.

50. STEINGO, L, DANSKY, R, POCOCK, WA, AND BARLOW, JB: *Apical hypertrophic nonobstructive cardiomyopathy.* Am Heart J 104:635–637, 1982.

51. YAMAGUCHI, H, ISHIMURA, T, NISHIYAMA, S, NAGASAKI, F, NAKANISHI, S, TAKATSU, F, MISHIJO, T, UMEDA, T, AND MACHII, K: *Hypertrophic non-obstructive cardiomyopathy with giant negative T waves (apical hypertrophy): Ventriculographic and echocardiographic features in 30 patients.* Am J Cardiol 44:401–412, 1979.

52. PANTANO, JA AND ORIEL, RJ: *Prevalence and nature of cardiac arrhythmias in apparently normal well-trained runners.* Am Heart J 104:762–768, 1982.

53. COBBS, BW, JR: *Clinical recognition and medical management of rheumatic heart disease and other acquired valvular disease.* In HURST, JW AND LOGUE, RB (EDS): *The Heart,* ed 2. McGraw-Hill, New York, 1970, p 813.

54. JERESATY, RM: *Mitral valve prolapse-click syndrome.* Progr Cardiovasc Dis 15:623–652, 1973.

55. POCOCK, WA AND BARLOW, JB: *Post-exercise arrhythmias in the billowing posterior mitral leaflet syndrome.* Am Heart J 80:740–745, 1970.

56. GIBSON, DG AND BROWN, DJ: *Abnormal left ventricular wall movement in patients with chest pain and normal coronary arteriograms. Relation to inferior T wave changes and mitral prolapse.* Br Heart J 41:385–391, 1979.

57. JERESATY, RM: *Mitral valve prolapse.* Raven Press, New York, 1979, pp 142–209.

58. JERESATY, RM, EDWARDS, JE, AND CHAWLA, SK: *Mitral valve prolapse and ruptured chordae tendineae.* Am J Cardiol 55:138–142, 1985.

59. WIT, AL, FENOGLIO, JJ, WAGNER, BM, AND BASSETT, AL: *Electrophysiological properties of cardiac muscle in the anterior mitral valve leaflet and the adjacent atrium in the dog. Possible implications for the genesis of atrial dysrhythmias.* Circ Res 32:731–745, 1973.

60. TRENT, JK, ADELMAN, AC, WIGLE, ED, AND SILVER, MD: *Morphology of a prolapsed mitral valve leaflet.* Am Heart J 79:539–543, 1970.

61. BHARATI, S, GRANSTON, AS, LIEBSON, PR, LOEB, HS, ROSEN, KM, AND LEV, M: *The conduction system in mitral valve prolapse syndrome with sudden death.* Am Heart J 101:667–670, 1981.

62. JAMES, TN: *Pathology of small coronary arteries.* Am J Cardiol 20:679–691, 1967.

63. MCKIBBIN, JK, POCOCK, WA, BARLOW, JB, SCOTT MILLAR, RN, AND OBEL, IWP: *Sotalol, hypokalaemia, syncope, and torsade de pointes.* Br Heart J 51:157–162, 1984.

64. HANCOCK, WD AND COHN, K: *The Syndrome associated with midsystolic click and late systolic murmur.* Am J Med 41:183–196, 1966.

65. MOTULSKY, AG: *Biased ascertainment and the natural history of .diseases.* N Engl J Med 298:1196–1197, 1978.

66. POCOCK, WA, BOSMAN, CK, CHESLER, E, BARLOW, JB, AND EDWARDS, JE: *Sudden death in primary mitral valve prolapse.* Am Heart J 107:378–382, 1984.

4

MITRAL REGURGITATION

SECTION 1: CLINICAL AND HEMODYNAMIC FEATURES, CAUSES, AND MEDICAL MANAGEMENT

In addition to the many underlying conditions that can result in mitral valve billow and regurgitation listed in Table 3-1, the complex valve mechanism may become incompetent from other causes that produce pathological or functional changes in one or more components of the valve. The leaflets may be fibrosed and shortened as a result of rheumatic carditis. Alternatively, leaflet tissue may be excessive owing to myxomatous degeneration and thus fail to maintain coaptation. Myxomatous degeneration may also produce dilatation and impaired contraction of the anulus, which is a feature of the floppy valve and Marfan's syndromes. Marked dilatation of the anulus occurs in severe rheumatic carditis with resultant significant mitral regurgitation. Failure of the normal contraction of the anulus, which we have called anular dysfunction, probably contributes in some patients to mild mitral regurgitation in early active rheumatic carditis and in primary mitral valve prolapse. Mitral regurgitation may sometimes be associated with calcification of the anulus. Elongated or ruptured chordae tendineae will allow one or more leaflets to become flail and may result from rheumatic carditis, infective endocarditis, myxomatous degeneration, or idiopathic causes. Lastly, the papillary muscles may not contract normally and thus fail to maintain coaptation of the leaflet edges. Papillary muscle dysfunction may be due to other causes but is most commonly a consequence of occlusive coronary artery disease, which may also cause these muscles to rupture. Marked enlargement of the left ventricle, such as occurs in chronic aortic regurgitation, results in lateral displacement of the papillary muscles, which diminishes the desirable vertical force of their contraction on the chordae tendineae. Lateral tension on the chordae and the leaflets does not allow adequate coaptation of the leaflet edges, and so-called functional mitral regurgitation may supervene. This is not usually severe.

PHYSICAL SIGNS

Mitral incompetence is diagnosed predominantly by the presence of a mitral regurgitant systolic murmur. In mild incompetence, this will be the only abnormal clinical sign. With moderate or severe mitral regurgitation, there will be other abnormalities.

THE PULSE

In 1959, Paul Wood[1] pointed out that the pulse in mitral regurgitation is of small volume and is *rapid rising*. These features contrast with the slow-rising, small-volume pulse of aortic stenosis. Pulse character is most accurately assessed by palpating larger vessels such as the brachial, carotid, or femoral arteries.

THE JUGULAR VENOUS PULSE

It was again Paul Wood[1] who commented on the slightly raised and prominent wave form of the jugular venous pulse in significant mitral regurgitation. These features probably reflect compression of the right atrium owing to bulging of the interatrial septum by the enlarged tense left atrium. This sign is clinically helpful, provided the many other reasons for a raised jugular venous pressure are excluded. Occasionally, when the mitral regurgitation is very severe, and especially when the heart is "restricted" by mediastinal or pericardial adhesions (see Chapter 8, Section 2), we have observed the marked bulging of the interatrial septum to result in a prominent right atrial systolic wave, palpable in both the jugular pulse and the liver, which thus simulated tricuspid regurgitation (see Chapter 10, Section 2).

PALPATION OF THE PRECORDIUM

The presence of a "left atrial lift" is an invaluable clinical sign of severe mitral regurgitation. This occurs during the ascending limb of the V wave of the left atrial pressure tracing. The left atrium is situated posterior to the rest of the heart and expands prior to and at the time of the V wave with the spine posterior to it and the right ventricle anterior. Palpation with the ball of the hand over the sternum, or preferably slightly to the left of it, will detect a double impulse. The first impulse occurs when the right ventricle contracts (that is, the time of the first heart sound) and the second when the left atrium expands (that is, near the time of the second heart sound). This sign of mitral regurgitation is elicited most easily in children, young adults, or asthenic patients. It is particularly helpful if the systolic murmur is soft despite the severity of the regurgitation, as may occur, for example, with a ring leak of a mitral prosthetic valve. Moreover, the sign is virtually 100 percent specific. The exception is a submitral aneurysm, which can result in a similar impulse and from a similar mechanism but without significant mitral regurgitation (see Chapter 6, Section 2). A dyskinetic segment of the left ventricle may mimic a left atrial lift but can usually be differentiated in that it is felt more laterally and is both a less diffuse and a less forceful impulse.

AUSCULTATORY FEATURES

THE SYSTOLIC MURMUR

The configuration and length of mitral systolic murmurs (Fig. 4-1) depend not only on the pressure difference between the left ventricle and left atrium but also on functional anatomical factors, which determine the time of maximal regurgitation. The murmur of mitral regurgitation is typically pansystolic and may be plateau shaped, have maximal accentuation in early or late systole, or be crescendo-decrescendo with maximal intensity in mid-systole. A murmur of mild mitral regurgitation can be confined to late or early systole. The decrescendo nonpansystolic murmur, which is quite frequently associated with tight mitral stenosis, may be difficult to differentiate from a short ejection murmur. We have observed early decrescendo nonpansystolic

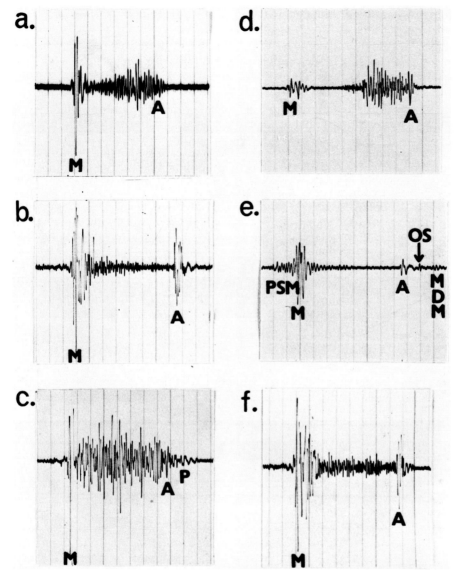

FIGURE 4-1. Six types of mitral regurgitant murmurs: *a*, pansystolic, late accentuation; *b*, pansystolic decrescendo; *c*, crescendo-decrescendo pansystolic; *d*, late systolic; *e*, early, non-pansystolic; *f*, plateau-shaped, pansystolic. A = aortic component of second heart sound; P = pulmonary component of second heart sound; M = mitral component of first heart sound; MDM = mid-diastolic murmur; OS = opening snap; PSM = presystolic murmur. (From Barlow, JB: *The diagnosis and treatment of mitral incompetence.* S Afr Med J 42:400–403, 1968, with permission.)

murmurs to change spontaneously to late systolic murmurs (see Chapter 3). Other murmurs of mitral regurgitation are usually easily recognized by their pansystolic nature or typical cadence in the case of the late systolic murmur. Information derived from hemodynamic alterations produced by posture, amyl nitrite inhalation, or phenylephrine injection may be contributory (see Section 2). In some instances there is difficulty in assessing an apical systolic murmur when an aortic ejection murmur is heard at the base or where hypertrophic cardiomyopathy (HCM) is suspected. Both an aortic ejection murmur and the systolic murmur of HCM invariably increase in intensity and length in the beat after the compensatory pause following a ventricular extrasystole. On the other hand, the pansystolic murmur of mitral regurgitation, presumably because of functional anatomical factors, seldom becomes louder under those circumstances.

MUSICAL MITRAL SYSTOLIC MURMURS (SO-CALLED WHOOPS OR HONKS)

Musical mitral systolic murmurs reflect free vibration at a uniform frequency of the leaflet or part thereof, usually the edge. Most musical mitral systolic murmurs do not denote severe mitral regurgitation. Musical murmurs may be extremely loud and may lose their musical intonation during respiration or with changes of posture. It is unusual for a flail mitral leaflet, with or without infective endocarditis, to produce a musical systolic murmur when severe regurgitation is present. Whereas most musical mitral systolic murmurs are relatively benign and are associated with mild regurgitation, a musical systolic murmur of mitral regurgitation in a porcine valve, whether Hancock or Carpentier-Edwards, is an ominous sign. Whether the mitral regurgitation is severe or not, further disruption of the porcine leaflets is inevitable (see Chapter 8, Section 2).

Minimal or mild mitral regurgitation should be diagnosed by auscultation alone, by the presence of a systolic murmur. Echocardiography is often completely normal. With hemodynamically significant mitral regurgitation, alterations of other auscultatory features become relevant.

THE SECOND HEART SOUND

The pattern of the reduplication of the two components of the second sound falls into three main groups in mitral regurgitation.

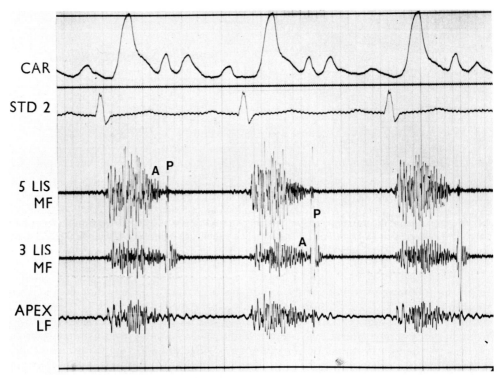

FIGURE 4-2. Phonocardiograms and external carotid tracing (CAR) of a 49-year-old man with severe mitral regurgitation due to ruptured chordae tendineae. The murmur is crescendo-decrescendo with mid-systolic accentuation, and the second heart sound is split 0.04 sec in expiration.

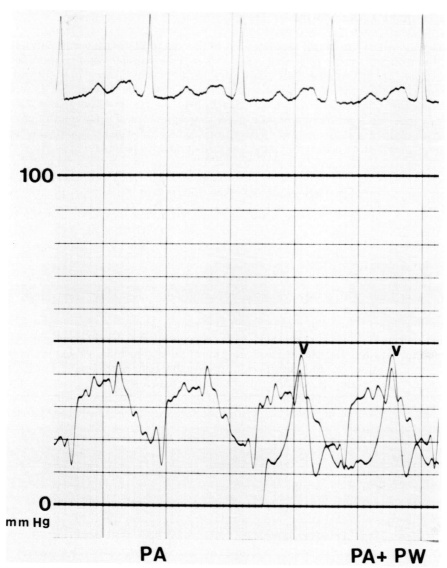

100 ──────────────────────────

0 ──────────────────────────

mm Hg

PA   **PA+ PW**

FIGURE 4-3. Pulmonary artery (PA) and simultaneous pulmonary artery and pulmonary capillary wedge (PW) pressures in a 22-year-old woman with severe rheumatic mitral regurgitation, anular dilatation, and a flail anterior mitral leaflet. The V wave of the pulmonary wedge pressure exceeds the pulmonary systolic pressure and is reflected in the pressure tracing of the PA.

1. In mild mitral regurgitation, the second sound is normal.
2. With more significant regurgitation, left ventricular ejection is shortened and the aortic valve closes earlier. The second sound is widely split and remains reduplicated in expiration (Fig. 4-2). Splitting usually ranges from about 0.02 second in expiration to 0.05 second in inspiration. A2 tends to be soft. If the pulmonary artery pressure rises, P2 increases in intensity. This wide splitting of the second sound is important clinical evidence that the extent of mitral regurgitation is hemodynamically significant.
3. In some patients with severe acute mitral regurgitation, the extremely high V wave of the left atrial tracing is transmitted to the pulmonary artery and causes early closure of the pulmonary valve (Fig. 4-3). This may result in reversed splitting of the second sound, which clinically will often appear single because the relatively loud pulmonary component precedes a soft A2.

THE THIRD HEART SOUND

All patients with pure mitral regurgitation of at least moderate severity will have an apical third heart sound. In severe cases, this may be palpable as a sound vibration rather than as an impulse. Although apex cardiography shows a slight outward movement at the time of the third heart sound, I have never been able to feel this and the clinical impression is one of retraction of the apex at the time of the third heart sound. The third heart sound in mitral regurgitation reflects rapid filling of the left ventricle from the over-filled left atrium. A true third heart sound due to this mechanism will not occur if significant mitral stenosis is present.

It should be remembered that at least 95 percent of subjects under the age of about 18 years have a prominent physiological third heart sound. A third heart sound in a person of that age group therefore does not, in itself, imply that the regurgitation is severe.

MID-DIASTOLIC MURMUR

In many patients with pure severe mitral regurgitation, a mid-diastolic murmur follows the third heart sound. In nonrheumatic mitral regurgitation this is usually extremely short. When the mid-diastolic murmur is longer, it often indicates some leaflet abnormality, most commonly fibrosis, associated with rheumatic thickening of the mitral leaflet. The mid-diastolic murmur will also be long if there is significant aortic regurgitation, but this results from the Austin-Flint mechanism. The presence of a third heart sound precludes the possibility that a long mid-diastolic murmur indicates significant mitral stenosis. In addition, an Austin-Flint murmur never has the typical presystolic accentuation of tight mitral stenosis with pliable leaflets.

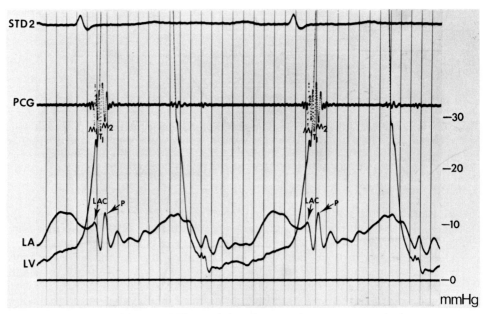

FIGURE 4-4. Standard lead 2 (STD 2) of the electrocardiogram, external phonocardiogram (PCG), left atrial (LA), and left ventricular (LV) pressure in a patient with a pericardial patch in the posterior leaflet and stenosis of the valve. The left atrial C (LAC) wave is bifid, and the second peak, P, coincides with a third major vibration of the first heart sound, M2. (Q-M1 [LAC] = 0.085 sec). Paper speed 100 mm/sec.

THE FIRST HEART SOUND

It is frequently stated that the mitral component (M1) of the first sound is soft in pure severe mitral regurgitation. This is often not so, and the first sound may be loud when the leaflets and chordae are pliable. There are four principal factors that contribute to an increased intensity of the first sound. These are (1) the position of the leaflets at the time of onset of ventricular contraction; (2) the rate of ventricular contraction; (3) the mobility and size of the leaflets; and (4) the adequacy of the leaflets to halt regurgitant flow. It is only the latter that is significantly affected in patients with pure severe mitral incompetence and mobile voluminous leaflets, and the majority therefore have a loud M1. The loud first sound is not infrequently heard outside the apex and may be localised to a small area. Simultaneous phonocardiography and left atrial pressure tracings will show a large left atrial C wave at the peak of which the loud M1 occurs. Confirmation that the mobility and size of the leaflets are directly related to the intensity of M1 and height of the left atrial C (LAC) wave is derived from both experimental and clinical evidence. Lakier and co-workers[2] increased the size of the anterior mitral leaflet in baboons by insertion of a fascia lata patch and demonstrated increase in the amplitude of LAC waves and delay of its peak. Phonocardiograms were not done in that study but were recorded in two patients who had had large pericardial patches inserted into their posterior leaflets for correction of mitral regurgitation. Both had loud delayed M1 components, which coincided with very large amplitude LAC waves (Fig. 4-4).

A useful auscultatory sign of a partially flail leaflet or of an aneurysm of a mitral leaflet is the presence of two left-sided components of the first heart sound (Fig. 4-5). This is analogous to the double tricuspid component of the first heart sound, which occurs in Ebstein's anomaly (Fig. 4-6). Early nonejection systolic clicks can usually be differentiated from a double mitral component of the first heart sound in that the timing is less constant. Furthermore, nonejection systolic clicks seldom occur with severe mitral regurgitation.

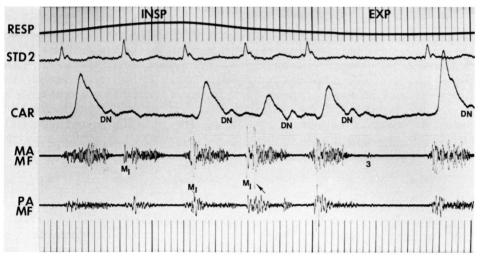

FIGURE 4-5. A 64-year-old man with severe mitral regurgitation due to prolapse of both leaflets and extensive chordal rupture to the posterior leaflet. The mitral component of the first sound (M1) is varying in intensity with the atrial fibrillation, and at times a second loud component of the first heart sound (*arrow*) was recorded. This was clearly audible. MA = mitral area; MF = medium frequency; PA = pulmonary area; DN = dicrotic notch; 3 = third heart sound. (From Barlow, JB and Pocock, WA: *The problem of nonejection systolic clicks and associated mitral systolic murmurs: Emphasis on the billowing mitral leaflet syndrome. Am Heart J* 90:636–655, 1975, with permission.)

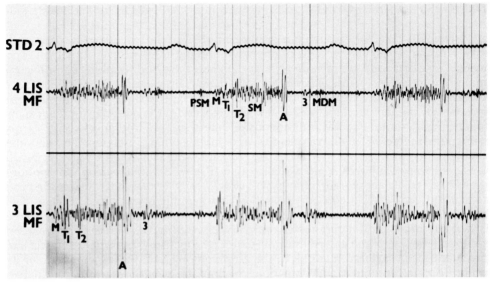

FIGURE 4-6. Phonocardiograms of a 21-year-old man with mild Ebstein's anomaly. Tricuspid valve closure has two components, T1 and T2. The markedly delayed T2, also known as a "sail sound," is thought to arise from the voluminous anterior cusp of the tricuspid valve after the slack has been taken up. Right-sided third sound (3), systolic (SM), and diastolic (MDM) murmurs are shown. 4LIS = 4th left intercostal space; 3LIS = 3rd left intercostal space. (From Pocock, WA, Tucker, RBK, and Barlow, JB: *Mild Ebstein's anomaly.* Br Heart J 31:327–366, 1969, with permission.)

In mitral incompetence with fibrosed and rigid leaflets, which mainly results from rheumatic heart disease, the first heart sound is usually soft, particularly if the anterior leaflet is affected. In most such instances, there is associated stenosis.

THE FOURTH (ATRIAL) SOUND

An atrial sound is an important physical sign in conditions when there is resistance to ventricular filling because of decreased compliance of the myocardium. A left-sided atrial sound is therefore common in systemic hypertension, ischemic heart disease, and hypertrophic cardiomyopathy. Provided the PR interval is normal, the presence of an atrial sound is always pathological. Contrary to the experience of others, I have not detected an atrial sound in pure severe mitral regurgitation, irrespective of whether it is chronic or acute. The presence of an atrial sound in ischemic heart disease and hypertrophic cardiomyopathy when mitral regurgitation may be associated implies that the regurgitation is not severe.

CAUSES

Mitral regurgitation caused by mitral valve prolapse, infective endocarditis, and rheumatic heart disease is discussed in detail in other chapters. Ruptured chordae tendineae, papillary muscle dysfunction, and prosthetic valve incompetence will be discussed here.

RUPTURED CHORDAE TENDINEAE

Rupture of chordae tendineae may involve chordae inserting into either leaflet. The causes are diverse and include infective endocarditis, acute rheumatic carditis, Marfan's syndrome, and direct or indirect trauma. In a large percentage of cases there is no identifiable cause, so-called idiopathic rupture of chordae tendineae. It is strange that the course of "idiopathic" rupture has still to be clarified. All cardiologists are familiar with the presentation of a patient with recent onset of severe breathlessness due to idiopathic chordal rupture. The patients are usually middle-aged or elderly males with no previous cardiac history, and the usual finding at surgery is that one or more chordae to the posterior leaflet are ruptured. The leaflet itself is often ballooning as well as flail. The billowing may be localised to the middle scallop of the leaflet. Both leaflets may be voluminous and compatible with the so-called floppy valve syndrome (Fig. 4-7). Based on the available evidence, it seems unlikely that the majority of these cases are a sequel to longstanding mitral valve billow and prolapse. Mitral valve billow is more common in women, and it is rare to observe progression to ruptured chordae in men with mitral valve billow and late systolic murmurs. Furthermore, a number of men with pansystolic murmurs due to mild or moderate mitral regurgitation remain unchanged for many years and are seldom observed suddenly to rupture their chordae. However, Jeresaty and co-workers[3] have recently reported four patients with ruptured chordae in whom mitral valve prolapse had been documented 4 to 11 years earlier. From pathological examination of the mitral valve in 25 cases of chordal rupture, they concluded that mitral valve prolapse was the underlying morphologic abnormality in 23 (88 percent). It is important to emphasize that *sudden* onset of mitral regurgitation, albeit fairly mild, will result in acute breathlessness that responds well to medical management. Surgery need not be indicated for many years, if at all.

The syndrome of acute severe mitral regurgitation due to idiopathic chordal rupture should be readily recognized clinically. The patient is usually in sinus rhythm, and the heart is only slightly enlarged. Chest radiographs, electrocardiography, and echocardiography show mild left atrial dilatation, and evidence of left ventricular hypertrophy is frequently absent. Auscultatory signs comprise a normal,

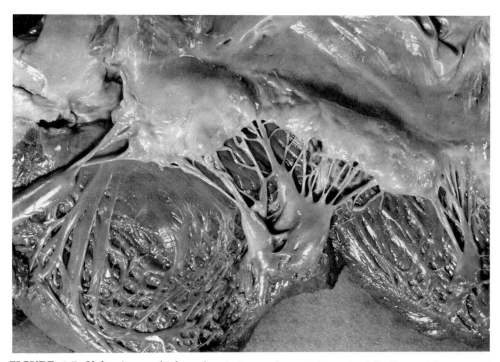

FIGURE 4-7. Voluminous thickened anterior and posterior mitral leaflets with ruptured chorda tendinea to the posterior leaflet. The patient was a 59-year-old man who died from carcinoma of the pancreas.

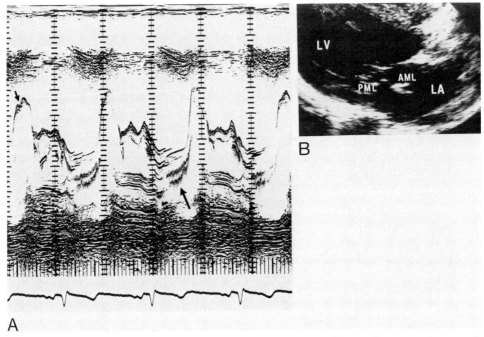

FIGURE 4-8. Severe mitral regurgitation with ruptured chordae tendineae to the anterior mitral leaflet. *A*, M-mode echocardiogram shows systolic flutter *(long arrow)* of both leaflets and diastolic flutter *(short arrow)* of the anterior leaflet. *B*, 2-D echocardiogram, long-axis view, during systole shows the flail anterior mitral leaflet (AML). LA = left atrium; LV = left ventricle; PML = posterior mitral leaflet.

loud, or reduplicated mitral component of the first heart sound, a loud crescendo-decrescendo pansystolic murmur (which in the case of posterior leaflet chordal rupture often radiates to the base of the heart and even to the carotid arteries), a relatively widely split second heart sound with increased intensity of the pulmonary component, a third heart sound, and an absent or very short mid-diastolic murmur. The configuration and radiation of the murmur resemble that found in aortic stenosis, but the rapid rising pulse and the widely reduplicated second sound should serve to differentiate the two conditions. Echocardiography should confirm the diagnosis and shows a markedly prolapsed or a flail leaflet (Fig. 4-8). Diastolic fluttering of the leaflet may be observed but is not invariable. Left ventricular contraction is "supernormal." Cardiac catheterization is seldom necessary to confirm the diagnosis but when performed will show normal or slightly raised left ventricular end-diastolic pressures and a typical late-onset high-pressure V wave in the left atrial (Fig. 4-9) or pulmonary capillary wedge pressure tracing. Left ventricular cineangiocardiography confirms gross regurgitation of dye into the relatively small left atrial cavity and demonstrates systolic expansion of the left atrium contrasting with the contracting left ventricle. A very mobile or flail leaflet can sometimes be observed. Postangiography, there is a striking increase in the height of the left atrial V wave (Fig. 4-9).

These patients respond well to diuretic and vasodilator therapy. Surgical intervention is unnecessary and undesirable (see Chapter 8) in the acute stage while severe pulmonary edema is still present. A mitral valvuloplasty is often possible, but it is crucial that the surgeon completely corrects the mitral regurgitation.

PAPILLARY MUSCLE DYSFUNCTION

Any condition that involves the myocardium may result in papillary muscle dysfunction and mitral regurgitation. This includes dilated cardiomyopathy and viral

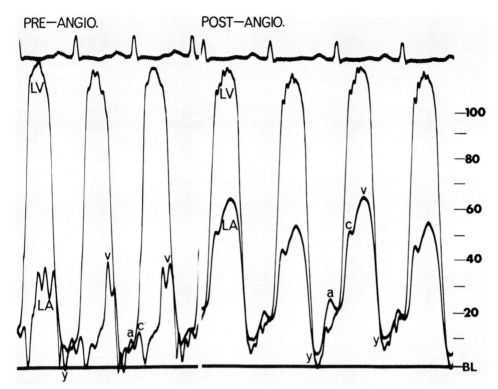

FIGURE 4-9. Simultaneous left atrial (LA) and left ventricular (LV) pressures in a 49-year-old woman with severe pure mitral regurgitation. Postangiography, the V wave starts earlier and reaches a pressure of 65 mmHg, and the LV end-diastolic pressure is higher (see also Figs. 4-14, 4-15).

myocarditis, but the most important cause is occlusive coronary artery disease. The regurgitation is seldom severe, and valve replacement or valvuloplasty are rarely indicated except when the principal reason for operation is coronary artery bypass surgery. Marked mitral regurgitation in a patient with chronic occlusive coronary artery disease may reflect double pathology.

Intermittent severe mitral regurgitation resulting from papillary muscle dysfunction is occasionally observed and may coincide with ischemic chest pain. Such intermittent regurgitation should be suspected in any patient with a history of transient, severe dyspnea despite examination revealing a small heart with minimal left ventricular dysfunction and mild regurgitation.

Functional mitral regurgitation resulting from horizontal displacement of the papillary muscles in patients with dilated left ventricles that are otherwise normal is seldom hemodynamically significant. A cause of this is severe, sometimes acute, aortic regurgitation. The mitral valve only occasionally needs to be repaired or replaced at the time of surgery for the aortic valve.

PROSTHETIC VALVE INCOMPETENCE

Significant or severe mitral regurgitation resulting from degeneration of the leaflets of a tissue prosthetic valve is invariably accompanied by a fairly loud systolic murmur and other evidence of degeneration such as a mid-diastolic murmur. Severe regurgitation in patients with prosthetic valves such as the Björk-Shiley, St. Jude, and Medtronic-Hall valves is nearly always due to a paravalvular leak. Clinical detection of this may be difficult in that the systolic murmur is usually soft, seldom louder than Grade 2 and may be only Grade 1. I have never encountered a patient, with or without a prosthetic valve, who has hemodynamically significant mitral regurgitation that is completely silent. A prosthetic ring leak is diagnosed by the symptoms, the presence of a soft apical systolic murmur and of signs of severe mitral regurgitation such as a left atrial lift, widely split second sound, and evidence of pulmonary artery and venous hypertension. Echocardiography is contributory in such cases, because good contraction of the left ventricle is detected. Other clinical and echocardiographic features specific to the particular prosthesis are discussed in Chapter 8.

ELECTROCARDIOGRAM OF SIGNIFICANT MITRAL REGURGITATION

If the patient is in sinus rhythm, there is usually some evidence of left atrial enlargement, although this is seldom as marked as in most cases with tight mitral stenosis. The time of onset of atrial fibrillation depends more on the age of the patient and the degree of dilatation of the left atrium than on the severity of mitral regurgitation. Dilatation of the atrium is largely determined by the extent of the disease involving the left atrial wall. Thus, patients with rheumatic mitral regurgitation generally have larger left atrial cavities than do nonrheumatic patients with a comparable severity of regurgitation. Nevertheless, children and young adults with gross mitral regurgitation and greatly enlarged left atrial cavities, with or without active rheumatic carditis, usually remain in sinus rhythm. Conversely, elderly patients with relatively mild mitral regurgitation frequently have atrial fibrillation.

Evidence of left ventricular hypertrophy is usually absent in patients with acute mitral regurgitation but may also be unimpressive in some of those with chronic regurgitation. Children with severe mitral regurgitation sometimes develop marked pulmonary arterial hypertension, in which case the axis shifts to the right of 90° and considerable clockwise rotation may occur. Left ventricular voltages are inconspicuous but may sometimes be detected if leads V_7 and V_8 are recorded, or if V_4 to V_6 are recorded in the sixth intercostal space. Schamroth and associates[4] recently observed that the ECG signs of left ventricular hypertrophy differ in chronic mitral and aortic regurgitation in that there is an absence of deep S waves in V_1 in the former, whereas tall left precordial R waves are present in both. They consider that this is due to a change in the direction of the vectors because of the altered position of the heart, which in turn results from the left atrial dilatation. The precordial T waves may be relatively normal with severe mitral regurgitation and considerable pulmonary venous hypertension.

CHEST RADIOGRAPHS

The most important confirmatory sign of mitral regurgitation on the chest radiograph is left atrial enlargement. This is best seen as a "double density" in the slightly overpenetrated posteroanterior projection. With more marked left atrial enlargement the left main bronchus may be elevated. Associated pulmonary venous hypertension may be apparent from dilatation of upper lobe veins, interstitial edema, Kerley B lines, interlobar effusions, or frank pulmonary edema. It is important to emphasize, however, that the lung fields may appear normal (Fig. 4-10). Furthermore, most notably in acute severe mitral regurgitation of nonrheumatic etiology, there may be no definite evidence of left atrial enlargement. Enlargement of the left ventricle in mitral regurgitation cannot usually be assessed reliably on chest roentgenograms. Posterior displacement of the cardiac shadow just above the diaphragm in the left lateral view

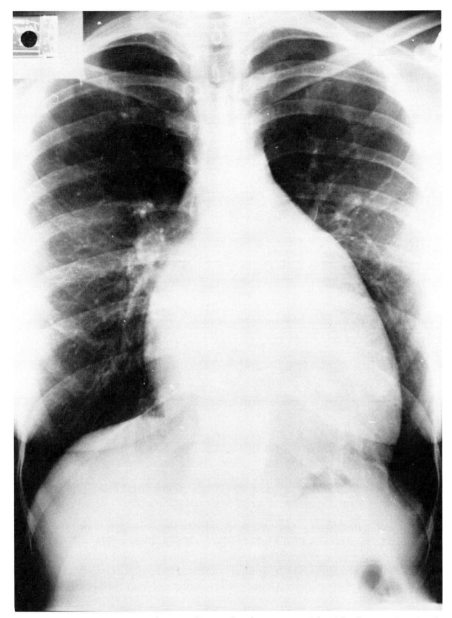

FIGURE 4-10. Posteroanterior chest radiograph of a young girl with rheumatic mitral valve disease and severe regurgitation. The heart is enlarged and the left atrium prominent, but the lung fields are unremarkable.

is compatible with left ventricular enlargement, but even this sign may be unreliable if marked right ventricular and right atrial dilatation are associated.

ECHOCARDIOGRAPHY

Although abnormalities of the mitral leaflets may be detected, perhaps the most important echocardiographic feature of significant mitral regurgitation is the combi-

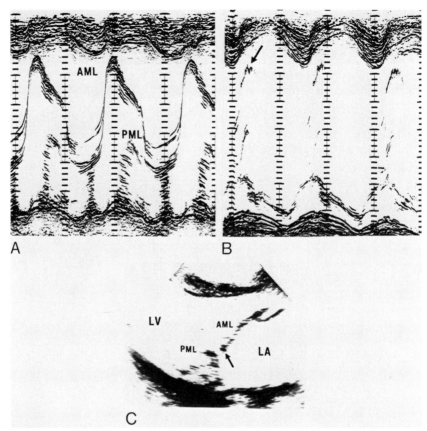

FIGURE 4-11. M-mode (*A, B*) and 2-D echocardiograms (*C*) of the same patient as in Figure 4-10. *A,* The anterior mitral leaflet is thickened with a reduced E-F slope. The posterior leaflet is also thickened and has mild anterior motion. These features are compatible with chronic rheumatic valvular disease. *B,* Flutter *(arrow)* of the anterior leaflet. *C,* Long-axis view, systolic frame. The tip of the flail anterior mitral leaflet *(arrow)* points to the left atrium.

nation of a well-contracting left ventricle and some left atrial enlargement in a patient who has symptoms and clinical signs of pulmonary venous hypertension. Even patients with marked cardiomegaly, both clinically and on chest radiograph, due to chronic mitral regurgitation will show these features. The echocardiographic evidence of a well-contracting left ventricle is sometimes out of accord with the clinical impression of a dilated, poorly contracting left ventricle. The size of the left ventricular cavity provides some indication of whether the regurgitation is acute or chronic.

Leaflet abnormalities depend on the underlying pathology. Marked billowing, flail leaflets, and fibrosed and thickened leaflets may be detected (Fig. 4-11). Vegetations attached to the valve may be observed in infective endocarditis. Diastolic flutter will be present in some instances of mitral regurgitation due to floppy valves or flail leaflets. It is important to emphasize that echocardiographic alterations relating to the leaflets may be unimpressive in cases of severe mitral regurgitation.

CARDIAC CATHETERIZATION

A pulmonary arterial wedge pressure will often suffice to provide the height of the V wave and the mean left atrial pressure. Difficulties in wedging the catheter and obtaining an adequate tracing may arise in cases of severe pulmonary arterial hypertension. Moreover, diastolic events are sometimes not accurately reflected in a wedge pressure. We generally prefer to obtain a left atrial pressure through a Brockenbrough catheter. This technique is relatively safe in experienced hands, but technical difficulties may be encountered when the right atrium is very dilated or the left atrial wall is lined with organized thrombus. The procedure is contraindicated in the presence of a very dilated proximal aorta.

The height and timing of the left atrial C wave contribute to the assessment of the mobility and size of the mitral leaflets, especially of the anterior leaflet. A double kick of the left atrial C wave may be detected with an aneurysm of a mitral leaflet, a flail leaflet, or with leaflets in which a pericardial patch has been inserted (see Fig. 4-4).

It is important to appreciate that evaluation of the severity of mitral regurgitation on the height of the left atrial V wave alone may be misleading, as there are a number of factors that modify the level of this pressure. These factors will now be briefly discussed.

LEFT ATRIAL CAVITY SIZE AND WALL COMPLIANCE

In the presence of a normal mitral valve, the left atrial V wave reflects passive filling of the left atrium from the lungs. One of the functions of the left atrium is that of a storage chamber. If the atrial cavity is abnormally small, the height of the V wave will increase. Many years ago, we inserted homograft aortic valves in several patients as a method of mitral valve replacement. The technique involved placing the homograft above the mitral anulus, thereby unavoidably diminishing the size of the left atrial cavity. Even with normal function of the homograft, this resulted in an abnormally high left atrial V wave (Fig. 4-12). This was undesirable and I suspect was a factor in some of the early postoperative deaths when mitral regurgitation was associated. Another circumstance in which an abnormally high left atrial V wave will occur is when a thrombus has filled the left atrial cavity. In the presence of significant mitral regurgitation, the left atrial V wave will be higher if the left atrial cavity is relatively small and the wall noncompliant (Fig. 4-13) than in a dilated chamber with a diseased and more compliant wall. Left atrial pressures in patients with severe mitral regurgitation but dilated left atrial cavities may be entirely normal.

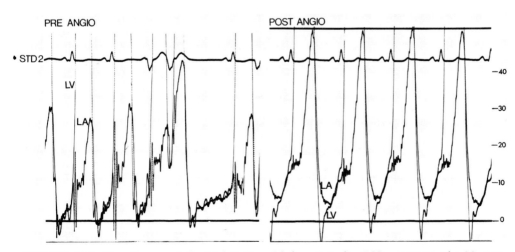

FIGURE 4-12. Simultaneous left atrial (LA) and left ventricular (LV) pressures of a 39-year-old woman with an aortic homograft above the mitral anulus. Very mild mitral regurgitation was present. The markedly elevated left atrial V wave is the result of the small left atrial cavity.

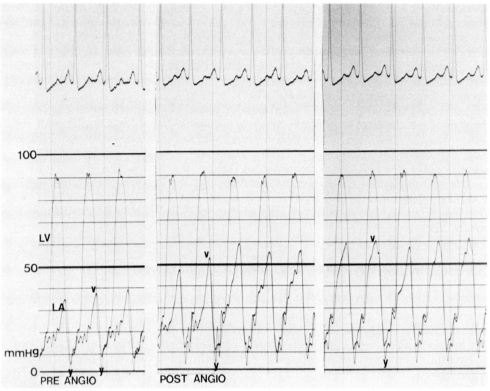

FIGURE 4-13. Simultaneous left atrial (LA) and left ventricular (LV) pressures in a 23-year-old woman with severe, pure mitral regurgitation. Postangiography, there is a progressive increase in height and an earlier onset of the V wave. In addition, the left ventricular end-diastolic pressure is higher postangiography.

CIRCULATING BLOOD VOLUME

Patients with severe mitral regurgitation who have been dehydrated from excessive diuretic therapy may have normal left atrial pressures but will develop tall V waves immediately after the injection of radio-opaque dye. Radio-opaque dye decreases left ventricular function but, more importantly in this context, it also increases circulating blood volume. It has therefore been our policy for more than two decades to report left atrial and other pressures both prior to and immediately after such injection.

LEFT VENTRICULAR END-DIASTOLIC PRESSURE

Even in the absence of mitral regurgitation, the V wave and mean left atrial pressure increase if the left ventricular end-diastolic pressure is raised. The V wave will be raised further if mitral regurgitation is associated. My surgical colleague, Robin Kinsley, devised a ratio of the left ventricular end-diastolic pressure to V wave height in order to assess the relative roles of left ventricular dysfunction and mitral regurgitation. If the ratio was more than 0.5, he concluded that the mitral regurgitation was not hemodynamically significant. His observations were made from pressures obtained at surgery for aortic valve replacement, and they influenced his decision as to whether the mitral valve should be replaced.

ASSOCIATED MITRAL STENOSIS

If there is associated mitral stenosis, the left atrium may not have emptied completely at the end of diastole. Mitral regurgitation will then produce a higher left atrial pressure than if there were no mitral stenosis. Both the left ventricular end-diastolic pressure and mitral stenosis, or a combination of the two, will not only affect the height of the V wave but will also influence the configuration of the left atrial pressure. With pansystolic mitral regurgitation, the left atrial pressure may start rising immediately after the first heart sound if the left atrial pressure was already relatively high because of a raised left ventricular end-diastolic pressure or incomplete emptying of the left atrium. This contrasts with the late onset of rise of the V wave in patients with pure mitral regurgitation and no stenosis and in patients with a relatively low left ventricular end-diastolic pressure (Fig. 4-14; see also Figs. 4-9, 4-13).

Patients with severe aortic regurgitation can maintain a low left atrial pressure relative to the raised left ventricular end-diastolic pressure, provided the mitral valve is competent. If there is mitral regurgitation and the valve is also incompetent in diastole, the left atrial pressures will be potentially higher.

EXTENT OF MITRAL REGURGITATION

Although the severity of the mitral regurgitation clearly affects the left atrial pressure tracing, it should always be remembered that other factors always require consideration.

MEDICAL MANAGEMENT

In the absence of complications, the amount of mitral regurgitation may not change for many years, particularly if mild. There is some evidence that "mitral insufficiency begets mitral insufficiency"[5] and that, with the passage of time, the anulus progressively dilates, increasing the amount of regurgitation. This may occur if the regurgitation is at least moderate and especially if a connective tissue or other disorder, notably rheumatic carditis, is present, which weakens the posterior mitral anulus. The most definitive treatment of mitral regurgitation is open heart surgery, and the timing, indications, and types of procedure will be discussed in Chapter 8. It is here pertinent to mention briefly several broad principles of the management of patients with mitral regurgitation.

PROPHYLAXIS AGAINST INFECTIVE ENDOCARDITIS

All patients with permanent, as opposed to transient, mitral regurgitation are at risk of developing infective endocarditis. Prophylactic antibiotics are thus recommended, and the various regimens are discussed in Chapter 9.

ATRIAL FIBRILLATION AND OTHER ARRHYTHMIAS

Atrial fibrillation may supervene in patients with mitral regurgitation, especially in the elderly. Unless there is a specific contraindication, long-term anticoagulant therapy with Coumadin derivatives is recommended for patients who have chronic atrial fibrillation, in order to prevent systemic embolism. Recent-onset fibrillation or recur-

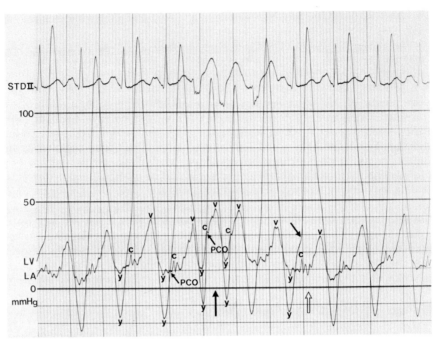

FIGURE 4-14. Left atrial (LA) and left ventricular (LV) pressure tracings of a 53-year-old woman with significant mitral regurgitation and stenosis. A number of interesting features are demonstrated. Pressure crossover (PCO) of LA and LV is readily apparent but is indicated (*upsloping small dark arrows* in two complexes. The patient has a sinus tachycardia with a rate of about 116 beats per minute. Three consecutive ventricular ectopic beats occur. With the first four sinus beats, there is a pressure difference of about 25 mmHg at the y point and throughout the short diastole. The V waves of the LA tracing rise late and reach about 40 mmHg in the last two sinus beats before the ventricular ectopics. With the first ventricular ectopic beat *(large dark arrow)*, the mitral leaflets are caught in the "open position" and their movement towards closure results in LA pressure rising with, but preceding, the LV pressure, to a c wave almost simultaneous with the PCO *(second upsloping small dark arrow)* of about 32 mmHg. The V wave of the first ventricular ectopic beat has an early onset and reaches about 45 mmHg. With the next ventricular ectopic beat, LA pressure is still high, hence the V wave again rises early because of mitral regurgitation into a high pressure and "full" LA. Note that the left ventricular systolic pressures of the first two ventricular ectopic beats are relatively low. With the third ventricular ectopic beat, left ventricular systolic pressure is higher and the V wave late in onset and only about 35 mmHg. This could be partly due to a functional anatomical factor of the mitral valve allowing less mitral regurgitation. With the first sinus beat after the ventricular ectopics *(open arrow)* the slow rise of the left ventricular pressure until the time of the left atrial C wave is well shown *(downsloping small dark arrow)*. The left ventricular pressure rises more quickly once the mitral leaflets have reached the peak of their billow into the left atrium. With that first sinus beat, the V wave is again of late onset and only 30 mmHg, presumably owing mainly to a functional anatomical factor. With the two subsequent sinus beats, the V wave rises to a higher level, presumably because left atrial emptying is less despite no impressive change in left atrial end-diastolic pressure. C = C wave of left atrial tracing.

rent attacks of other supraventricular tachyarrhythmias may respond well to sotalol, which, in addition to its beta-receptor blocking activity, has a Class III antiarrhythmic effect. Verapamil, especially when administered intravenously, is highly effective in this context. Quinidine would also be effective, but we very seldom use this drug for fear of its unpredictable and dangerous side effects. Most patients with chronic atrial fibrillation require their ventricular rates to be decreased. It was traditional to prescribe digoxin, but in many instances we now prefer a beta-receptor blocking agent. Beta-blockers, especially sotalol, are also contributory in patients who develop ventricular ectopy. When symptoms are troublesome or Holter monitoring reveals intractable multifocal ventricular ectopy, amiodarone therapy is indicated despite a high incidence of troublesome side effects.

PULMONARY VENOUS HYPERTENSION

Many patients with moderate pure mitral regurgitation remain asymptomatic for years. Tiredness or abnormal breathlessness may occur with exercise, and strenuous exercise should be avoided by patients with moderate or greater degrees of mitral regurgitation. Breathlessness may improve on diuretic treatment alone or when this is combined with long-term vasodilator therapy. The timing of surgical intervention remains a difficult problem, which is discussed in Chapter 8.

Acute-onset mitral regurgitation, albeit moderate or even fairly mild, may cause extreme breathlessness and pulmonary edema. Medical management with diuretics and vasodilators invariably achieves considerable improvement, and surgical treatment may not ever be necessary or can be postponed for many years.

SECTION 2: MITRAL AND OTHER SYSTOLIC MURMURS

with WENDY A. POCOCK

If auscultation is to continue to be practiced, then the recognition and assessment of systolic murmurs will remain a meaningful and common challenge. The most important physical sign in the diagnosis of mitral regurgitation is the presence of a systolic murmur. Very mild regurgitation, especially if intermittent, can only be diagnosed on auscultation. Echocardiography, cineangiocardiography, electrocardiography, and x-ray films of the chest may be completely normal or inconclusive. The role of Doppler ultrasound requires clarification. Mild mitral regurgitation is therefore diagnosed by the correct assessment of an "isolated" systolic murmur. The term "isolated" systolic murmur refers to one which is associated with minimal or no other clinical, electrocardiographic, echocardiographic, or radiological signs of heart disease.

In this section a general approach to the assessment of all systolic murmurs will be briefly discussed and then the problem of the isolated systolic murmur considered in more detail.

CLASSIFICATION OF SYSTOLIC MURMURS

In 1933, Levine[1] introduced his now widely accepted classification of systolic murmurs based on intensity alone. This classification is excellent for record purposes but is of limited value in deciding whether a murmur is innocent and whether the lesion is a severe one. The six grades are as follows:

Grade 1—A very soft murmur detected only after listening to several cardiac cycles

Grade 2—A soft murmur that is heard immediately

Grade 3—Moderately loud

Grade 4—Loud

Grade 5—Very loud but audible only with the stethoscope in contact with the chest wall

Grade 6—Extremely loud and audible with the stethoscope away from the chest wall

Levine did not discuss associated systolic thrills in his original classification, but later workers have assumed that a systolic thrill is detected with Grade 5 and

Grade 6 murmurs. Although Grade 5 and 6 murmurs invariably denote pathology, this is not necessarily severe. On the other hand, a Grade 1/6 systolic murmur of mitral regurgitation is always pathological, and very severe mitral regurgitation may occur with murmurs no louder than Grade 2.

In 1955, Leatham[2] divided systolic murmurs into the two main groups of ejection or regurgitant. This classification, which is based on anatomical and hemodynamic considerations, was a major contribution to the clinical assessment of systolic murmurs and has been widely adopted.

EJECTION SYSTOLIC MURMURS

An ejection systolic murmur results from forward flow of blood through the left or right ventricular outflow tracts and can theoretically occur in one or a combination of the following circumstances:

1. Increased rate of ejection
2. Valvular, subvalvar, or supravalvular stenosis
3. Valvular damage or anomaly without obstruction
4. Dilatation of the vessel distal to the valve

An aortic or pulmonary ejection systolic murmur starts after the component of the first sound and ends before the component of the second sound of the side of the heart in which it arises. An ejection systolic murmur is crescendo-decrescendo in shape but is longer and accentuates later when caused by obstruction to the ventricular outflow as opposed to other mechanisms of production (Fig. 4-15). In severe

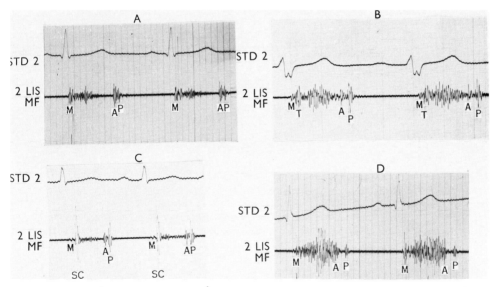

FIGURE 4-15 Pulmonary ejection systolic murmurs. A, Normal heart. The murmur is short and accentuates early, and the second sound is normal. The phonocardiogram is recorded during inspiration, and the second sound is split 0.03 to 0.04 second. B, Atrial septal defect. A similar short ejection murmur is present, but the second sound is split 0.06 second with accentuation of P. Recorded during expiration. C, Idiopathic dilatation of the pulmonary artery. The murmur is soft and short and an ejection click (SC) is present. The second sound is split 0.03 second and P accentuated. Recorded during expiration. D, Pulmonary stenosis. The murmur accentuates in mid-systole and extends to A. The second sound is split 0.06 second, and P is soft. The gradient across the pulmonary valve was 55 mmHg. Recorded during expiration. M, T = mitral and tricuspid components of first heart sound; 2LIS = 2nd left intercostal space. Time interval between the heavy vertical lines is 0.2 second. (From Barlow, JB and Pocock, WA: *The isolated systolic murmur.* S Afr Med J 39:909–918, 1965, with permission.)

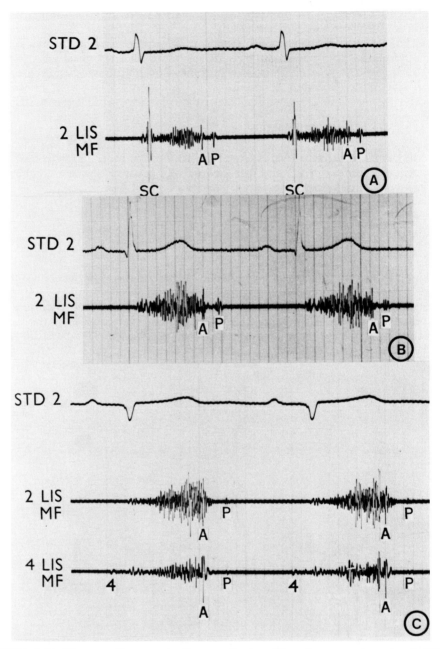

FIGURE 4-16. Phonocardiograms in three patients with pulmonary stenosis of different severity. The pulmonary ejection murmur is longer and accentuates later in the more severe degrees of stenosis. Pulmonary valve closure (P) is correspondingly softer and more delayed.

    A. Gradient 45 mmHg. A–P = 0.05 sec.
    B. Gradient 55 mmHg. A–P = 0.06 sec.
    C. Gradient 150 mmHg. A–P = 0.10 sec.

(From Barlow, JB and Pocock, WA: *The isolated systolic murmur.* S Afr Med J 39:909–918, 1965, with permission.)

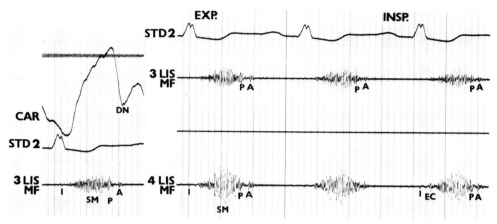

FIGURE 4-17. Tight aortic stenosis with complete left bundle branch block in a 54-year-old woman. There is marked reversed splitting with P preceding A in all phases of respiration. The long aortic ejection murmur (SM) extends past pulmonary valve closure. The dicrotic notch (DN) of the external carotid tracing (CAR) identifies aortic valve closure (A). A soft ejection click (EC) is present.

outflow obstruction, the long ejection murmur will extend up to or beyond the normal semilunar valve closure sound of the unaffected side of the heart but ends before its own delayed and soft second sound component. In severe pulmonary stenosis, for example, the long, harsh pulmonary ejection systolic murmur extends through the aortic closure sound but stops before the very delayed, soft pulmonary component of the second sound (Fig. 4-16). Similarly, in tight aortic stenosis, especially if reversed splitting is exaggerated by associated left bundle branch block (Fig. 4-17), the long aortic ejection murmur extends up to or beyond the pulmonary component. It is important that these long ejection murmurs are not confused with a pansystolic murmur.

REGURGITANT SYSTOLIC MURMURS

Regurgitant systolic murmurs are caused by regurgitation of blood through an incompetent atrioventricular valve or through a defect in the ventricular septum from a high-pressure chamber to one at a lower pressure. Because a pressure gradient is usually present throughout systole, regurgitant murmurs are frequently pansystolic. Thus, the systolic murmur of mitral regurgitation most commonly starts with the mitral component of the first sound and extends just past the aortic closure sound. When a regurgitant systolic murmur is not pansystolic, the explanation has to lie in a modification by pressure or anatomical factors. The late systolic murmur of mitral regurgitation reflects competence of the valve in the early part of systole, because of functional anatomical factors. In fact, if the duration and configuration of a mitral regurgitant systolic murmur depended only on the systolic pressure gradient between left ventricle and left atrium, the murmur would always be crescendo-decrescendo with maximal accentuation in mid-systole, when the largest pressure difference between the two chambers potentially exists (Fig. 4-18). It is therefore apparent that the configuration of all other murmurs of mitral regurgitation must depend on functional anatomical factors, which affect the time of maximal regurgitation (Fig. 4-18). The murmur of a ventricular septal defect is typically pansystolic (Fig. 4-19A, B) reflecting regurgitation of blood throughout left ventricular systole. The murmur may be confined to the earlier part of systole by two mechanisms. First,

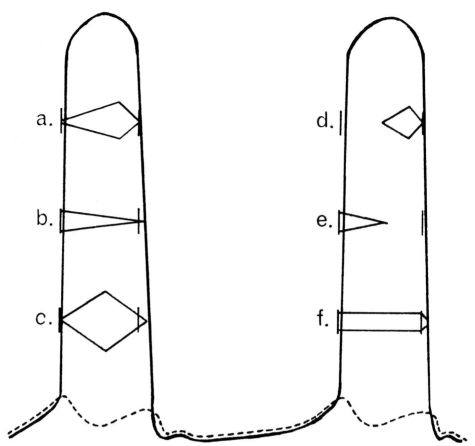

FIGURE 4-18. Diagrammatic representation of the normal left atrial and left ventricular pressures and the six different types of mitral systolic murmur. The configuration of the pansystolic crescendo-decrescendo murmur (C) is the only one that can be explained on a pressure basis. Functional anatomical factors must be responsible for the late accentuating pansystolic (*a*), decrescendo pansystolic (*b*), late systolic (*d*), decrescendo nonpansystolic, (*e*) and plateau-shaped pansystolic (f) murmurs. (From Barlow, JB: *The diagnosis of mitral incompetence.* S Afr Med J 42:400–403, 1968, with permission.)

if the defect is very small and situated in the muscular septum it will close during the latter half or third of systole, giving the so-called atypical systolic murmur of ventricular septal defect (Fig. 4-19C). Second, when considerable pulmonary hypertension is present there is audible left-to-right shunting in early systole only.

The intensity of any murmur depends largely on the velocity, as opposed to the volume, of blood flow and on the nature of the abnormality at the site of origin of the murmur. Thus, a small ventricular septal defect with a high velocity of flow will usually produce a louder murmur than a large defect. Similarly, gross functional tricuspid regurgitation is often silent, because little turbulence is set up by the large volume of blood flowing through a dilated, but otherwise normal, tricuspid valve. The force of ventricular contraction will also significantly affect the velocity of blood flow through the relevant outflow tract. For example, in severe aortic stenosis with left ventricular failure, the velocity of flow is relatively reduced, and the aortic ejection murmur is soft or may be nearly inaudible. Factors affecting the intensity of a murmur are reflected in Figure 4-20.

So-called musical murmurs, which may be systolic or diastolic, were defined by McKusick as "the improved ability to represent the murmur by conventional

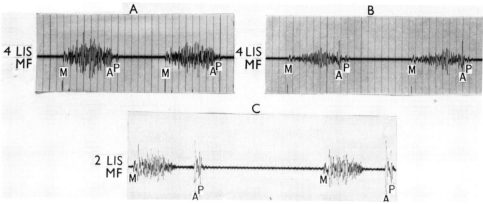

FIGURE 4-19. Three murmurs of a ventricular septal defect. *A,* Pansystolic crescendo-decrescendo murmur with mid-systolic accentuation. *B,* Pansystolic crescendo-decrescendo murmur with maximal accentuation later in systole. *C,* Short "atypical" murmur. Abbreviations as in previous figures. (From Barlow, JB and Pocock, WA: *The isolated systolic murmur.* S Afr Med J 39:909–918, 1965, with permission.)

musical notation."[3] The factors that determine the musical intonation of a murmur are not always apparent, but there is frequently a structure such as an everted aortic cusp, an aberrant chorda tendinea, or other tissue that is "set into vibration in a specifically periodic, and therefore musical, manner."[3] Musical murmurs are of a single frequency and in this way produce a quality suggestive of a musical tone.

It is not unusual for an individual patient to have systolic murmurs arising at more than one site. Thus, an aortic ejection murmur due to aortic stenosis is not infrequently associated with an apical pansystolic murmur of mitral regurgitation. Some conditions (for example, hypertrophic cardiomyopathy) may have a systolic murmur that is partly ejection, with the earlier vibrations arising in the left ventricular outflow tract, and partly regurgitant due to associated mitral incompetence. Assessment of the splitting of the second heart sound is essential to the correct diagnosis of the site of origin of a systolic murmur. Postural maneuvers, amyl nitrite inhalation, and phenylephrine injection are aids that are sometimes employed (Fig. 4-21).

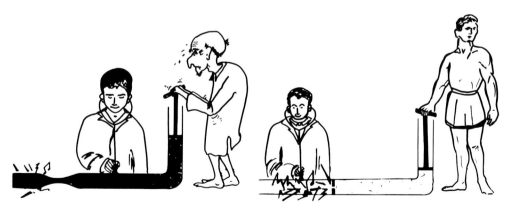

FIGURE 4-20. Factors that affect the intensity of a systolic murmur. The velocity of blood flow is determined by the force of the pump (ventricular contraction), the orifice size, and blood viscosity. The nature of the obstruction (abrupt or gradual) and the site of auscultation are other factors that determine the loudness of a murmur.

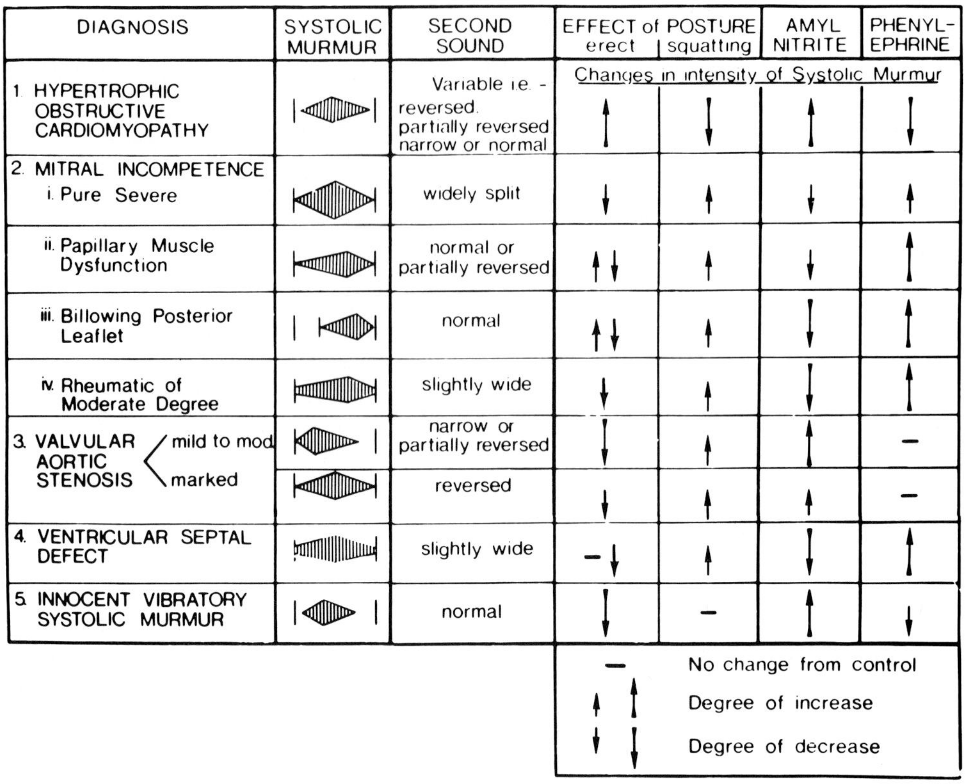

DIAGNOSIS	SYSTOLIC MURMUR	SECOND SOUND	EFFECT of POSTURE erect / squatting		AMYL NITRITE	PHENYL-EPHRINE
			Changes in intensity of Systolic Murmur			
1. HYPERTROPHIC OBSTRUCTIVE CARDIOMYOPATHY	◁▭▷	Variable i.e. – reversed, partially reversed narrow or normal	↑	↓	↑	↓
2. MITRAL INCOMPETENCE i. Pure Severe	◁▭▷	widely split	↓	↑	↓	↑
ii. Papillary Muscle Dysfunction	◁▭▷	normal or partially reversed	↑↓	↑	↓	↑
iii. Billowing Posterior Leaflet	◁▭▷	normal	↑↓	↑	↓	↑
iv. Rheumatic of Moderate Degree	◁▭▷	slightly wide	↓	↑	↓	↑
3. VALVULAR AORTIC STENOSIS — mild to mod	◁▭	narrow or partially reversed	↓	↑	↑	–
— marked	◁▭▷	reversed	↓	↑	↑	–
4. VENTRICULAR SEPTAL DEFECT	▭▥▭	slightly wide	–↓	↑	↓	↑
5. INNOCENT VIBRATORY SYSTOLIC MURMUR	◁▭▷	normal	↓	–	↑	↓

–	No change from control
↑ ↑	Degree of increase
↓ ↓	Degree of decrease

FIGURE 4-21. Diagrammatic representation of the character of the systolic murmur and of the second heart sound in five conditions. The effects of posture, amyl nitrite inhalation, and phenylephrine injection on the intensity of the murmur are shown.

THE ISOLATED SYSTOLIC MURMUR

An isolated systolic murmur may be completely innocent, but it may be pathological. The differentiation is of the utmost importance. Isolated systolic murmurs occur commonly in children and young adults and are often detected when auscultation is performed as part of a routine examination at school or during an unrelated illness. In such instances, young patients and their parents need positive reassurance that there is no organic cardiac lesion present. An incorrect assessment of a heart as being "pathological" may result in unnecessary limitation of activities, over-protective parental attitudes, difficulty in obtaining employment, heavily loaded insurance policies, and even the development of a cardiac neurosis. In addition, the incorrect diagnosis of valvular heart disease may condemn some children to a prolonged antibiotic regimen as prophylaxis against rheumatic fever, and also to the inconvenience of having to take antibiotics as prophylaxis against infective endocarditis at times of dental therapy or other risk. For similar reasons, the failure to recognize organic heart disease is also undesirable.

INNOCENT SYSTOLIC MURMURS

There are two types of systolic murmur that may be associated with a completely normal heart. These are the vibratory murmur and the pulmonary ejection murmur.

Vibratory Systolic Murmur

This murmur was first described in 1909 by George Still[4] as a physiological bruit. The characteristic feature is the low-pitched buzzing quality, which has resulted in a variety of descriptive terms including "musical," "groaning," "buzzing," "fiddle string," and "vibratory." The vibratory murmur appears as regular, low-frequency vibrations on a phonocardiogram (Fig. 4-22) and is frequently associated with a physiological third heart sound. It may be audible over the entire precordium but is commonly of maximum intensity just inside the apex or at the left sternal border (Fig. 4-23). The murmur may be as loud as Grade 4 in intensity but is usually Grade 1 or 2. It is louder with exercise, anxiety, or pyrexia and may disappear as the subject becomes less anxious during an examination. The vibratory murmur has a fairly characteristic behavior with posture, becoming softer or disappearing on standing and then reappearing on squatting. In a large epidemiological survey conducted by us more than a decade ago, of Black schoolchildren with an age range of 2 to 18 years, a vibratory systolic murmur was present in approximately 70 percent. This number is in accord with the prevalence of 85 percent found by Fogel[5] in a study of 146 children. The murmur is also heard in young adults, especially when physically fit. In an earlier study, we heard vibratory systolic murmurs in at least 10 percent of normal young adults and 25 percent of pregnant women.

The mechanism of production of this prevalent systolic murmur remains unexplained. Stuckey[6] postulated in 1957 that it was of "aortic origin." Vibration of part of the heart muscle, an extracardiac origin, or a pulmonary valve origin are other theories that have been put forward. The response of the murmur to the Valsalva maneuver was shown by us to be compatible with a left-sided origin and this was confirmed by Wennevold[7] in 1967, using intracardiac phonocardiography. The vibratory murmur should not be referred to as an innocent *aortic* ejection murmur. It is often associated with an innocent pulmonary ejection murmur and, particularly in epidemiological studies, it may be preferable to use the term "innocent systolic murmur" to include both pulmonary ejection and vibratory systolic murmurs.

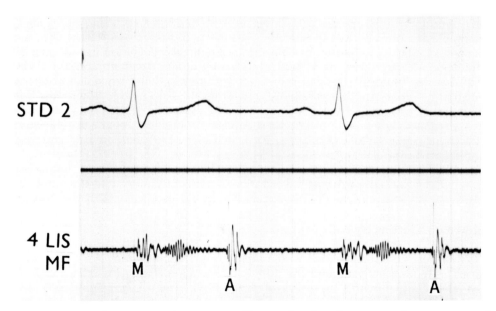

FIGURE 4-22. Vibratory systolic murmur. The regular, low-frequency vibrations are well demonstrated. (From Barlow, JB and Pocock, WA: *The isolated systolic murmur.* S Afr Med J 39:909–918, 1965, with permission.)

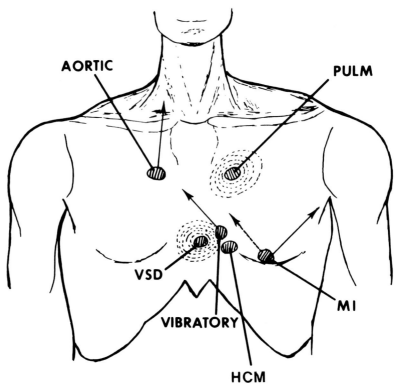

FIGURE 4-23. Maximal intensity and radiation of six isolated systolic murmurs. HCM = hypertrophic cardiomyopathy; MI = mitral incompetence; PULM = pulmonary; VSD = ventricular septal defect.

A short mid-diastolic murmur with no other evidence of heart disease is occasionally heard in children with vibratory systolic murmurs. We heard such mid-diastolic murmurs in 32 children (0.27 percent) in our large epidemiological study among Black schoolchildren in Soweto.[8] This entity of short mid-diastolic murmurs in apparently healthy children has not received general recognition in textbooks on cardiology, although they have been detected by others. Leatham and associates[9] favor that the "murmur" results from a left- and right-sided third sound occurring one after the other. Another possibility is that they arise from rapid flow across normal mitral or tricuspid valves. We have followed children with this murmur, and it has sometimes disappeared despite no rheumatic prophylaxis. In at least one child, a loud nonejection systolic click appeared, which suggested that there was a minimal abnormality of the mitral valve.

A vibratory systolic murmur is recognized by auscultation alone. Echocardiography will be normal; cardiac catheterization is not contributory and should not be necessary. The murmur usually disappears during adolescence or early adulthood.

Pulmonary Ejection Systolic Murmur

This murmur is often associated with a vibratory systolic murmur, but it may occur alone. It is loudest in the second and third left interspaces (Fig. 4-23) and is relatively high pitched and blowing. It presumably has a similar origin to the pulmonary ejection murmur associated with an atrial septal defect or anomalous pulmonary venous drainage. Significant left-to-right shunts at atrial level due to an atrial septal defect or anomalous venous drainage are differentiated by the associated features of wide fixed splitting of the second sound, a loud pulmonary closure sound, loud tricuspid component of the first heart sound, and a tricuspid mid-diastolic murmur. Difficulty may be encountered, however, with a very small atrial septal defect (pulmonary to systemic flow ratio of less than 1.5:1) or an isolated anomalous pulmonary vein. These may be clinically indistinguishable from a normal heart with a physiological pulmonary ejection murmur and an unusually widely split second sound.

Some patients with "straight-back syndrome" have prominent pulmonary ejection systolic murmurs and may be difficult to distinguish from patients with atrial septal defect. The tricuspid component of the first sound may be delayed and the second heart sound widely split in both conditions. Although the second sound varies with respiration in the straight-back syndrome, it can also move with respiration in small atrial septal defects. In some instances of straight-back syndrome, the second sound seems to move very little with respiration, possibly owing to compression on the right ventricle not allowing increased filling of that chamber during inspiration. The systolic murmur of straight-back syndrome probably arises high in the right ventricular outflow tract, and the murmur will become considerably louder and longer if firm pressure is applied to the sternal area during auscultation. We have, in fact, produced a pressure gradient of approximately 30 mmHg with this maneuver at cardiac catheterization.

So-called idiopathic dilatation of the pulmonary artery may also have a fairly prominent pulmonary ejection murmur. The condition is often associated with an early systolic pulmonary click and the second sound may be widely split with a relatively loud pulmonary component. In our view, this condition is probably associated with a congenital bicuspid pulmonary valve or other valve abnormality, but this postulate has not, to our knowledge, been confirmed by echocardiography or pathology. The condition may be associated with mild pulmonary regurgitation in about 30 percent of cases.

Pulmonary stenosis, albeit mild, is characterized by a harsher and longer systolic murmur with some delay and decreased intensity of the pulmonary component of the second sound. The length of the murmur and the degree of delay and softness of P2 correlate with the severity of the outflow obstruction (see Fig. 4-16). Obstruction may be above, below, or at valve level. Pulmonary valve stenosis is almost invariably congenital, but acquired conditions such as carcinoid or a myxomatous tumour of the valve may occasionally be the cause. Rheumatic involvement reputedly occurs but has never been encountered by us. Right-sided infective endocarditis, whether or not the valve was originally abnormal, occasionally causes a prominent pulmonary ejection systolic murmur, but signs of organic pulmonary regurgitation invariably predominate. Subvalvar obstruction is almost always congenital in origin and is most often at infundibular level. A double-chambered right ventricle in which the site of the obstruction is in the body of the ventricle is another congenital cause. Hypertrophic cardiomyopathy reputedly may involve the right side of the heart only, but other signs of that condition would be expected. Supravalvular pulmonary obstruction is uncommon but may be produced by external pressure on the pulmonary artery from a mediastinal tumour, aortic aneurysm, pericardial cyst, or localised constrictive pericarditis. Congenital stenosis, or coarctation, of the main pulmonary trunk is another cause of right ventricular outflow obstruction. In that condition, the closing pressure of the pulmonary valve is low, and the pulmonary component of the second sound is therefore soft but not appreciably delayed.

Echocardiography is useful in confirming a significant left-to-right shunt at atrial level, in that the right ventricle is dilated and there is paradoxical movement of the septum. With small shunts we have found that echocardiography is inconclusive, and even contrast echocardiography has not always been of assistance to us.

AORTIC EJECTION SYSTOLIC MURMUR

A truly innocent ejection systolic murmur that is without any absence of pathology of the aortic valve is very rare if it occurs at all. A left-sided ejection murmur, often loudest at the apex, is frequent in hypertension but may arise in the left ventricular outflow tract. Ejection murmurs associated with anemia, thyrotoxicosis, complete heart block, and other high-output states are probably entirely or mainly right-sided in origin. The innocent vibratory systolic murmur, also of left-sided origin, should not be referred to as an aortic ejection murmur. Although aortic ejection systolic murmurs are often audible over the entire precordium and may be maximal at the apex, base, or left sternal border in about the fourth left interspace, an important distinguishing feature from pulmonary murmurs is that they are louder at the second right intercostal space (Fig. 4-23) than at the corresponding space on the left. Furthermore, a characteristic feature is their specific radiation to the carotid arteries. Pulmonary ejection murmurs may be audible in the neck, particularly on the left side, but they do not radiate specifically into the carotid arteries.

Isolated aortic systolic murmurs are not unusual in the older age group and are caused by atherosclerotic thickening of the base of a cusp. In our experience, the most common cause of an aortic ejection murmur is rheumatic heart disease; but an early diastolic murmur is often associated, and most of those patients also have mitral valve involvement. A congenital bicuspid aortic valve may indeed have an ejection murmur, but there is almost always an associated aortic ejection click. Other causes of aortic valve pathology have obvious associated features. These include rheumatoid arthritis, ankylosing spondylitis, Hunter's polydystrophy, lupus erythe-

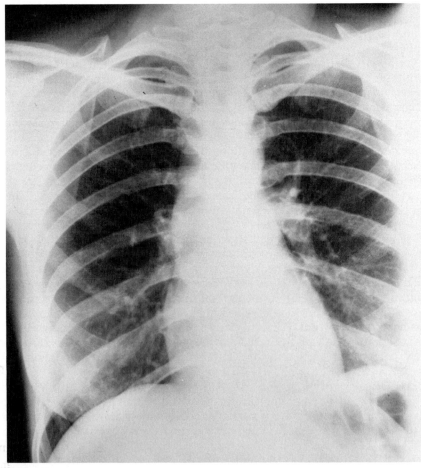

FIGURE 4-24. Posteroanterior chest radiograph of a 26-year-old woman with dilated ascending aorta and mild aortic regurgitation. The dilatation increased after a pregnancy, probably owing to medionecrosis in an aorta with medial hypoplasia. There were no skeletal features of Marfan's syndrome.

matosus, Marfan's syndrome, syphilis, familial hypercholesterolemia, and Ehlers-Danlos syndrome. Infective endocarditis involving the aortic valve will also have an aortic ejection murmur and may occasionally cause severe stenosis.

Thus, although isolated aortic ejection systolic murmurs due to atherosclerosis are common in the elderly, a true aortic ejection murmur as the only evidence of pathology of the aortic valve is rare in children and young adults.[10] Congenital bicuspid aortic valves invariably also produce an aortic ejection click as may an abnormally dilated aortic root (Fig. 4-24). Aortic valve pathology due to rheumatic heart disease or other pathological process has ancillary evidence of the relevant underlying condition.

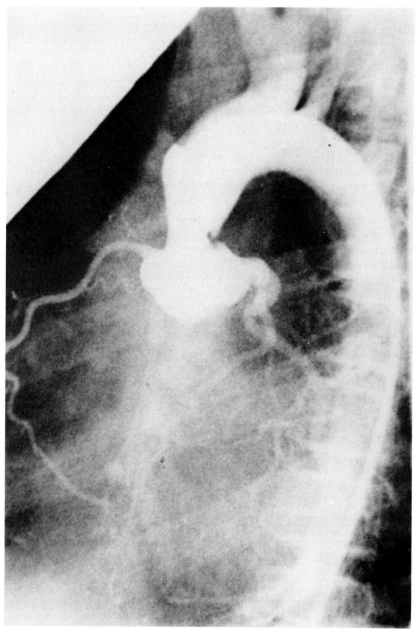

FIGURE 4-25. Aortogram in the left anterior oblique projection in a 14-year-old boy with supravalvular aortic stenosis. The narrowing of the lumen immediately distal to the origin of the coronary arteries is clearly demonstrated.

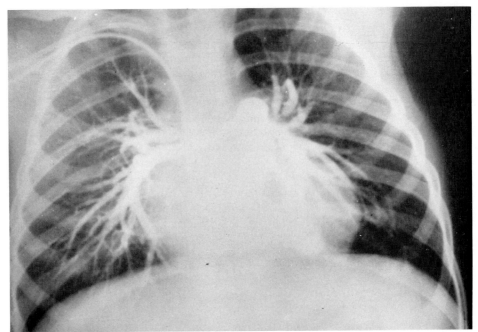

FIGURE 4-26. Pulmonary angiogram in a 2-year-old boy with supra-aortic stenosis showing bilateral multiple peripheral pulmonary artery stenoses.

Hemodynamically significant valvular aortic stenosis has a longer murmur with decreased intensity and delay of A2 resulting in reversed or partially reversed splitting of the components of the second heart sound. Mild, discrete congenital subaortic stenosis will also exhibit an isolated left-sided ejection murmur, which may be loudest at a lower interspace than in congenital valvular stenosis and is usually not associated with an ejection click. Mild aortic regurgitation, due to secondary pathology of the aortic leaflets, may supervene. Supra-aortic stenosis (Fig. 4-25) may be detected by an isolated aortic ejection systolic murmur, which may be loudest high in the first right interspace. Associated features such as hypercalcemia, pulmonary artery stenosis (Fig. 4-26), mental retardation, a characteristic facies (see Fig. 2-17) may be apparent. Inequality of upper limb pulses, due to narrowing of the origin of an artery or the so-called Coanda effect, should be sought. Familial homozygous hypercholesterolemia is a cause of acquired and sometimes severe, supra-aortic stenosis. Several such children or adolescents in our experience have required surgical management.

The importance of correctly identifying an isolated aortic ejection murmur lies in appreciating that the heart is pathological and that the patient is at risk for developing infective endocarditis.

Echocardiography may be of assistance in confirming a bicuspid valve. Dilatation of the aorta immediately above the valve may be detected in patients with medial hypoplasia, whether or not there is an associated bicuspid valve. Mild thickening of aortic leaflets may be demonstrated in rheumatic aortic valve involvement in the absence of significant stenosis. The detection of a membrane under the aortic valve may be possible in mild subaortic stenosis. In more severe cases of subaortic stenosis, early closure of the aortic leaflets is a helpful sign.

REGURGITANT SYSTOLIC MURMUR OF MITRAL INCOMPETENCE

The isolated apical systolic murmur of mitral regurgitation has been discussed in Section 1 of this chapter and in Chapter 3. Correct evaluation is crucial, because the

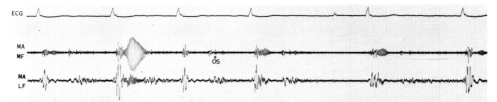

FIGURE 4-27. Musical mitral systolic murmur showing marked variation in length and intensity. The patient has tight mitral stenosis, atrial fibrillation, and very mild mitral regurgitation. An opening snap (OS) and long mid-diastolic murmur are demonstrated.

murmur may be the only sign of mild or minimal mitral regurgitation. The typical murmur is pansystolic in that it starts with the mitral closure sound and extends up to, or just beyond, the aortic component of the second sound. Mitral regurgitant murmurs are frequently constant in intensity throughout systole but may accentuate in late systole or be confined to that period. The murmur is loudest at the apex and best heard with the patient in the left lateral position. It may radiate to the axilla, to the back, or, particularly with posterior leaflet incompetence, medially and towards the base of the heart. A musical mitral systolic murmur (Fig. 4-27), the so-called honk or whoop, may be early, late, or holosystolic, but the extent of the mitral regurgitation is usually mild.

REGURGITANT SYSTOLIC MURMUR OF VENTRICULAR SEPTAL DEFECT

The isolated systolic murmur of a fairly small ventricular septal defect is typically pansystolic, is often accompanied by a thrill, and is usually loudest in the third or fourth intercostal space (see Fig. 4-23). It is crescendo-decrescendo in shape with maximal accentuation in mid-systole (see Fig. 4-19A). Late systolic accentuation (see Fig. 4-19B) is sometimes encountered in small defects. The murmur is often harsh but may have a high-pitched blowing quality. In small left-to-right shunts, the second heart sound is normal in all respects. An apical mid-diastolic flow murmur is seldom present if the shunt is less than 2:1. If the second sound is considered normal or is difficult to assess, and if a pulmonary ejection click is absent, the murmur of mild pulmonary stenosis may be confused with that of a ventricular septal defect. Under such circumstances, the response to vasoactive drugs such as amyl nitrite and phenylephrine or the Valsalva maneuver may be contributory. The pulmonary ejection murmur becomes louder with amyl nitrite inhalation as the venous return to the right side of the heart increases, whereas the regurgitant murmur of a ventricular septal defect will soften (see Fig. 4-21). After phenylephrine injection, the ejection murmur shows little or no change, whereas regurgitant murmurs become louder. There may be difficulty in distinguishing the murmur of a small ventricular septal defect from that of mitral regurgitation. Although the murmur of mitral regurgitation is usually loudest at the apex with radiation to the axilla, these features may not be easy to elicit in children, in whom the precordial area is small. Furthermore, the quality of the murmurs is similar, and both may accentuate in late systole. The presence of an apical mid-diastolic murmur and accurate assessment of the second sound are contributory in differentiating mild mitral regurgitation from a small ventricular septal defect. Whereas a normal second sound and a short mid-diastolic murmur are common in mild mitral incompetence, often following a third heart sound, a mid-diastolic murmur is not present in a ventricular septal defect unless the shunt is significant. In such cases the second sound is more widely split, P2 increased in intensity, and clinical evidence of some right ventricular hypertrophy apparent. Thus, a left-sided regurgitant systolic murmur with a mid-diastolic murmur and normal second sound favor mild mitral incompetence; whereas in the absence of a mid-diastolic murmur the diagnosis is likely to be that of a small ventricular septal defect. Aus-

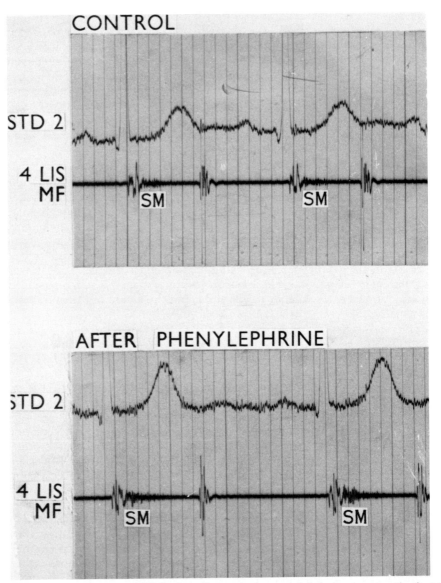

Figure 4-28. Atypical murmur (SM) of small ventricular septal defect occupying the first third of systole only. Phonocardiograms before and after the injection of phenylephrine show the increase in intensity of the regurgitant murmur during the period of hypertension. (From Barlow, JB and Pocock, WA: *The isolated systolic murmur.* S Afr Med J 39:909–918, 1965, with permission.)

cultation in the standing position may also be contributory (see Fig. 4-21). The murmur of a ventricular septal defect usually remains unchanged or becomes slightly softer, whereas that of mitral incompetence, particularly if due to prolapse, may become louder in the standing position.

The differentiation of a pansystolic murmur of ventricular septal defect from the regurgitant systolic murmur of tricuspid incompetence is seldom a problem in view of the rarity of tricuspid regurgitation as an isolated entity.

Very small defects of the ventricular septum cause a crescendo-decrescendo murmur that ends well before the second heart sound (see Fig. 4-19C) and is therefore not pansystolic. This "atypical" murmur is maximal at the fourth left interspace or lower sternal area and may have a high-pitched blowing quality. The murmur may be very short and last for only the first third of systole. After phenylephrine injection, the murmur will become louder (Fig. 4-28). Theoretically, it is important to detect a small ventricular septal defect because of prophylaxis for infective endocarditis. In practice, however, we have encountered only two cases of infective endocarditis on a small muscular ventricular septal defect. Infective endocarditis on larger defects with pansystolic murmurs is more common, and prophylactic measures are mandatory.

REGURGITANT SYSTOLIC MURMUR OF TRICUSPID INCOMPETENCE

Isolated organic tricuspid regurgitation is most commonly a sequel of trauma or infective endocarditis. The regurgitation is usually marked, and other signs, notably a distended liver and raised venous pressure, are obvious. Rheumatic involvement of the tricuspid leaflets as an isolated lesion does occur, but an associated mid-diastolic murmur is invariably present. Isolated tricuspid valve billowing or prolapse seems of little clinical importance unless, for any reason, the right ventricular systolic pressure becomes raised. The systolic murmur of tricuspid regurgitation sometimes increases in intensity with inspiration, but this sign may be unreliable.

SYSTOLIC MURMUR OF IDIOPATHIC HYPERTROPHIC CARDIOMYOPATHY

The systolic murmur of hypertrophic cardiomyopathy is usually loudest at the left sternal border, is somewhat late starting (Fig. 4-29), and may continue past the aortic component of the second sound. The murmur increases in intensity with amyl nitrite inhalation, on standing, and during the straining phase of the Valsalva maneuver. It tends to diminish in intensity during squatting (see Fig. 4-21). The second heart sound is often abnormal, and inconstant or variable partially reversed splitting can be detected on careful auscultation over several minutes. The electrocardiogram is rarely normal, but other clinical features of the condition are invariably present. It is rare in our experience for patients with hypertrophic cardiomyopathy to present with a truly isolated systolic murmur.

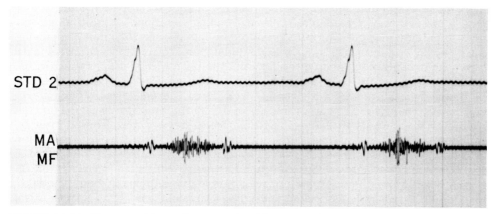

FIGURE 4-29. Hypertrophic cardiomyopathy. The onset of the murmur is 0.08 second after the first heart sound and 0.15 second after the Q of the electrocardiogram. (From Barlow, JB and Pocock, WA: *The isolated systolic murmur.* S Afr Med J 39:909–918, 1965, with permission.)

VASCULAR MURMURS

Extracardiac murmurs arising in vessels of the neck and thorax require attention, since they may mimic intracardiac murmurs and be misassessed. For example, an innocent pulmonary ejection murmur associated with a cervical arterial bruit is sometimes mistakenly diagnosed as an aortic ejection murmur.

Innocent Vascular Murmurs

VENOUS HUM. Over 75 percent of children and young adults are reputed to have a venous hum. This bruit is particularly common in high-output states, and, although characteristically a continuous murmur, in the supine position it is frequently confined to systole. Inspiration, the upright posture, or rotation of the neck to the opposite side may increase the intensity of the murmur. Audible on one or both sides of the neck, a venous hum may radiate as far down as the third intercostal space. Differentiation from an intracardiac murmur is made by its disappearance with pressure on the jugular veins.

ARTERIAL BRUIT. Innocent cervical arterial bruits are also prevalent in children and young adults and possibly arise at the aortic arch or the bifurcation of the innominate artery. They may be audible over the precordium and are distinguished from an intracardiac ejection murmur, with which they may be coincidentally associated, by their delayed onset, short duration, greater intensity above the clavicles, and different quality.

MAMMARY SOUFFLE. In some pregnant women, blood flow through dilated mammary vessels produces a murmur known as a mammary souffle. This bruit may be continuous or confined to systole. It is abolished by firm pressure with a finger adjacent to the end-piece of a stethoscope and thus easily distinguished from all intracardiac murmurs.

Pathological Vascular Murmurs

Murmurs produced by a communication between the systemic and pulmonary circulations, such as a patent ductus arteriosus, are continuous unless the diastolic component is abolished by a raised pulmonary vascular resistance. The systolic murmur is then, however, accompanied by signs of severe pulmonary hypertension.

A murmur can be regarded as continuous when vibrations extend through the second sound into diastole. Murmurs produced by reduction in the internal diameter of an artery are continuous or systolic in timing, depending on the extent of narrowing and the distance of the site of origin from the heart. Thus, a tight constriction will result in a large pressure gradient in both systole and diastole, and the murmur may then be heard throughout the cardiac cycle. Even with milder narrowing, however, the distance from the heart of the site of origin of a murmur produced only in systole may result in its extending past the second heart sound. The murmur of coarctation of the aorta may be heard at the apex, second left intercostal space, and back. The onset of the murmur is delayed in relation to the first heart sound, and it may be confined to systole or flow over into diastole. A similar late-onset systolic or continuous murmur is found in pulmonary artery stenosis or coarctation. Although this condition is generally associated with other congenital cardiac anomalies, such as ventricular septal defect, pulmonary stenosis, or supravalvular aortic stenosis, it is occasionally an isolated lesion and may involve the proximal or peripheral pulmonary arteries. The murmur may be loudest on either side of the sternum, the lateral chest wall, or posteriorly over the back.

REFERENCES

SECTION 1

1. WOOD, P: *Diseases of the Heart and Circulation,* ed 2. Eyre & Spottiswoode, London, 1959, pp 484, 507.
2. LAKIER, JB, KINSLEY, RH, POCOCK, WA, AND BARLOW, JB: *Left atrial C wave and mitral leaflet size.* Cardiovasc Res 6:585–588, 1972.
3. JERESATY, RM, EDWARDS, JE, AND CHAWLA, SK: *Mitral valve prolapse and ruptured chordae tendineae.* Am J Cardiol 55:138–142, 1985.
4. SCHAMROTH, L, SCHAMROTH, CL, SARELI, P, AND HUMMEL, D: *The electrocardiographic differentiation of the causes of left ventricular diastolic overload.* Chest 89:95–99, 1986.
5. EDWARDS, JE AND BURCHELL, HB: *Pathologic anatomy of mitral insufficiency.* Mayo Clin Proc 33:497–509, 1958.

SECTION 2

1. LEVINE, SA: *The systolic murmur. Its clinical significance.* JAMA 101:436–438, 1933.
2. LEATHAM, A: *A classification of systolic murmurs.* Br Heart J 17:574, 1955.
3. MCKUSICK, VA: *Cardiovascular Sound in Health and Disease.* Williams & Wilkins, Baltimore, 1958, pp 137, 202.
4. STILL, GF: *Common disorders and diseases of childhood.* H. Frowde, London, 1909.
5. FOGEL, DH: *The innocent systolic murmur in children: A clinical study of its incidence and characteristics.* Am Heart J 59:844–855, 1960.
6. STUCKEY, D, DOWD, B, AND WALSH, H: *Cardiac murmurs in schoolchildren.* Med J Aust 1:36–68, 1957.
7. WENNEVOLD, A: *The origin of the innocent 'vibratory' murmur studied with intra-cardiac phonocardiography.* Acta Med Scand 181:1–5, 1967.
8. MCLAREN, MJ, LACHMAN, AS, POCOCK, WA, AND BARLOW, JB: *Innocent murmurs and third heart sounds in Black schoolchildren.* Br Heart J 43:67–73, 1980.
9. LEATHAM, A, SEGAL, B, AND SCHAFTER, H: *Auscultatory and phonocardiographic findings in healthy children with systolic murmurs.* Br Heart J 25:451–459, 1963.
10. BARLOW, JB AND POCOCK, WA: *The significance of aortic ejection systolic murmurs.* Am Heart J 64:149–158, 1962.

BIBLIOGRAPHY

SECTION 1

ARMSTRONG, TG, MEERAN, MK, AND GOTSMAN, MS: *The left atrial lift.* Am Heart J 82:764–769, 1971.

BOLEN, JL AND ALDERMAN, EL: *Ventriculographic and hemodynamic features of mitral regurgitation of cardiomyopathic, rheumatic and nonrheumatic etiology.* Am J Cardiol 39:177–183, 1977.

BRODY, W AND CRILEY, JM: *Intermittent severe mitral regurgitation. Hemodynamic studies in a patient with recurrent acute left-sided heart failure.* N Engl J Med 283:673–676, 1970.

GROSE, R, STRAIN, J, AND COHEN, MV: *Pulmonary arterial V waves in mitral regurgitation: Clinical and experimental observations.* Circulation 69:214–222, 1984.

RAFTERY, EB, OAKLEY, CM, AND GOODWIN, JF: *Acute subvalvar mitral incompetence.* Lancet 2:360–365, 1966.

ROBERTS, WC AND PERLOFF, JK: *Mitral valvular disease. A clinicopathologic survey of the conditions causing the mitral valve to function abnormally.* Ann Intern Med 77:939–975, 1972.

TEI, C, TANAKA, H, NAKAO, S, YOSHIMURA, H, MINAGOE, S, KASHIMA, T, AND KANEHISA, T: *Motion of the interatrial septum in acute mitral regurgitation. Clinical and experimental echocardiographic studies.* Circulation 62:1080–1088, 1980.

VEYRAT, C, AMEUR, A, BAS, S, LESSANA, A, ABITBOL, G, AND KALMANSON, D: *Pulsed Doppler echocardiographic indices for assessing mitral regurgitation.* Br Heart J 51:130–138, 1984.

WALLER, BF, MORROW, AG, MARON, BJ, DEL NEGRO, AA, KENT, KM, McGRATH, FJ, WALLACE, RB, McINTOSH, CL, AND ROBERTS, WC: *Etiology of clinically isolated, severe, chronic, pure mitral regurgitation: Analysis of 97 patients over 30 years of age having mitral valve replacement.* Am Heart J 104:276–288, 1982.

SECTION 2

BARLOW, JB AND POCOCK, WA: *The isolated systolic murmur.* S Afr Med J 39:909–918, 1965.

LEATHAM, A: *Auscultation of the Heart and Phonocardiography,* ed 2. Churchill-Livingstone, Edinburgh, 1975.

5

MITRAL STENOSIS

with JEFFREY B. LAKIER and WENDY A. POCOCK

For practical purposes, mitral stenosis is a sequel of rheumatic carditis. Congenital mitral stenosis, especially as an isolated lesion, is extremely rare. Severe mitral anular calcification and constrictive pericarditis have been reported to cause a holodiastolic pressure difference across the mitral valve, but the obstruction is seldom severe unless there is associated pathology.

The functional anatomy of rheumatic mitral stenosis can be divided into the three main groups that follow. They may occur singly or in combination.

Commissural Fusion

When this occurs on its own, the leaflets remain mobile and pliable and the chordae tendineae are nearly normal. Surgical relief of the commissural fusion should result in a virtually normal mitral valve mechanism.

Leaflet Fibrosis, Thickening, and Calcification

These pathological changes are almost invariably associated with commissural fusion, but the leaflet disease predominates. Obstruction to left atrial emptying results from an inability of the thickened and rigid leaflets to open. Mitral valves of this type are often found after a previous commissurotomy where the commissures have remained "open," but tight functional stenosis is present because of the immobility of the rigid leaflets.

Subvalvar Stenosis

Thickened and fused chordae may cause considerable obstruction to flow. Subvalvar stenosis is not always associated with nonpliable leaflets.

SYMPTOMS AND COURSE OF MITRAL STENOSIS

These can be extremely variable. Although the majority of patients have experienced increasing breathlessness on exertion for the previous 10 or more years, a number present with recent-onset pulmonary edema or right ventricular failure and deny existence of previous symptoms. It is possible that some of the latter patients were unaware of gradually increasing breathlessness, because they did not have a normal standard for comparison. Unless the physician is aware of the presentation of pulmonary edema or right ventricular failure in patients who deny previous disability, mitral stenosis may be overlooked.

PULMONARY EDEMA

This may be precipitated by the recent onset of atrial fibrillation or another arrhythmia with a rapid ventricular rate. Thrombi or vegetations associated with infective endocarditis (which partially occlude the mitral valve orifice) and thrombi in the left atrium (which results in a smaller cavity) are other causes of an extremely high left atrial pressure. Pregnancy may precipitate pulmonary edema, especially in women in whom mitral stenosis was previously unsuspected. The mitral stenosis in any patient presenting with pulmonary edema may not be critical, and exercise tolerance may have been hitherto excellent. Excessive physical exertion is another factor that may produce severe pulmonary venous congestion and edema. In many patients the sudden onset of pulmonary edema is unexplained.

SUDDEN ONSET OF RIGHT VENTRICULAR FAILURE

Paul Wood[1] commented years ago that breathlessness in some patients with mitral stenosis became less marked when severe pulmonary arterial hypertension with right ventricular failure supervened. Although many patients who present with right ventricular failure have been aware of increasing breathlessness, some have not. Causes for deterioration and sudden onset of right ventricular failure are the same as for pulmonary edema. In other instances, pulmonary embolism or infection may be responsible, but a cause cannot always be identified.

THE CLINICAL SIGNS OF MITRAL STENOSIS

MITRAL FACIES

This sign is not as readily apparent in deeply pigmented races. "Highly coloured" cheeks are of two types. The cheeks may be red in a few patients (probably less than 10 percent) who do not have marked pulmonary hypertension. Patients with pulmonary hypertension, particularly when complicated by functional tricuspid regurgitation, have cyanosis of the cheeks. Peripheral vasoconstriction and cyanosis are frequently associated. This appearance has been referred to as "tricuspid facies" and is a nonspecific sign that may occur in any patient with severe pulmonary arterial hypertension. It presumably reflects high systemic venous pressure and a low cardiac output. It is also encountered in patients with severe organic tricuspid valve disease, especially when the stenotic element predominates.

THE PULSE

The pulse volume is normal or slightly reduced. Atrial fibrillation is the arrhythmia that is most frequently encountered with mitral stenosis, but this is rare in children and young adults, even in the presence of severe stenosis.

PALPATION OF THE PRECORDIUM

In most patients with mitral stenosis, an abnormally forceful right ventricular impulse can be felt along the lower left sternal border. This should be palpated with the ball of the hand. The extent of the abnormality depends on the presence and severity of pulmonary hypertension and associated tricuspid regurgitation. A forceful pulmonary artery pulsation in the second left interspace may be detectable with the tips of the fingers. Patients with tight pliable mitral stenosis without pulmonary arterial hypertension have a normally situated or only slightly displaced apical impulse. The apex may have a snapping quality owing to an easily palpable, loud first heart sound. An apical mid-diastolic or presystolic thrill may be detected. Pulmonary arterial hypertension without tricuspid regurgitation seldom causes more than mild cardiac enlargement. Whether or not tricuspid regurgitation develops probably depends on an elevated pulmonary arterial resistance and an abnormal right ventricular myocardium, including principally the tricuspid anulus (see Chapter 10). Gross functional tricuspid regurgitation is far more prevalent in patients with mitral stenosis than in patients with pulmonary arterial hypertension due to other causes. This favors a myocardial factor, presumably a result of the original rheumatic process. When tricuspid regurgitation supervenes, considerable cardiac dilatation may occur with the apex beat displaced to the anterior axillary line. In the absence of mitral regurgitation or other cause of left ventricular enlargement, the apical impulse will have an outwards and upwards direction which contrasts with the outwards and downwards direction of the apical impulse of left ventricular enlargement. The functional tricuspid regurgitation associated with tight mitral stenosis causes a marked parasternal heave. In addition, readily palpable systolic pulsation of the distended liver and a large systolic wave in the jugular venous pulse are apparent. The tricuspid "rock" discussed by Chesler[2] occurs in some patients, and this is described in more detail in Chapter 10. It is noteworthy that many patients with mitral stenosis and functional tricuspid regurgitation do not have marked pulmonary arterial hypertension as assessed by cardiac catheterization. In such instances, the pulmonary vascular resistance is raised, but the pulmonary artery pressure has dropped as a result of a reduction in pulmonary arterial flow secondary to right ventricular dysfunction and tricuspid regurgitation.

Mitral stenosis alone, irrespective of the height of the left atrial V wave, will not cause a left atrial lift. This sign does not reflect the height of the V wave but the extent of volume expansion of the left atrial cavity at that time. The presence of a left atrial lift in a patient with mitral stenosis is therefore strong evidence in favor of accompanying significant regurgitation. It must be remembered, however, that mitral regurgitation and stenosis augment each other. In other words, an incompetent mitral valve narrowed to 1.5 cm will be functionally more stenotic, because of the over-filled left atrium from the mitral regurgitation, than a similar degree of stenosis without incompetence. Similarly, a severe amount of regurgitation will result in a higher left atrial mean pressure if the valve is narrowed to 2.5 cm than it would in one that is not stenosed.

AUSCULTATION OF MITRAL STENOSIS

This section discusses auscultation in "pure" mitral stenosis or stenosis with some regurgitation. Organic disease of the tricuspid valve also influences the auscultatory features of mitral valve disease, but these will be considered in Chapter 10. Auscultation remains an accurate, convenient, practicable, and inexpensive method of diagnosing mitral stenosis. Objectives of auscultation include (1) evaluation of the degree of stenosis and of the pliability of leaflets and chordae tendineae; (2) detection of the presence and severity of associated mitral regurgitation; and (3) evaluation of pulmonary arterial hypertension and functional tricuspid regurgitation.

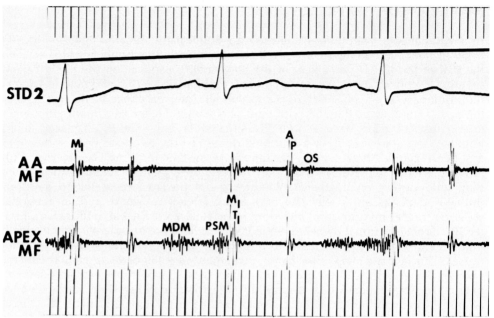

FIGURE 5-1. The auscultatory signs of tight mitral stenosis with a pliable valve. The opening snap (OS) has recorded best at the aortic area (AA). In this and subsequent tracings time lines measure 0.04 sec. M1 = mitral component of the first heart sound; A,P = aortic and pulmonary components of the second heart sound; MDM = mid-diastolic murmur; PSM = presystolic murmur.

In mitral stenosis the cardiac cycle is best timed by detecting the first heart sound and then timing other events from that. Auscultatory features of mitral stenosis are heard mainly at the apical area and are best assessed with the bell of the stethoscope applied very lightly to the skin of the chest wall. Pressure on the bell must be only firm enough to make a seal. Too-firm pressure will decrease the intensity of the low-pitched mid-diastolic murmur. The tube, or tubes, of the examiner's stethoscope must not be in contact with the patient's clothing or bedclothes, and it is sometimes necessary to depress the mattress away from the stethoscope in order to avoid such contact. For the assessment of mitral stenosis to be complete, it is mandatory that auscultation be carried out in the left lateral position. With gross tricuspid regurgitation and marked cardiomegaly, the left ventricle is rotated far posteriorly, and a mid-diastolic murmur directed into that chamber will be audible only if the auscultator listens at the appropriate site, which may be on the anterior, mid-, or even the posterior axillary line. Auscultation must be undertaken all around the apical area with the objective of assessing sounds and murmurs at their optimal sites. The first heart sound may be loudest at one area, the mid-diastolic murmur at another, presystolic accentuation of the diastolic murmur at a third, and a mitral regurgitant systolic murmur at a fourth. An opening snap may be loudest or only audible at virtually any area of the precordium including the apex or the base of the heart. Occasionally, an opening snap may be audible at the aortic area only.

The classic features of pliable, pure, tight mitral stenosis are (1) a loud first heart sound; (2) a loud, high-pitched opening snap; and (3) a long mid-diastolic murmur with presystolic accentuation (Fig. 5-1). Systole is silent. Usually stenotic mitral valves are neither completely "pliable" nor "rigid," and all gradations from ideally pliable to totally rigid exist. If auscultation is to continue to be useful in the assessment of mitral stenosis, it should be practised skillfully and the signs correctly interpreted. It is therefore pertinent to consider in some detail the mechanism of production of heart sounds and murmurs in pure or predominant mitral stenosis.

First Heart Sound

The site of maximal intensity of the mitral component of the first sound must be sought. This is often outside the apex and at a different area to the site of maximal intensity of the diastolic murmur. Factors such as associated mitral regurgitation, the PR interval, and the force of left ventricular contraction play relatively minor roles

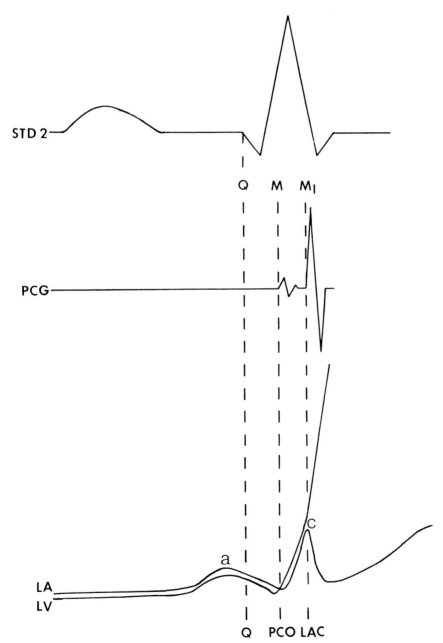

FIGURE 5-2. Diagrammatic representation of simultaneous standard lead II of the ECG (STD2), external phonocardiogram (PCG), left atrial (LA), and left ventricular (LV) pressures. The early vibration M coincides with the point of crossover (PCO) of LV and LA pressures. M1 occurs after PCO at the time of the peak of the left atrial C (LAC) wave. The Q-M1 interval can thus be subdivided into Q-M plus M-M1, which is the same as Q-PCO plus PCO-LAC. a = left atrial A wave. (From Lakier et al,[3] with permission.)

in affecting the intensity of the first heart sound in mitral stenosis. The severity of the stenosis contributes to the valve orifice remaining "open" at the onset of left ventricular systole, but this feature also is relatively unimportant. The most important factor producing a loud first heart sound is mobility of the leaflets and chordae, particularly the anterior leaflet; but because some patients with rigid leaflets have a loud first sound, we believe that tensing of chordae tendineae also contributes to the sound. Nevertheless, mobility of at least part of the anterior leaflet is probably the most important factor. Closure of the mitral valve, both in normal subjects and in patients with mitral stenosis, occurs when the rising left ventricular pressure exceeds the left atrial pressure (Fig. 5-2). This point marks the end of the pre-isovolumetric phase, the onset of the isovolumetric phase of ventricular systole, and time at which the leaflet edges appose. After this pressure crossover, the coapted mitral leaflets continue to ascend into the left atrial cavity, contributing to the left atrial C wave, at the peak of which the mitral leaflets and chordae are maximally tensed and the mitral component of the first heart sound (M1) occurs.[3] In patients with mitral stenosis who have mobile and relatively voluminous leaflets, the left atrial C wave is large and its peak delayed. The mitral component of the first sound is thus also delayed and loud. With very tight stenosis and mobile leaflets, the Q-M1 interval may be as long as 0.12 second, resulting in reversed splitting of the major components of the first heart sound (Fig. 5-3). With rigid leaflets, the left atrial C wave will be small and the mitral component of the first sound relatively soft (Figs. 5-4, 5-5). Stenosis due entirely to commissural fusion, with pliable leaflets and mobile chordae, will result in a loud, high-pitched first heart sound, and the valve will remain competent. Some thickening of the leaflets or immobility of chordae produces a lower-pitched, albeit still loud, first heart sound, and there may also be a Grade 1 or 2 systolic murmur of mild mitral regurgitation. When the valve mechanism is very rigid, the mitral component of the first sound is soft. In such instances there is usually associated mitral regurgitation. Two components of the mitral first sound may be present with dominant mitral stenosis if part of a leaflet billows asynchronously. In such instances, the left atrial C wave will have a double peak.

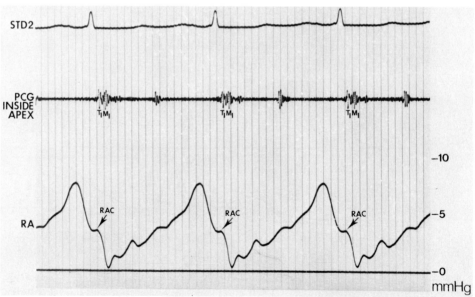

FIGURE 5-3. Standard lead II of the ECG, external phonocardiogram, and right atrial tracing in a patient with tight mitral stenosis. A high frequency vibration (T1) occurs 0.07 second after Q, the onset of which coincides with right atrial C (RAC) wave. T1 precedes M and the first sound is thus reversed. Paper speed 150 mm/sec.

MITRAL STENOSIS WITH SHORTENED CHORDAE & RIGID LEAFLETS

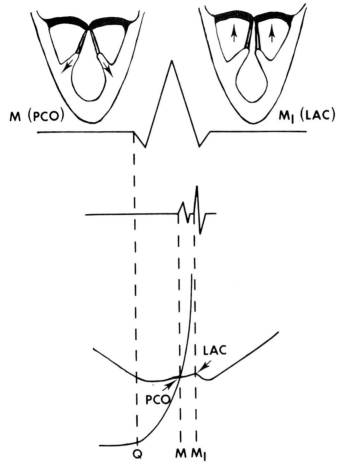

FIGURE 5-4. Diagrammatic representation of the LV and LA pressures and prolonged Q-M1 (LAC) interval in mitral stenosis with rigid leaflets. M and PCO are delayed because of the high left atrial pressure but the M (PCO)–M1 (LAC) interval is short and LAC small since little ascent of the rigid leaflets is possible.

Left Ventricular Systole

In pure mitral stenosis, left ventricular systole is silent. The presence of an apical systolic murmur, whether nonpansystolic or pansystolic, implies some fibrosis or tethering of a leaflet by shortened chordae.

A nonejection systolic click, often variable in timing and intensity, may occur with mitral stenosis and is probably due to functional inequality of chordae. This auscultatory feature may be present before or after mitral commissurotomy. In at least one instance in our experience, a "postvalvotomy" nonejection systolic click was associated with iatrogenic rupture of a papillary muscle after closed commissurotomy (Fig. 5-6).

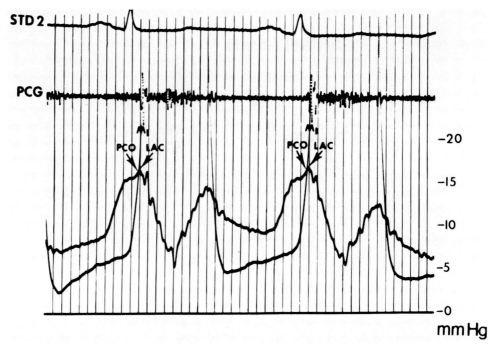

FIGURE 5-5. Simultaneous ECG, phonocardiogram, left atrial, and left ventricular pressures in a patient with tight mitral stenosis in sinus rhythm. The Q-M1 (LAC) interval is prolonged to 0.08 second, the major cause of the prolongation being a Q-PCO (M) interval of 0.07 second. M1 (LAC) occurs 0.01 second after PCO. LAC is of small amplitude indicating a rigid valve mechanism. Paper speed 100 mm/sec. (From Lakier et al,[3] with permission.)

Second Heart Sound

The second sound is variable in mitral stenosis. In many cases, the splitting remains physiologically normal. The pulmonary component (P2) may be increased in intensity when pulmonary arterial hypertension is present. Functional tricuspid regurgitation often supervenes early in patients with pulmonary hypertension secondary to mitral stenosis and affects the splitting of the second sound as well as the intensity of P2. Because the pulmonary artery pressure tends to drop with severe tricuspid regurgitation, P2 will not be very loud. Furthermore, the right ventricular ejection period decreases in some cases of severe tricuspid regurgitation, analogous to the shortening of the left ventricular ejection period in mitral regurgitation. This may result in a relatively earlier P2 with consequent partially reversed, or even reversed, splitting of the second sound.

Mitral Opening Snap

Although there is some correlation between the A-OS interval, as measured on a phonocardiogram, and the degree of valve narrowing, this feature no longer has much clinical relevance. The opening snap does have some bearing on the assessment of leaflet pliability. The sound can occur at any site over the precordium and is best heard with the diaphragm of the stethoscope. In extremely tight mitral stenosis the A-OS interval is very short (±0.5 second), and the opening snap may not be heard with the patient in the supine position, because it falls inside the "auscultatory gap" of the human ear. The A-OS interval becomes slightly longer if the patient is auscultated immediately after adopting the upright position. The presence

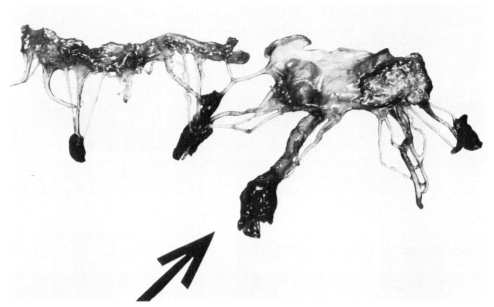

FIGURE 5-6. Excised rheumatic mitral valve with an avulsed papillary muscle *(arrow)*. Immediately after closed mitral commissurotomy an intermittent loud nonejection click was heard. Mitral regurgitation developed, and the patient required valve replacement. (From Marchand, P, Barlow, JB, du Plessis, LA, and Webster, I: *Mitral regurgitation with rupture of normal chordae tendineae.* Br Heart J 28:746–758, 1966, with permission.)

of an opening snap implies that the anterior leaflet or part thereof is mobile. Since much of the mitral valve mechanism may be rigid, this sign has limited clinical significance. When the opening snap is very high pitched, it is more likely than when lower pitched to be associated with pliable leaflets. An opening snap is not in itself a sign of severe mitral stenosis and may occur in patients with predominant mitral regurgitation. The *absence* of an opening snap in a patient with mitral stenosis has more relevance and indicates that both leaflets are rigid. In such instances, closed mitral commissurotomy is contraindicated, open commissurotomy unlikely to be successful, and either an extensive valvuloplasty or valve replacement will be required (see Chapter 8).

Third Heart Sound

Although the exact mechanism of production of a third heart sound remains uncertain, rapid left ventricular filling or at least insignificant obstruction to ventricular filling is a prerequisite for its production. Consequently, it has been accepted for many years that a left ventricular third heart sound will not occur with moderate or severe mitral stenosis, and in our view, this is essentially correct. A third heart sound will not be heard or recorded in mitral stenosis with a pliable valve mechanism. However, a low-pitched vibration simulating a third heart sound does occur in two circumstances:

1. It may be part of a loud starting mid-diastolic murmur, often associated with mitral regurgitation. At an optimal site, this sounds like a loud starting mid-diastolic murmur, but if the auscultator moves the stethoscope away from this site, the softer mid-diastolic vibrations of the murmur will become inaudible. The "loud start" simulates a third heart sound and will be recorded as such on a phonocardiogram.

2. Some patients with a rigid valve mechanism, particularly with subvalvar involvement, have a loud-starting, very short mid-diastolic murmur, even though the mitral stenosis is functionally tight. The mitral vibrations may resemble a third heart sound.[4]

Fourth Heart Sound (Atrial Sound)

An atrial sound does not occur in patients with significant mitral stenosis. This is important when the possibility of mitral stenosis occurring in association with conditions such as aortic stenosis, left ventricular dysfunction, or systemic hypertension arises. The echocardiogram of the mitral valve in such patients may show a flat EF slope that simulates mitral stenosis. When an atrial sound is palpable or audible, mitral stenosis is precluded.

Mid-Diastolic and Presystolic Murmurs

Provided the mitral valve mechanism is fairly pliable, a rumbling mid-diastolic murmur is invariably present and may be heard with little difficulty. The optimal site for detection of the murmur varies, and it may be far out on the left chest wall. When the mitral valve is pliable and the stenosis tight, the diastolic murmur is holo-diastolic.

It has been generally accepted that patients with mitral stenosis in sinus rhythm frequently have presystolic accentuation of the murmur following atrial systole. It was also believed that this "presystolic" murmur disappeared with the onset of atrial fibrillation. In 1971 Criley and co-workers,[5,6] using high-speed cineangiography, correlated leaflet movement with simultaneously recorded left atrial and left ventricular pressures and external phonocardiograms and clarified the mechanism of production of a "presystolic murmur." Working independently from Criley, we reached similar conclusions.[7] Identification of a presystolic murmur is not only of academic interest, because, in our experience, it is the single most reliable auscultatory sign of a pliable leaflet mechanism in cases of pure mitral stenosis. It is therefore relevant to review the mechanism of production in some detail.

The postulated changes in the functional anatomy of the mitral valve and left heart chambers from the onset of left atrial (LA) systole until M1, in patients with mitral stenosis in sinus rhythm, are shown diagrammatically in Figure 5-7 in relation to the pressures and auscultatory features. Immediately before the LA contracts, a pressure difference is still present across the mitral valve but has been decreasing. The stenosed mitral valve orifice is fully "open," but the mid-diastolic murmur is decreasing slightly in intensity because of the diminishing gradient and hence reduced volume and velocity of flow through the valve. When the LA contracts, the resulting a wave increases the LA-LV gradient, with a consequent increase in both the volume and velocity of flow through the stenosed mitral orifice, and true presystolic accentuation of the mid-diastolic murmur occurs (interval A). During this period, the more rapid flow is due entirely to the increased LA-LV gradient caused by atrial contraction. Following the onset of LV contraction (point B) and throughout the pre-isovolumetric phase of LV systole (interval B-PCO), a change in the mitral valve mechanism occurs. The stenosed orifice decreases in size until the leaflets appose, and the valve is "closed," at point of crossover (PCO). This reduction of the mitral valve orifice during the pre-isovolumetric phase of LV systole may depend in part on functional anatomical factors; but it almost certainly results predominantly from the rising LV pressure, which decreases and eventually abolishes the LA-LV gradient, "closing" the valve orifice, at PCO. Despite this pressure difference decreasing throughout the pre-isovolumetric phase, the diminishing valve orifice

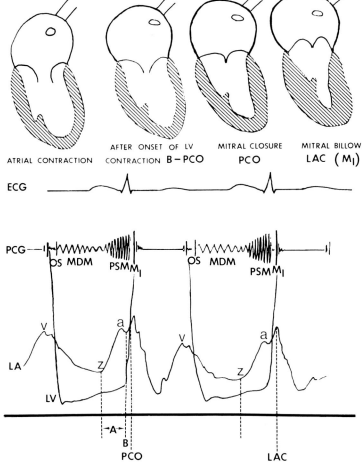

FIGURE 5-7. Diagrammatic representation, based on simultaneously recorded tracings at cardiac catheterization, of LA and LV pressures, external phonocardiogram and electrocardiogram of a patient with tight mitral stenosis in sinus rhythm. Schematic diagrams of the two left heart chambers and the mitral leaflets correlate with the hemodynamic and sound events. Thus, diagram "atrial contraction" represents the functional anatomical status during interval A when the mitral leaflets are "wide open;" "after onset of LV contraction" illustrates the period B-PCO during which the valve orifice progressively decreases because of the rising LV pressure until it is occluded at "mitral closure" (PCO). At "mitral billow" the leaflets are billowed further up to produce LAC and the sound M1. Note the undetectable "silent" period between PSM and M1 during the interval PCO-LAC.

would result in a progressive *increase in velocity* but a *decrease in volume* of blood flow across the valve. The presystolic murmur thus accentuates further until PCO, after which the orifice is occluded and the valve "closed." In addition to being the end of the pre-isovolumetric phase, PCO is the start of the isovolumetric phase. After PCO, the LV pressure continues to rise rapidly, and the apposed mitral leaflets are billowed up into the LA cavity forming the LAC, at the peak of which the sudden tension on the chordae and leaflets produces a loud M1. During the period PCO-LAC (M1), no murmur should be produced at the mitral valve (Fig. 5-7); but this time interval is extremely short in mitral stenosis, and the silent period is not detectable. Both clinically and phonocardiographically, the mitral diastolic murmur appears to crescend from the onset of the left atrial A wave to the sound M1 producing typical "presystolic accentuation."

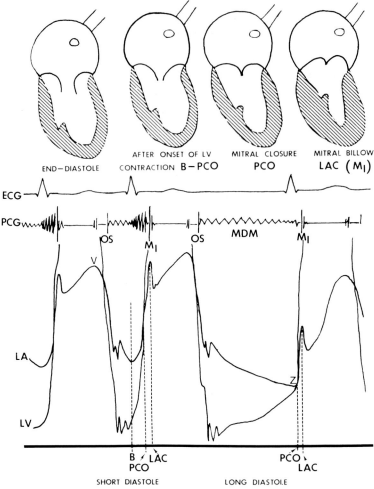

FIGURE 5-8. Diagrammatic representation of events in a patient with mitral stenosis and atrial fibrillation. The rise in LA pressure and accentuation of the diastolic murmur are seen only after a short diastole. (From Lakier et al,[7] with permission.)

The situation is essentially similar in mitral stenosis with atrial fibrillation after a short diastolic pause (Fig. 5-8). In the absence of any LA contraction, the LA-LV pressure difference is still decreasing prior to the onset of the pre-isovolumetric ventricular systolic phase (Fig. 5-8, point B); thus, the volume and velocity of flow through the stenosed mitral valve orifice are also decreasing slightly and the mid-diastolic murmur is becoming a little softer. When the LV contracts, and throughout the pre-isovolumetric ventricular contraction phase (Fig. 5-8, interval B-PCO), the mitral orifice must again diminish in size until it is occluded at PCO. As in mitral stenosis with sinus rhythm, the diminution of the valve orifice may depend partly on functional anatomical factors, but the rising LV pressure is likely to be the most important factor in decreasing the orifice size. Accentuation of the diastolic murmur thus occurs with the progressive *increase in velocity* of flow produced by the diminishing mitral orifice, although the *volume* is again *decreased*. While the leaflets are moving towards the closed position (Fig. 5-8, interval B-PCO) and thus towards the LA chamber, the volume of that cavity must decrease. Because the LA pressure is relatively high at this time and the chamber continues to receive blood from the pulmonary venous system, the small elevation of the LA pressure during the pre-

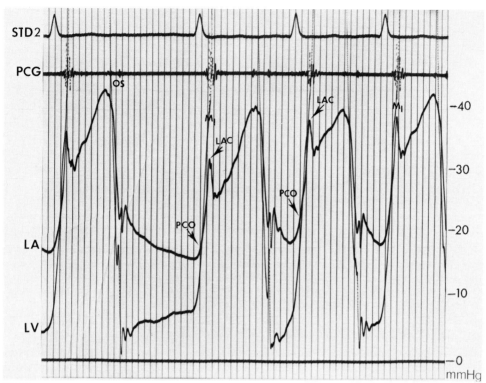

FIGURE 5-9. Standard lead II of the ECG, external phonocardiogram, left atrial, and left ventricular pressure tracings in a patient with mitral restenosis after insertion of a pericardial patch into the posterior leaflet. The atrial pressure rises during the pre-isovolumetric contraction phase, before PCO. The delayed (Q-LAC = 0.12 sec) and large amplitude LAC coincides with a similarly delayed M1. Paper speed 75 mm/sec. (From Lakier et al,[7] with permission.)

isovolumetric contraction phase (Fig. 5-8, interval B-PCO; Fig. 5-9) is understandable. After the mitral orifice has been occluded at PCO, the leaflets will, as with sinus rhythm, move farther up into the LA cavity to produce LAC and the sound M1. The very short PCO-LAC (M1) interval is again undetectably silent.

After a long diastolic pause these hemodynamic events are very different and are similar to those in atrial fibrillation without mitral stenosis. Since LA and LV pressures now either approach equalization or have already equalized at the end of ventricular diastole (Fig. 5-8, point Z), the velocity of flow across the mitral valve is relatively low and the diastolic murmur is soft or absent (Figs. 5-8, 5-9, 5-10). After the onset of LV contraction, PCO and valve closure take place almost immediately; the pre-isovolumetric phase of LV systole is thus extremely short, no rise in LA pressure prior to PCO is seen, and no accentuation of the diastolic murmur is produced.

The PR interval and the severity of the mitral stenosis will influence the configuration of an atrial systolic murmur. The contention that an increasing velocity of flow through the closing mitral valve orifice during the LV pre-isovolumetric contraction phase is the cause of the crescendo of the diastolic murmur in tight mitral stenosis with atrial fibrillation, and the explanation of the associated and synchronous rise in LA pressure *before* PCO, are compatible with observations we have made in cases of tight mitral stenosis in sinus rhythm and a relatively long PR interval. In such instances, the left atrial a wave occurs earlier in diastole, and the LA-LV gradient is significantly decreasing just before the onset of left ventricular contraction (Fig. 5-11, *right*). For these reasons the atrial systolic murmur has a crescendo-decrescendo configuration at this time. With the onset of the LV pre-isovolumetric con-

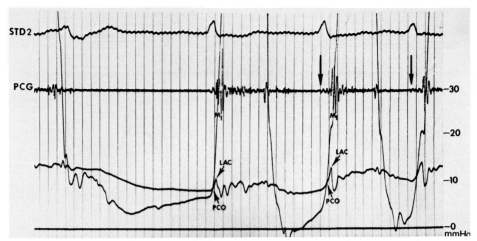

FIGURE 5-10. Accentuation *(long arrows)* of a mid-diastolic murmur and a simultaneous rise in LA pressure are shown after the short diastolic pauses and precede the point (PCO) at which the LV pressure exceeds that of the LA. Following the long diastolic pause, no such vibrations are recorded and the LA pressure does not rise before PCO. LAC (the peak of the left atrial C wave) coincides with the onset of M1. Paper speed 150 mm/sec. (From Lakier et al,[7] with permission.)

traction phase, the stenosed mitral orifice decreases in size as the leaflets are moved towards the LA cavity, the murmur accentuates again (Fig. 5-12), and the LA pressure rises before PCO (see Fig. 5-11).

Thus, in patients with mitral stenosis and a presystolic murmur the mitral orifice progressively narrows throughout the pre-isovolumetric period. The situation is

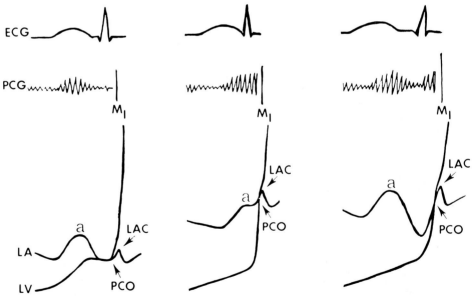

FIGURE 5-11. Diagrammatic illustration of the influence of the PR interval and the severity of the mitral stenosis on the configuration of a presystolic murmur. With mild mitral stenosis *(left panel)* the LA-LV pressure gradient equalizes before the onset of LV contraction and the murmur is crescendo-decrescendo. With more significant stenosis or a relatively short PR interval *(center panel)*, the murmur is entirely crescendo. With tight mitral stenosis, but a relatively long PR interval *(right panel)*, the murmur is crescendo-decrescendo at the time of the early A wave but then accentuates again during pre-isovolumetric LV contraction.

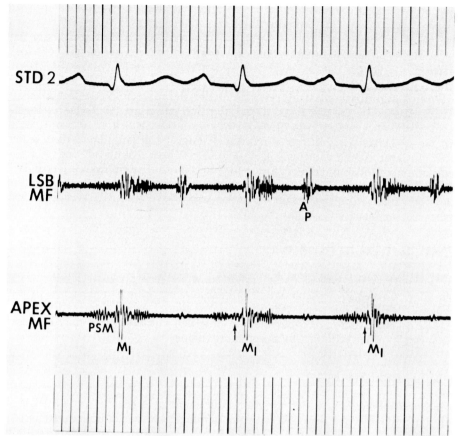

FIGURE 5-12. Phonocardiogram of a patient with tight mitral stenosis in sinus rhythm (PR interval = 0.22 sec). A crescendo-decrescendo presystolic murmur is present, which again accentuates *(arrow)* immediately before M1. Paper speed 75 mm/sec.

analogous to closing the door of a house in the face of a strong wind. As the door is forced towards closure, the volume of air entering the house decreases whereas the velocity of the air flow increases, as does the intensity of the sound vibrations of the wind passing through the narrowing aperture. There must be some mobility of the valve mechanism for a murmur of mitral stenosis to crescendo during the pre-iso-volumetric contraction phase, because the accentuation depends on a progressive decrease in size of the mitral valve orifice. With a completely rigid valve mechanism in which such a decrease cannot take place, the velocity of blood flow would not increase when the LV pressure rises to reduce and eventually to abolish the LA-LV pressure gradient and the volume of flow through the fixed, stenosed valve orifice. Such a valve is unlikely to be completely competent. Since its rigid mechanism does not allow the leaflets to billow up into the LA cavity, the LAC is small and M1 relatively soft.

Clarification of the term "presystolic" is relevant. The onset of mechanical systole is identified in the clinical situation by the first heart sound, and it is appropriate that accentuation of a murmur that immediately precedes that sound should be regarded as "presystolic," despite the fact that the vibrations have been shown to occur during the pre-isovolumetric phase of left ventricular contraction. In patients with mitral stenosis in sinus rhythm and a relatively short PR interval, the "presystolic" accentuation does start prior to the onset of ventricular contraction, but an increasing intensity of the murmur continues throughout the pre-isovolumetric phase. In patients with mitral stenosis and a relatively long PR interval, the left atrial a wave occurs earlier in diastole with a resultant increase in the LA-LV pressure difference at that time. This pressure difference then decreases prior to the onset of left ventricular contraction. For these reasons, the atrial systolic murmur may have a crescendo-decrescendo configuration. However, with the onset of left ventricular contraction, the ventricular pressure rises and as the leaflets move towards closure, the murmur accentuates again. Thus, even with sinus rhythm, this latter part of the "presystolic" murmur is not truly presystolic, but, because the onset of clinical systole is determined by the first heart sound, this nomenclature should be retained.

Presystolic accentuation is often heard only in a small area and not always where the mid-diastolic murmur is loudest. It must be differentiated from a mid-diastolic murmur, which continues up to a loud first heart sound but does not have definite accentuation immediately prior to that sound. The mitral leaflets may be fairly rigid despite a loud first sound, and we have found presystolic accentuation highly contributory in that context. When definite presystolic accentuation is detected, the leaflets are invariably mobile.

"SILENT" MITRAL STENOSIS

By far the most common cause of "silent" mitral stenosis is poor auscultation. In the examination of over 3000 patients with mitral stenosis during the last two or more decades, we have encountered "silent" or near-"silent" mitral stenosis in no more than 10. However, there are circumstances in which mitral stenosis may be missed or the severity underestimated by auscultation alone.

Very Mild Mitral Stenosis

Very mild mitral stenosis of definite rheumatic etiology is rare, and the leaflets are usually fairly pliable. A presystolic murmur is almost always audible in the left lateral position if the patient is in sinus rhythm. Mild mitral stenosis is detected more frequently in the elderly patient with atrial fibrillation. A short mid-diastolic murmur is audible and mild mitral regurgitation is often associated. Some of these cases presumably reflect secondary atherosclerotic or degenerative changes superimposed on minimal leaflet lesions of rheumatic or other etiology. Others may be analogous to the degenerative process, which is manifested as calcification of the anulus. It is rarely necessary to exercise patients in order to detect a mid-diastolic or presystolic murmur in mild stenosis. Most patients are apprehensive during a clinical examination, and careful auscultation is more meaningful than increasing the cardiac output further with exercise.

Marked Pulmonary Arterial Hypertension

Severe pulmonary hypertension decreases flow through the mitral valve, but the mitral murmurs are readily audible in the absence of pulmonary thromboembolic disease and of marked tricuspid regurgitation. Severe pulmonary thromboembolic disease that may be accompanied by cyanosis and secondary polycythemia makes the murmurs of underlying mitral stenosis difficult to hear. In some instances, the mitral stenosis is the less significant disease entity. It has already been emphasized that auscultation in the mid- or posterior axillary line is mandatory when there is marked tricuspid regurgitation and considerable cardiac enlargement.

Left Atrial Thrombus

Thrombus formation in the left atrium may interfere with the flow of blood through the mitral valve especially if it partially occludes the mitral orifice (Figs. 5-13, 5-14).

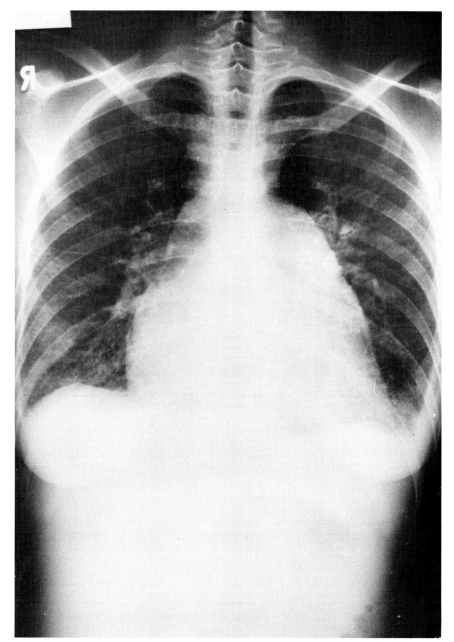

FIGURE 5-13. Posteroanterior chest radiograph of a patient with tight mitral stenosis and left atrial thrombus, showing cardiomegaly, left atrial enlargement, and pulmonary venous hypertension.

Postcommissurotomy Rigid Valve Leaflets

Mitral stenosis with rigid leaflets seldom occurs without associated commissural fusion and in these patients a long mid-diastolic murmur is readily audible. After mitral commissurotomy, however, the stenosis may remain, or later become, functionally severe despite the fact that the commissures have been well split. Not much turbulence is created by the thickened, immobile leaflets with a fixed orifice; and the mid-diastolic murmur may be short. The hemodynamic severity of such cases should be suspected from the symptoms and other clinical signs.

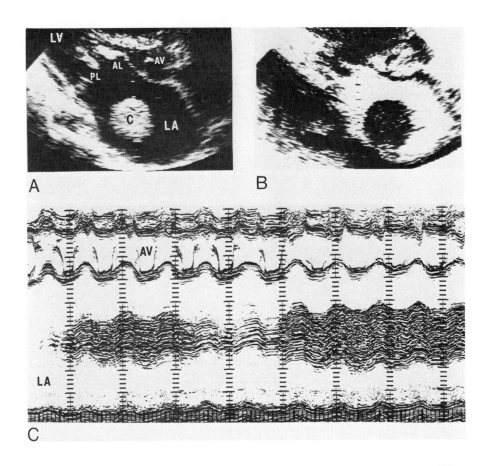

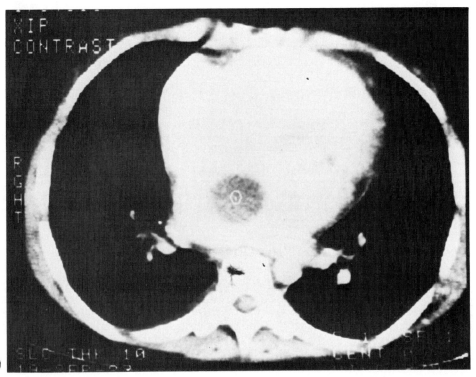

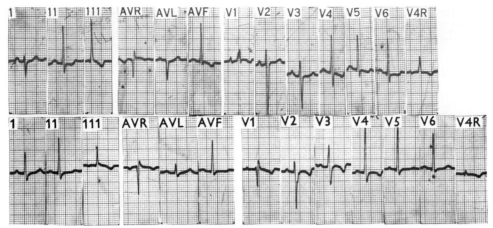

FIGURE 5-15. *Upper tracing,* ECG of a patient with tight mitral stenosis, pulmonary hypertension, and right ventricular hypertrophy. *Lower tracing,* Six months postcommissurotomy, the signs of right ventricular hypertrophy have regressed.

Subvalvar Stenosis

It is also very rare to have dominant subvalvar stenosis without leaflet involvement and commissural fusion, except in patients who have had a commissurotomy. Surgeons have not always accurately assessed the subvalvar mechanism during closed commissurotomy. Many such patients have severe functional stenosis from the fusing of chordae. Because a "watering-can" effect results, and there is not a single jet of blood with a rapid velocity of flow, a mid-diastolic murmur may be inaudible.

THE ELECTROCARDIOGRAM IN MITRAL STENOSIS

Left atrial enlargement can usually be detected when the patient is in sinus rhythm. When pulmonary arterial hypertension develops, left atrial enlargement may be less obvious. The mean frontal plane QRS axis usually moves to the right. If the pulmonary hypertension is marked, there may be definite evidence of right ventricular hypertrophy with clockwise rotation and dominant R waves in the right chest leads, usually V_1 and V_{4R} (Fig. 5-15, *upper tracing*). Frequently, evidence of right ventricular hypertrophy will occur in lead V_{4R} only. A dominant R in that lead, even if less than 5 mm, is associated with right axis deviation in most instances. These changes regress (Fig. 5-15, *lower tracing*) when the left-sided hemodynamics normalise after surgery and associated pulmonary thromboembolic disease is absent.

Changes in the ST segment suggestive of ischemia may be recorded in the left precordial leads despite anatomically normal coronary arteries. After closed mitral commissurotomy, there may be large QRS voltages and marked ST-T wave changes in the left precordial leads. These changes have not been widely recognized and are often misinterpreted as indicating considerable left ventricular hypertrophy or is-

←_____

FIGURE 5-14. Echocardiograms (*A–C*) and contrast computed tomography scan (*D*) of the same patient as in Figure 5-13. *A, B (negative images),* 2-D long-axis views in diastole show thickened rigid mitral leaflets (AL and PL) and intra-atrial clot (C), which measured 30 mm. The left atrium (LA) is dilated. *C,* M-mode echocardiogram shows dense laminated echoes in the dilated left atrium (LA). AV = aortic valve. *D,* Thrombus is visible as a dense nonopacified shadow in the region of the left atrium.

chemic heart disease. We attribute them to the proximity of the heart to the chest wall as a result of adhesions.

RADIOLOGICAL APPEARANCES OF MITRAL STENOSIS

The principal radiological sign of mitral stenosis is left atrial enlargement. This is detected in the posteroanterior view as a double density or prominent left atrial appendage, and in the lateral view as a protrusion above the left ventricular contour. Evidence of pulmonary venous hypertension (Figs. 5-16, 5-17) should also be sought. This includes prominence of the upper lobe venous markings, Kerley B lines, interlobar effusions, interstitial edema, and frank pulmonary edema. Pulmonary hemosiderosis is occasionally detected, more commonly in male subjects. When pulmonary arterial hypertension has supervened, the right ventricle and atrium may be enlarged (Fig. 5-17). Although the main pulmonary artery segment may become prominent, vascular changes in the lung fields are inconspicuous in the absence of associated pulmonary thromboembolic disease. The radiological signs of pulmonary thromboembolic disease are readily discernible and will be discussed in Chapter 10.

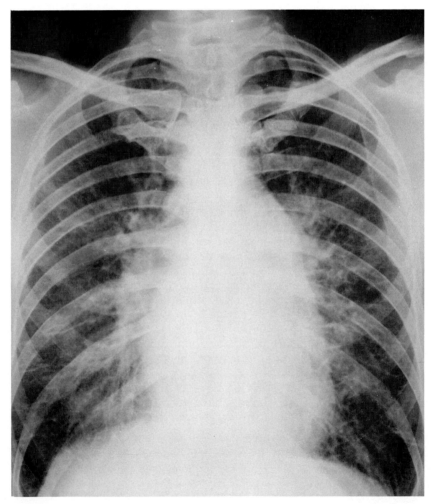

FIGURE 5-16. Posteroanterior chest radiograph of a patient with tight mitral stenosis and considerable pulmonary venous hypertension. There is interstitial pulmonary edema with Kerley B lines. The left atrium and main pulmonary artery segment are enlarged.

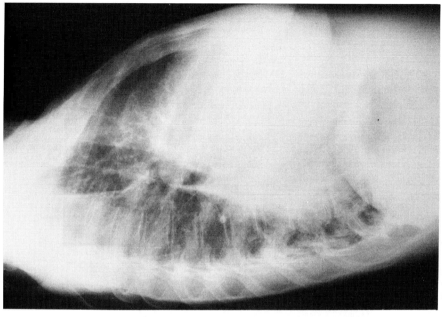

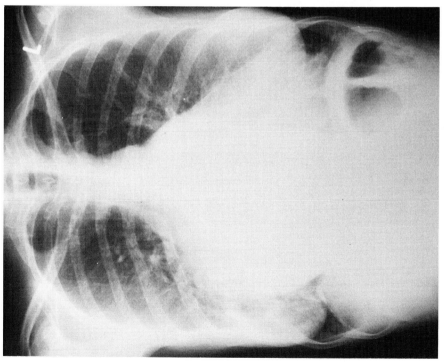

FIGURE 5-17. Posteroanterior (*A*) and lateral (*B*) chest radiographs of a 52-year-old woman with tight mitral stenosis, marked cardiac enlargement, a "giant" left atrium, and pulmonary venous hypertension. The upper lobe veins are dilated and the pulmonary artery segment is prominent. There is enlargement of the right atrium and ventricle.

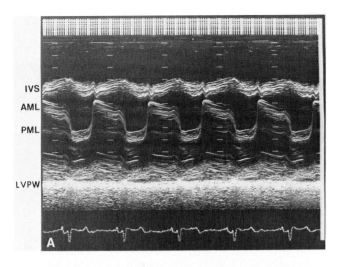

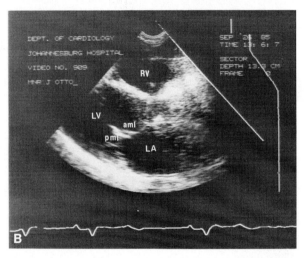

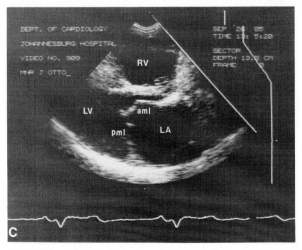

FIGURE 5-18. M-mode (*A*) and 2-D echocardiograms (*B*, systole; *C*, diastole) of a patient with tight mitral stenosis and a pliable valve. IVS = interventricular septum; AML = anterior mitral leaflet; PML = posterior mitral leaflet; LVPW = left ventricular posterior wall.

ECHOCARDIOGRAPHIC FEATURES OF MITRAL STENOSIS

Echocardiography, both M-mode and 2-D, is a highly contributory adjunct to clinical examination in the diagnosis and management of rheumatic mitral valve stenosis (Fig. 5-18). Correlation with findings at cardiac catheterization and at surgery has been good. Features on M-mode echocardiography include:

1. Prolonged and flattened E-F slope of the mitral valve
2. Loss of "A (wave) kick" on the mitral valve
3. Anterior movement of the posterior leaflet
4. Thickened valve echos
5. Left atrial enlargement
6. Features of pulmonary arterial hypertension (loss of "A (wave) kick" of pulmonary valve, reclosure movement of pulmonary leaflets during systole, right ventricular enlargement)

There are serious pitfalls in the assessment of the severity of the stenosis using M-mode echocardiography only. Conditions that decrease flow through the mitral valve, such as idiopathic pulmonary hypertension and aortic stenosis, may cause a flat E-F slope in the absence of mitral stenosis. Two-dimensional echocardiography should also be used. It has the advantage of allowing measurement of the diastolic orifice size (Fig. 5-19), and to an extent the subvalvular mechanism can be assessed.

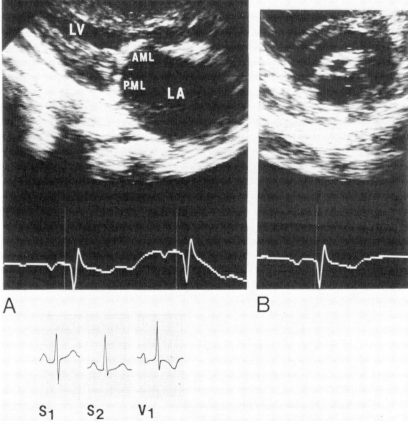

FIGURE 5-19. 2-D echocardiograms of a young woman with tight mitral stenosis and a rigid valve mechanism. *A,* Long-axis view shows thickened rigid leaflets and subvalvar chordal thickening. The left atrium (LA) is enlarged, and the left ventricular cavity (LV) is small. *B,* Short-axis view shows the small mitral valve orifice. Selected ECG complexes reflect right ventricular hypertrophy and left atrial enlargement.

In a recent double-blind study we conducted in 20 patients with mitral stenosis, we found a close correlation between the clinical assessment of tightness and pliability of the mitral valve and that found on 2-D echocardiography and at surgery.

CARDIAC CATHETERIZATION IN MITRAL STENOSIS

Although cardiac catheterization and cineangiocardiography have contributed immensely to our understanding of the hemodynamics, these investigations are seldom mandatory in the evaluation of patients with mitral stenosis. At most, we catheterize 10 percent of patients who are subjected to mitral valve surgery. The majority of these would have had other, including valvular, pathology that required clarification. Nonetheless, we also emphasize that unless correlated with clinical features and other factors, cardiac catheterization may provide misleading data in the assessment of a patient with mitral stenosis. Such factors include:

1. "Desiccation" of the patient with diuretics prior to catheterization
2. Small left atrial cavity due to intra-atrial thrombus or intramural calcified thrombus
3. Associated mitral regurgitation
4. The effects of conditions such as pulmonary thromboembolic or parenchymal disease, tricuspid regurgitation, aortic stenosis, and left ventricular dysfunction

Oft-neglected but interesting features, some of which have already been discussed, can be detected from the pressure tracings of left heart catheterization in mitral stenosis. Figure 5-20 illustrates the negative "suction" effect of the left ven-

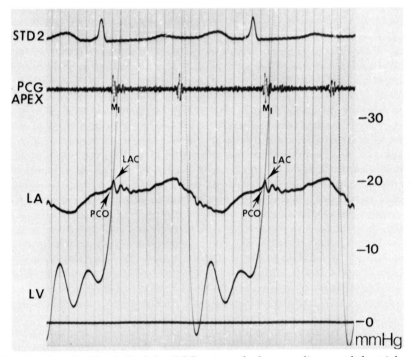

FIGURE 5-20. Standard lead II of the ECG, external phonocardiogram, left atrial, and left ventricular pressures in a patient with tight mitral stenosis. The left ventricular pressure drops below the zero point in early diastole. The patient is the same as in Figure 5-3. The Q-M1 (LAC) interval is 0.11 second. The major components of the first heart sound were reversed.

tricle, which is believed to aid diastolic filling. The different pressure configurations with varying degrees of stenosis and different PR intervals are illustrated in Figure 5-11. In patients with mobile leaflets, there is a change in the configuration of the left ventricular pressure at the peak of LAC (see Fig. 5-10). At this point, because the "slack" has been taken up in the mobile leaflet, the rate of rise of ventricular pressure is steeper.

LEFT VENTRICULAR FUNCTION IN MITRAL STENOSIS

The literature on left ventricular function in mitral stenosis has been contradictory. Some authors have found this normal, whereas others, using echocardiography, have often detected abnormalities.[8,9] We have not looked at this specific problem in a large number of patients. Nevertheless, we have encountered abnormalities of left ventricular function. These will be discussed in the following subgroups:

1. *"Double pathology" affecting the left ventricular myocardium.*
   In any Western society with a high prevalence of occlusive coronary artery disease, such as in South African Whites, there will be some patients with mitral stenosis who also have ischemic heart disease. We do not routinely perform selective coronary arteriography unless the patient has complained of angina or has electrocardiographic or other evidence to suggest myocardial ischemia. It must be remembered, however, that mild "ischemic" changes on the ECG are common in patients with tight mitral stenosis who have anatomically normal coronary arteries.
   South African Blacks have a high prevalence of idiopathic dilated cardiomyopathy and rheumatic heart disease, and it is inevitable that both conditions will sometimes occur in the same patient. In such instances, left ventricular enlargement is apparent on clinical examination, and there may be evidence of left ventricular hypertrophy on the ECG. Cardiac catheterization may show a pandiastolic gradient across the mitral valve and a raised left ventricular end-diastolic pressure. Mitral commissurotomy will improve symptoms by lowering the left atrial pressure, but the ultimate prognosis will depend on the course of the cardiomyopathy.

2. *The effects of right ventricular dilatation.*
   Right ventricular dilatation may be considerable in patients who develop tricuspid regurgitation, whether primarily organic, secondary to pulmonary hypertension, or a combination of both. This may result in compression of the left ventricle and a raised left ventricular end-diastolic pressure; but left ventricular systolic function, as assessed echocardiographically and cineangiocardiographically, appears normal. If the right ventricle remains dilated because of tricuspid regurgitation after otherwise successful mitral valve surgery, compression on the left ventricle may persist and the left ventricular end-diastolic pressure remain elevated. A "vicious cycle" ensues. This mechanism is discussed in more detail in Chapter 8, Section 2.

3. *Left ventricular dysfunction due to rheumatic carditis or mitral regurgitation.*
   Acute rheumatic carditis in a virulent form will directly and adversely affect myocardial function. Such patients may have dilated and poorly contracting left ventricles. Involvement of the mitral anulus by the carditis produces dilatation with resultant mitral regurgitation. It may be difficult or impossible to determine the relative roles of the rheumatic myocarditis and prolonged mitral regurgitation in causing the left ventricular dysfunction. Severe impairment of left ventricular systolic function persists, or more frequently becomes readily apparent, after correction of the mitral regurgitation. Although cases of acute rheumatic carditis with severe mitral regurgi-

tation will seldom survive without surgery, there must be less severe cases in which the regurgitation is moderate and surgery is not mandatory. We postulate that in some of these the mitral valve later becomes stenosed, resulting in a mixed mitral lesion or, in a few instances, pure mitral stenosis. We have encountered five adults with hemodynamically significant mitral stenosis and dilated, poorly contractile left ventricles. We suspect that these patients previously had mitral regurgitation with myocardial damage as a consequence of rheumatic carditis or of the mitral regurgitation itself and that the left ventricular dysfunction persisted after the development of mitral stenosis (Figs. 5-21, 5-22). Causally unrelated idiopathic dilated car-

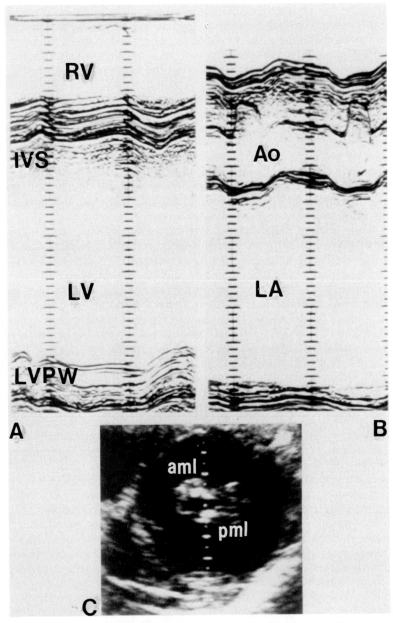

FIGURE 5-21. M-mode (*A, B*) and 2-D echocardiogram (*C*) of a 31-year-old woman with tight mitral stenosis and left ventricular dysfunction, probably on the basis of previous mitral regurgitation. *A,* Dilated, poorly contracting left ventricle. *B,* Dilated left atrial cavity. *C,* Short-axis 2-D view shows the narrowed, rigid orifice.

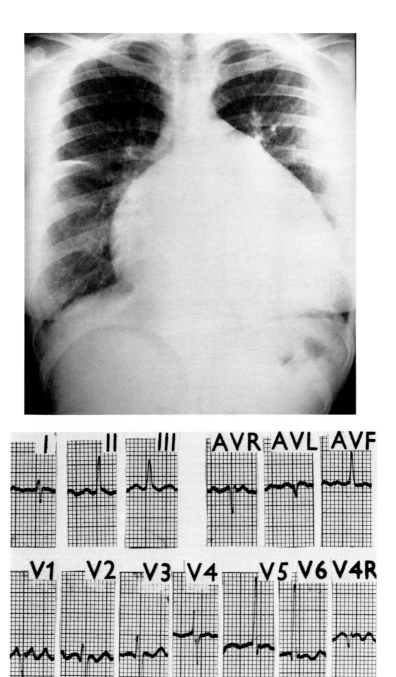

FIGURE 5-22. *A,* Posteroanterior chest radiograph of the same patient as in Figure 5-21 shows gross cardiomegaly. *B,* ECG demonstrates atrial fibrillation and no definite evidence of left ventricular hypertrophy.

diomyopathy is an unlikely explanation for their left ventricular dysfunction. Their ECGs do not suggest this, left ventricular end-diastolic pressures are normal, and only mild left ventricular hypertrophy is present on their echocardiograms. Less marked degrees of this "syndrome" may account for mild left ventricular dysfunction in other patients with mitral stenosis. The observation, which is discussed in Chapter 7, of a dilated anulus in a number of patients with pure or dominant mitral stenosis is compatible with this hypothesis.

MITRAL STENOSIS AND PREGNANCY

Pregnant women with mitral stenosis become increasingly dyspneic or may develop pulmonary edema at any time after 20 weeks' gestation. The vast majority can, and should, be treated medically at least until the fetus is viable but preferably until about 38 weeks' gestation. Patients with fairly mild or moderate stenosis respond well (as outpatients) to a diuretic and beta-receptor blocking agent taken on a daily basis. They are also given a supply of 40 mg furosemide tablets and are advised to take four to six of these should they become acutely short of breath, and then to come to the emergency room or seek other medical aid. Patients with more severe stenosis and those who have had pulmonary edema should be admitted to hospital and remain under observation until the pregnancy has reached 38 weeks. If the stenosis is very severe, cardiac surgery can be performed at that time, especially if a closed valvotomy is feasible. Even when open heart surgery is necessary, the baby usually does well. Labour is often but not invariably precipitated by the surgery. Unless the second stage is quick and easy, we expedite the delivery with forceps. Immediately after delivery we administer 40 mg or more of furosemide intravenously.

Very rarely, emergency surgery may be mandatory before the fetus is viable. A unique example, in our experience, was a woman with critically tight mitral stenosis and severe symptoms who had repeatedly refused operation prior to her pregnancy. At about 28 weeks' gestation, she was admitted with intractable pulmonary edema and hypotension. A closed valvotomy was attempted as a desperate lifesaving attempt, but the patient died.

Anticoagulation is not as crucial in pregnant women with mitral stenosis as in those with mechanical prosthetic valves. We usually prescribe 5000 units of subcutaneous heparin twice daily during the first trimester. Sodium warfarin may be used between 12 and 37 weeks' gestation. The likelihood of congenital abnormalities (nasal hypoplasia, epiphyseal stippling, optic atrophy) developing with anticoagulants of the coumarin group during the first trimester is unknown, but this risk is unjustifiable in patients with mitral stenosis. Warfarin should be stopped at 37 weeks' gestation because of the danger of hemorrhage in the fetus during labor. Heparin, which does not cross the placental barrier, is resumed until after delivery.

We have not encountered problems with beta-blocking agents in pregnancy or labour, nor have we observed serious side effects in the baby. Details of their use in patients with mitral stenosis is discussed in the subsequent section.

MEDICAL MANAGEMENT OF MITRAL STENOSIS

The principal symptom of mitral stenosis is breathlessness, which in many patients can be improved and controlled with diuretics for a number of years. Giuffrida and co-workers[10] showed that patients with mitral stenosis in sinus rhythm who were given intravenous propranolol had less of a tachycardia and consequently a smaller rise of pulmonary venous pressure during exercise than did the same patients before propranolol administration. For nearly a decade, it has been our policy to treat many patients with mitral stenosis, whether in sinus rhythm or atrial fibrillation, with a beta-receptor blocking agent. The development of right ventricular failure or significant hypotension in patients on beta blockers has seldom been a problem. We have had the most experience with propranolol, acebutolol, oxprenolol, and atenolol. Sotalol, which also has Class III antiarrhythmic effects, is also highly effective, especially in patients with supraventricular tachyarrhythmias. A disadvantage to sotalol is that it may predispose to ventricular tachycardia of the torsade de pointes variety, especially in the presence of hypokalemia. We are cautious about using beta-blocking agents in patients with right ventricular failure. There is still probably an indication for therapy with digoxin in patients with atrial fibrillation, but we seldom use this drug because of its side effects. A diuretic, usually a thiazide preparation, invariably improves the dyspnea. A more potent loop diuretic, such as furosemide, is sometimes necessary.

Although infective endocarditis is reputedly rare with pure mitral stenosis, it does occur and prophylaxis at times of risk is recommended.

Irrespective of whether the patient is in atrial fibrillation or sinus rhythm, systemic embolism is always a potential hazard. This is rare in children in the absence of infective endocarditis. Unless there is a specific contraindication or there are likely to be problems with control, we favor anticoagulation in all patients over the age of 20 years. Our problems with anticoagulant therapy are discussed in Chapter 8. In our experience, it is extremely rare for systemic embolism to occur if the anticoagulant control is good. On the other hand, it is not unusual for patients in their early twenties with tight mitral stenosis in sinus rhythm to present with a dense hemiplegia!

The timing of surgery in mitral stenosis and the types of procedure available are discussed in Chapter 8.

REFERENCES

1. WOOD, P: *Diseases of the Heart and Circulation*, ed 2. Eyre & Spottiswoode, London, 1959, pp 515–547.
2. CHESLER, E: *Schrire's Clinical Cardiology*, ed 4. John Wright & Sons, Bristol, 1981, p 15.
3. LAKIER, JB, FRITZ, VU, POCOCK, WA, AND BARLOW, JB: *Mitral components of the first heart sound*. Br Heart J 34:160–166, 1972.
4. GAMBLE, WH AND REDDY, PS: *Preservation of the third heart sound in mitral stenosis*. N Engl J Med 308:498–502, 1983.
5. CRILEY, JM, FELDMAN, IM, AND MEREDITH, T: *Mitral valve closure and the crescendo presystolic murmur*. Am J Med 51:456–465, 1971.
6. CRILEY, JM AND HERMER, AJ: *The crescendo presystolic murmur of mitral stenosis with atrial fibrillation*. N Engl J Med 285:1284–1287, 1971.
7. LAKIER, JB, POCOCK, WA, GALE, GE, AND BARLOW, JB: *Haemodynamic and sound events preceding first heart sound in mitral stenosis*. Br Heart J 34:1152–1155, 1972.
8. IBRAHIM, MM: *Left ventricular function in rheumatic mitral stenosis. Clinical echocardiographic study*. Br Heart J 42:514–520, 1979.
9. MACDONALD, IG: *Echocardiographic assessment of left ventricular function in mitral valve disease*. Circulation 53:865–871, 1976.
10. GIUFFRIDA, G, BONZANI, G, BETOCCHI, S, PISCIONE, F, GIUDICE, P, MICELI, D, MAZZA, F, AND CONDORELLI, M: *Hemodynamic response to exercise after propranolol in patients with mitral stenosis*. Am J Cardiol 44:1076–1082, 1972.

BIBLIOGRAPHY

CIESLINSKI, A, HUI, WKK, OLDERSHAW, PJ, GREGORATOS, G, AND GIBSON, D: *Interaction between systolic and diastolic time intervals in atrial fibrillation*. Br Heart J 51:431–437, 1984.
DEWAR, HA AND WEIGHTMAN, D: *A study of embolism in mitral valve disease and atrial fibrillation*. Br Heart J 49:133–140, 1983.

FLOYD, J, WILLIS, PW, AND CRAIGE, E: *The apex impulse in mitral stenosis: Graphic explanation of the palpable movements at the cardiac apex.* Am J Cardiol 51:311–314, 1983.

JOSWIG, BC, GLOVER, MU, HANDLER, JB, WARREN, SE, AND VIEWEG, WVR: *Contrasting progression of mitral stenosis in Malayans versus American-born Caucasians.* Am Heart J 104:1400–1403, 1982.

LACHMAN, AS AND ROBERTS, WC: *Calcific deposits in stenotic mitral valves. Extent and relation to age, sex, degree of stenosis, cardiac rhythm, previous commissurotomy and left atrial body thrombus from study of 164 operatively-excised valves.* Circulation 57:808–815, 1978.

LUTAS, EM, DEVEREUX, RB, BORER, JS, AND GOLDSTEIN, JE: *Echocardiographic evaluation of mitral stenosis: A critical appraisal of its clinical value in detection of severe stenosis and of valvular calcification.* J Cardiovasc Ultrason 2:131–139, 1983.

MORGAN, AA AND MOURANT, AJ: *Left vocal cord paralysis and dysphagia in mitral valve disease.* Br Heart J 43:470–473, 1980.

MOTRO, M, SCHNEEWEISS, A, LEHRER, E, RATH, S, AND NEUFELD, HN: *Correlation between cardiac catheterization and echocardiography in assessing the severity of mitral stenosis.* Int J Cardiol 1:25–34, 1981.

ROBERTS, WC, HUMPHRIES, JO, AND MORROW, AG: *Giant right atrium in rheumatic mitral stenosis. Atrial enlargement restricted by mural calcification.* Am Heart J 79:28–35, 1970.

THOMPSON, ME, SHAVER, JA, AND LEON, DF: *Effect of tachycardia on atrial transport in mitral stenosis.* Am Heart J 94:297–306, 1977.

UNVERFERTH, DV, FERTEL, RH, UNVERFERTH, BJ, AND LEIER, CV: *Atrial fibrillation in mitral stenosis: Histologic, hemodynamic and metabolic factors.* Int J Cardiol 5:143–152, 1984.

YAMAMOTO, T: *Two-dimensional echocardiographic assessment of mitral stenosis: Preoperative detection of organic change in the mitral valve apparatus.* J Cardiovasc Ultrason 2:273–283, 1983.

6

CONDITIONS INVOLVING THE MITRAL VALVE MECHANISM

SECTION 1: ANULAR CALCIFICATION

with WENDY A. POCOCK

Mitral anular calcification (Fig. 6-1) is a degenerative condition occurring mainly in older patients. It is reputedly more common in women, and most cases have associated mild mitral regurgitation. Roberts[1] emphasized the role of anular dilatation and failure of contraction as a mechanism of causation of the mitral regurgitation. Distortion of the posterior leaflet because of calcification as well as associated myxomatous mitral leaflet degeneration are other contributory factors.[2] Patients with mitral regurgitation are theoretically at risk of infective endocarditis, but we have not yet encountered such a case. Takamoto and Popp[3] demonstrated echocardiographically that conduction disturbances occur principally when the medial segment of the anulus or the anterior leaflet is involved in the calcific process. The frequent association of atrioventricular conduction disturbances with mitral anular calcification is sometimes referred to as Lev's disease.

When the calcification involves the mitral leaflets, a short mid-diastolic murmur is often heard. Rytand[4] in 1946 reported that this murmur may coincide with the varying timing of atrial systole in patients with complete atrioventricular dissociation. Hemodynamically significant mitral stenosis is uncommon but was detected by Doppler echocardiography in 8 percent of 51 patients with mitral anular calcification studied by Labovitz and colleagues.[5] Osterberger and co-workers[6] described six patients with mitral stenosis confirmed by cardiac catheterization. They considered that anular calcification alone, without significant leaflet involvement, can produce a holodiastolic mitral gradient by interfering with its normal diastolic relaxation.

Hemodynamically significant mitral stenosis due to anular calcification is extremely rare in our experience.

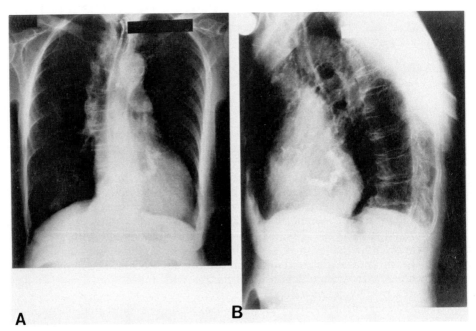

FIGURE 6-1. Posteroanterior *(A)* and left anterior oblique *(B)* chest radiographs in an elderly woman with extensive calcification of the mitral anulus. Calcification in the ascending aorta and arch of aorta is also present.

SECTION 2: SUBMITRAL LEFT VENTRICULAR ANEURYSM

with MANUEL J. ANTUNES, PINHAS SARELI, and WENDY A. POCOCK

The entity of nonischemic, submitral left ventricular aneurysms of unknown etiology is well recognized but is not mentioned in most standard textbooks. It occurs almost exclusively in Negroid peoples, particularly in Africa south of the Sahara, and has been documented mainly among Nigerians[1,2] and the Southern African Blacks.[3] Isolated instances among North American Blacks and West Indians have been reported. The aneurysms arise immediately below the posterior leaflet. Hemodynamic effects result from the diastolic overload of the aneurysm itself (Fig. 6-2A) and from interference with valve function producing mitral regurgitation (Fig. 6-2B). The myocardial blood supply may be impaired by compression and occlusion of the circumflex coronary artery, which runs in the atrioventricular groove close to the aneurysm.

CLINICAL FEATURES

Clinical features of submitral aneurysms include mitral incompetence, systemic embolism, angina pectoris, myocardial infarction, supraventricular and ventricular tachyarrhythmias, and cardiac failure. The condition may mimic rheumatic carditis or dilated cardiomyopathy, and in areas such as Southern Africa, where both are common causes of heart disease in the Blacks, the diagnosis of a submitral aneurysm may be difficult.

Mitral regurgitation is present in most patients and may be mild or extremely severe (Fig. 6-3A). The regurgitation results from dilatation or distortion of the posterior anulus, with loss of support of the posterior leaflet at its base and failure of leaflet apposition (see Fig. 6-2B). With increasing dilatation or distortion of the ring, chordae tendineae stretch or rupture with the production of a prolapsed or flail leaflet and gross mitral incompetence.

In Southern African Blacks, cardiomegaly without hemodynamically significant mitral regurgitation usually suggests the diagnosis of a dilated cardiomyopathy. The

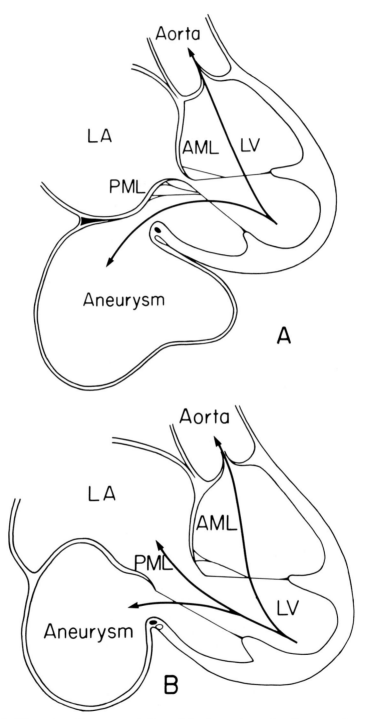

FIGURE 6-2. Diagrammatic representation of the hemodynamic effects produced by a submitral left ventricular aneurysm. For details see text.

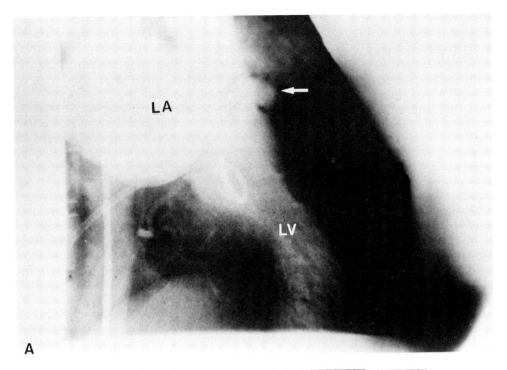

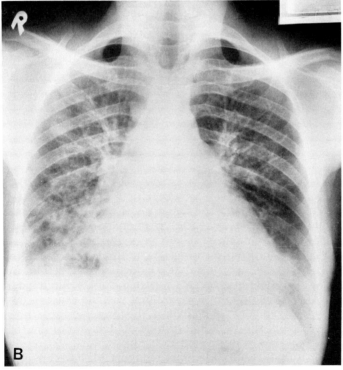

FIGURE 6-3. *A,* Left ventricular cineangiogram (RAO projection) in a 24-year-old Black woman (Case 8, Table 6-1) with a submitral aneurysm producing severe mitral regurgitation. The aneurysm *(arrow)* is small and is overshadowed by the large left atrial appendage. *B,* Posteroanterior chest radiograph showing cardiomegaly and infected pulmonary edema, most evident at the right base.

character of the left ventricular impulse is often of value in differentiating between this condition and a left ventricular aneurysm. Unlike the impulse of the dilated, poor myocardium in idiopathic cardiomyopathy, the apex beat is forceful owing to hypertrophy of a good myocardium in response to the diastolic overload produced by the aneurysm. In many cases a palpable impulse is present above the apex and along the left cardiac border. This impulse has a "double kick" and is a result of the aneurysm expanding in late systole. Because these aneurysms are posterior to the heart, the palpable double impulse is most often a referred pulsation analogous to a left atrial lift.

ETIOLOGY

The etiology of submitral ventricular aneurysms remains uncertain. Because of the predilection for the same anatomical sites and in the absence of evidence of other causes of a left ventricular aneurysm, such as atherosclerotic coronary artery diseases, syphilis, bacterial endocarditis, tuberculosis, and trauma, Abrahams and co-workers[1] suggested a congenital etiology. This postulate was supported by Chesler,[3] who stated that "a defect in the muscular fibrous junction below the intermediate portion of the left aortic cusp or the posterior leaflet of the mitral valve leads to a haematoma contained by the epicardium. Organization of this haematoma results in a fibrous walled epicardial aneurysm which may expand under the influence of the high pressure in the left ventricle." Submitral aneurysms are thus essentially false aneurysms. Evidence supporting a congenital theory is provided by the almost exclusive occurrence in Blacks; however, the occasional case among Whites has been described. An association with aneurysms of the abdominal aorta may occur, the histology of which suggests an arteritis, and a causal relationship of both of these conditions with active pulmonary tuberculosis has been postulated. If this is so, it is probably evidence supporting an "inflammatory" etiology for some of these ventricular aneurysms.

NATURAL HISTORY

Death is sometimes sudden, and the diagnosis is made only at necropsy. Sudden death may be due to an arrhythmia, acute pulmonary edema (Fig. 6-3B), or rupture of the aneurysm. In other patients, a severe work overload is produced by the aneurysm or by valvular incompetence and results in intractable cardiac failure to which associated myocardial ischemia contributes. Cockshott[2] divided his 50 patients into two groups: those in whom the aneurysm was an incidental finding during an admission for another condition, and those in whom it was the cause of the patient's presenting symptoms. Investigation of patients in the former group, who often have few or no symptoms, usually shows partial or total obliteration of the cavity by thrombus. Some of the patients who present in cardiac failure will respond to medical therapy, but they are not readily identified. Surgery in the acute phase is not indicated in such patients, and we have observed marked "spontaneous" improvement in several, presumably a result of partial or complete thrombosis in the aneurysm. Two patients previously reported[4] gave a history of a previous illness, compatible with cardiac failure, from which they had recovered. It is possible that a similar history could be obtained in other patients in whom an aneurysm has been detected as an "incidental" finding on radiological examination.

RADIOLOGICAL FEATURES

An abnormal bulge on the left border of the heart is a recognized feature of a subvalvar aneurysm (Fig. 6-4). Cockshott,[2] in his review of 50 patients encountered in Nigeria, stated that "in most cases the diagnosis is readily established by plain radiography. . . ." However, it has been our experience that an abnormal cardiac contour may be absent or may be masked by left atrial enlargement, and generalized, somewhat nonspecific cardiac enlargement is all that can be detected radiologically. In some patients, the aneurysm may be detected posterior to the cardiac silhouette in a lateral view. Calcification is a useful and very important diagnostic feature (Fig. 6-5) but will be present only if the aneurysm is not of recent origin.

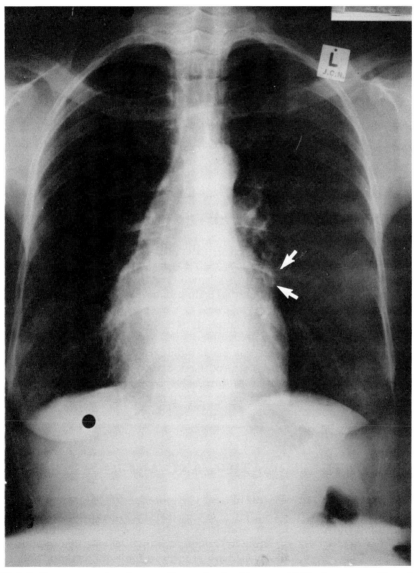

FIGURE 6-4. Posteroanterior chest radiograph of a 46-year-old Black woman (Case 2, Table 6-1) with submitral aneurysm and mild mitral regurgitation. The aneurysmal bulge (*arrows*) on the left heart border mimics the left atrial appendage.

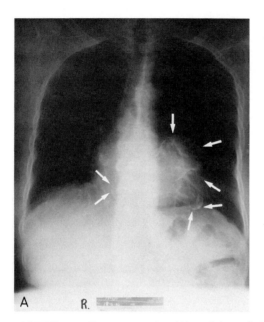 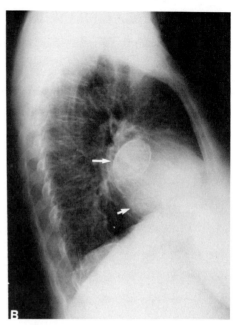

FIGURE 6-5. Posteroanterior *(A)* and lateral *(B)* chest radiographs of a 64-year-old Black woman (Case 1, Table 6-1), showing the large multiloculated calcified submitral aneurysm *(arrows)*.

ELECTROCARDIOGRAPHICAL FEATURES

Electrocardiographical evidence of left ventricular hypertrophy, out of proportion to the severity of the mitral regurgitation, may suggest the possibility of an additional hemodynamic load on the left ventricle. Low voltages, nonspecific ST-segment and T-wave changes and signs of myocardial ischemia or infarction may be encountered. A fairly common pattern is the presence of Q waves in leads I and aV_L. Electrocardiographical evidence of ischemia is often due to distortion or obstruction of the left circumflex coronary artery along its course in the atrioventricular groove. Conduction disturbances such as first-degree heart block are not uncommon and may also be related to myocardial ischemia produced by pressure on a coronary artery. Patients presenting with ventricular tachycardia or supraventricular tachycardia have also been encountered.[4] The ECG is normal in a minority of cases, and Chesler[3] found only one completely normal ECG in 15 patients with submitral aneurysms.

CARDIAC CATHETERIZATION AND ANGIOCARDIOGRAPHY

Until the advent of echocardiography and computerized tomography (CT), cardiac catheterization and angiocardiography were necessary to confirm the diagnosis, locate the origin of the aneurysm, and assess the severity of the hemodynamic disturbance. In our recent series (Table 6-1), angiography was positive in all nine cases in whom it was performed. Left ventriculography in the right anterior oblique position (Fig. 6-6) usually demonstrates the aneurysm, but multiple views may be required. Unless the diagnosis is suspected before the study is undertaken, the aneurysm may be overlooked, particularly if it is small and mitral regurgitation is present (see Fig. 6-3A). Large aneurysms are frequently loculated and may displace the car-

TABLE 6-1. Clinical Features, Diagnostic Methods, and Surgery in 12 Patients With Submitral Left Ventricular Aneurysms

CASE NUMBER	SEX	AGE (YRS)	CLINICAL NYHA	ASSESSMENT MR	CXR, Ca$^+$	ECHO-CARDIOGRAPHY	ANGIO-CARDIOGRAPHY	CT	SURGERY
1	F	64	II	–	+	–	+	+	–
2	F	46	II	+	+	–	Not done	+	–
3†	F	58	IV	+	–	–	Not done	+	Refused
4	M	31	IV	+	–	+	+	+	+**
5	F	61	IV	+	+	+	+	+	Refused
6	M	38	IV	+	–	+	+	+	+
7	M	31	IV	+	–	+	+	Not done	+
8	F	24	IV	++	–	–*	+	Not done	+
9	M	23	IV	++	–	+	Not done	Not done	+**
10	F	29	IV	++	–	+	Not done	Not done	+
11	F	35	IV	++	–	+	+	Not done	+
12	M	25	IV	++	–	+	+	+	+

+ = present; – = absent; MR = mitral regurgitation; ++ = significant mitral regurgitation; CXR, Ca$^+$ = calcification in aneurysm on chest radiograph; CT = computed tomography.

*Flail posterior leaflet

**Early mortality

†Recurrence of aneurysm two years after surgery

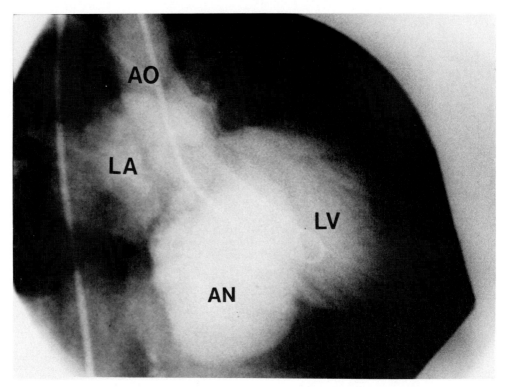

FIGURE 6-6. Left ventricular cineangiogram (right anterior oblique projection) of a 38-year-old Black man (Case 6, Table 6-1), demonstrating a large aneurysm (AN) and mitral regurgitation. There is delayed emptying of the aneurysm. LA = left atrium; AO = aorta; LV = left ventricle.

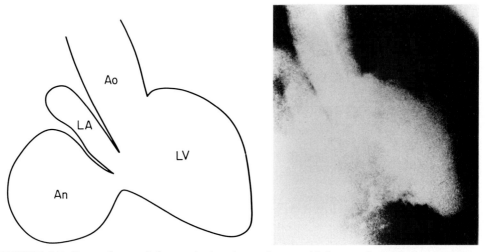

FIGURE 6-7. Frame from a left ventricular cineangiogram (right anterior oblique view) in a 56-year-old Black woman with a large submitral aneurysm (An). The left atrium (LA) is displaced superiorly and is compressed. LV = left ventricle; Ao = aorta. (From Davis et al,[5] with permission.)

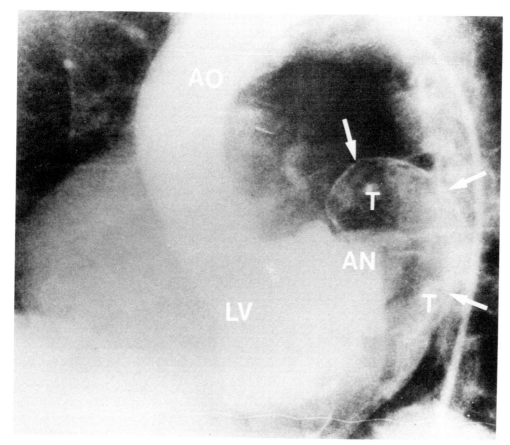

FIGURE 6-8. Left ventricular cineangiogram in the left anterior oblique projection in the patient in Table 6-1, Case 1. The large aneurysm (AN) communicates with the left ventricle (LV) but contains thrombus (T) and only opacifies partly. A thin rim of calcium (*arrow*) outlines the aneurysm.

diac shadow. In such instances, a left ventriculogram in the posteroanterior position is necessary to assess the position of the heart. In other cases, the left atrium is displaced superiorly and may be considerably compressed (Fig. 6-7). An aneurysm will only partially fill with dye, or will not fill at all, when it contains thrombus (Fig. 6-8). The catheter will enter a wide-necked aneurysm, which can be outlined by direct injection of contrast medium (Fig. 6-9).

ECHOCARDIOGRAPHIC FEATURES

In 1982, Davis and co-workers[5] from this Department studied a 56-year-old woman by 2-D echocardiography and demonstrated a submitral aneurysm as an echo-free space arising below the posterior mitral leaflet extending posteromedially and superiorly to compress the left atrial cavity (Fig. 6-10). A communication with the left ventricular cavity was seen in the region of the atrioventricular groove. We have studied 12 cases (including this patient, Case 3 in Table 6-1, who had a recurrence of the aneurysm after surgery) by 2-D echocardiography (Table 6-1). Two-dimensional echocardiography is superior to M-mode, but despite this, the aneurysm was

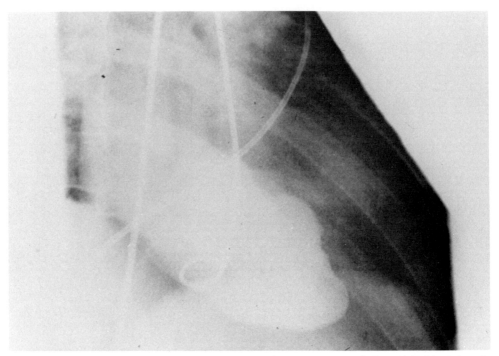

FIGURE 6-9. Direct injection into the aneurysm of contrast material; Case 7, Table 6-1, right anterior oblique view.

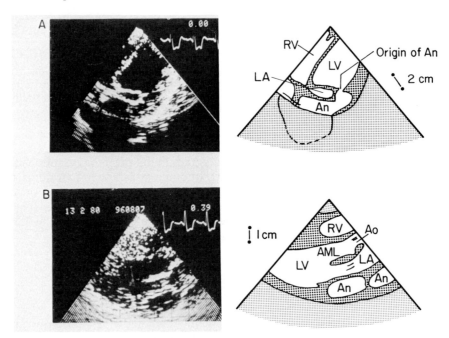

SUBMITRAL LV ANEURYSM

FIGURE 6-10. *A,* 2-D echocardiograms in the same patient as in Figure 6-7. Apical four-chamber view showing the aneurysm (An) as an echo-free space arising from the lateral aspect of the mitral valve area and extending posterosuperiorly and medially to compress the left atrium (LA). *B,* Parasternal long-axis view demonstrating the aneurysm as two echo-free spaces behind the mitral valve and left atrium. LV = left ventricle; RV = right ventricle; Ao = aorta; AML = anterior mitral leaflet. (From Davis et al,[5] with permission.)

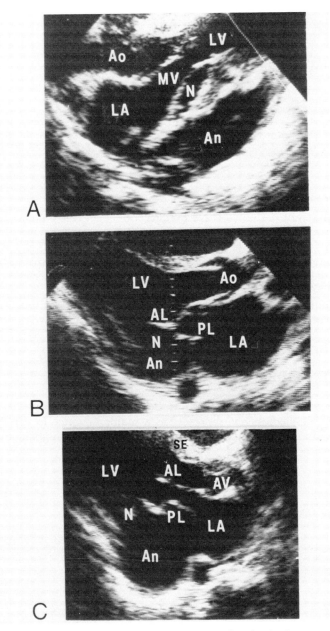

FIGURE 6-11. 2-D echocardiograms in three patients with submitral aneurysms. *A,* Case 7, Table 6-1. Modified long-axis view, diastolic frame, showing a large aneurysm (An) with the neck (N) below the mitral valve (MV). *B,* Case 9, Table 6-1. Long-axis view, systolic frame, demonstrating a shallow aneurysm with a wide neck behind the posterior mitral leaflet (PL). *C,* Case 10, Table 6-1. Long-axis view, diastolic frame, showing a large aneurysm (5 to 6 cm diameter).

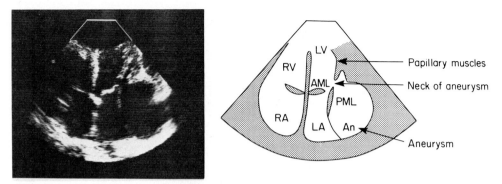

FIGURE 6-12. 2-D echocardiogram, apical four-chamber view, of the aneurysm in a 25-year-old Black man (Case 12, Table 6-1). The relationship of the aneurysm to the posterior mitral leaflet is clearly demonstrated.

detected in only eight patients (Table 6-1; Figs. 6-11, 6-12). Because of cardiac displacement and variable position of the aneurysms, unconventional views are sometimes necessary to demonstrate them. In three of the four patients in whom the aneurysm was not detected, echocardiography was technically unsatisfactory. Although the aneurysm was missed in Case 8, a flail posterior mitral leaflet was demonstrated (Fig. 6-13). A flail posterior leaflet provides important ancillary evidence of the existence of a submitral aneurysm, provided other causes such as trauma, infective endocarditis, and acute rheumatic carditis have been excluded.

COMPUTED TOMOGRAPHY (CT)

The use of CT and contrast CT in defining the position, size, presence, and extent of thrombus and calcification has represented a major advance in the diagnosis and assessment of submitral aneurysms (Figs. 6-14, 6-15). CT was positive in all seven

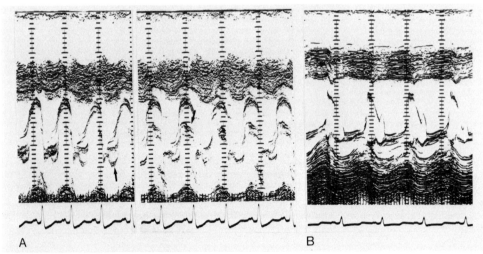

FIGURE 6-13. M-mode echocardiograms in the same patient as in Figure 6-3. *A,* Preoperatively. The posterior leaflet exhibits systolic prolapse *(bottom arrow)* and diastolic anterior movement *(top arrow)* compatible with a flail leaflet. *B,* Postoperatively. Normal movement of the mitral valve after resection of the aneurysm and valve repair.

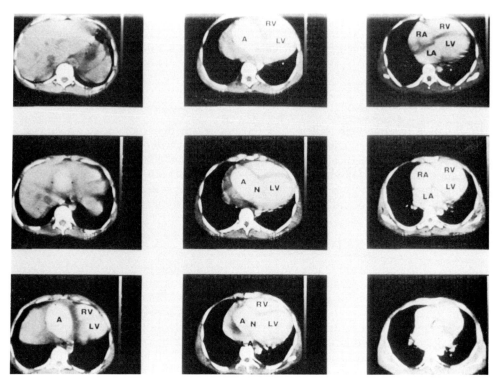

FIGURE 6-14. Consecutive computed tomography (CT) scan with injection of contrast material in a 31-year-old Black man (Case 4, Table 6-1), demonstrating the aneurysm (A) and its communication, via a wide neck (N), with the left ventricle (LV). There is extensive thrombus formation within the aneurysm.

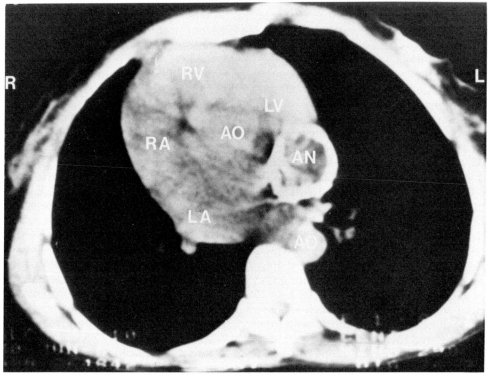

FIGURE 6-15. CT frame of Case 2, Table 6-1, showing the aneurysm (AN) surrounded by a ring of calcification. Abbreviations as in previous figures.

of our patients (Table 6-1) in whom it was performed, and the information obtained equalled or surpassed that derived from angiography. CT provides an excellent non-invasive method of investigation in suspected cases of submitral aneurysm.

MANAGEMENT

Conservative treatment is indicated if the aneurysm does not cause an excessive hemodynamic load on the left ventricle by virtue of its size or the presence of severe mitral regurgitation. Medical management comprises anticoagulation to prevent systemic embolization, prophylaxis against infective endocarditis in patients with mitral regurgitation, and antifailure therapy. In patients with severe volume overload and inadequate response to antifailure therapy, surgery is indicated.

PATHOLOGICAL ANATOMY AND SURGERY

The neck of the aneurysm is always situated beneath the posterior mitral leaflet, at any site between the anterolateral and posteromedial commissures, although it more commonly arises at the medial half of the anulus. The transverse diameter is variable, but it may replace up to two thirds of the anulus. Consequently, a large segment of the posterior leaflet is devoid of anular attachment. As the neck is circular, the vertical diameter is also large and gives a false impression of a deficiency in the left ventricular posterior wall. The unattached posterior mitral leaflet usually forms part of the roof of the aneurysm, which is contiguous with the floor of the left atrium (see Fig. 6-2). The direction of expansion of the aneurysm is extremely variable and influences the function of the mitral valve. In our experience, there is usually some protrusion into the left atrial cavity, which results in the posterior leaflet being pulled posteriorly, causing valve regurgitation (see Fig. 6-2B). Occasionally, the aneurysm may perforate into the left atrial cavity. Nevertheless, most of the aneurysmal sac lies behind the left ventricular posterior wall to which it is usually closely adherent. The cavity is often multiloculated and the different portions communicate through narrow orifices. These may be confused with the true neck of the aneurysm during surgery, if the aneurysm is approached from outside the heart.

For this reason, we favor an approach through the left atrium. This approach has the added advantage of providing a good exposure of the mitral valve, which is then amenable to valvuloplasty. If required, the procedure is performed under cardiopulmonary bypass. After entering the left atrium, the position of the neck of the aneurysm relative to the posterior anulus is identified by partially everting the free edge of the leaflet. A curved incision is then made in the floor of the left atrium parallel to the posterior anulus, about 2.5 cm from the free edge of the leaflet (Fig. 6-16). The aneurysm is thus entered through its roof, immediately above the neck, which can then be clearly visualized (Fig. 6-16). As there is no tissue deficiency, a direct closure of the neck is carried out. Occasionally, a redundant posterior leaflet may require quadrangular resection, using the technique described in Chapter 8, Section 1. In these cases, the repair is consolidated by the implantation of a Carpentier ring, which also helps to reshape the anulus. Finally, the continuity of the floor of the left atrium is re-established by suturing the two edges of the mitral incision, after excision of abnormal tissue forming part of the wall of the aneurysm. The remainder of the aneurysm is left as a blind sac, but large amounts of thrombus are removed prior to closure. This approach was used in the last six patients operated on (Table 6-1), all of whom had mitral regurgitation. The mitral valve could be preserved in all cases and there were no operative deaths related to the repair. One patient (Case 4, Table 6-1) died on the operating table of technical complications related to a different approach to the resection of the aneurysm. The other death (Case 9, Table 6-1) was due to uncontrollable hemorrhage from multiple adhesions.

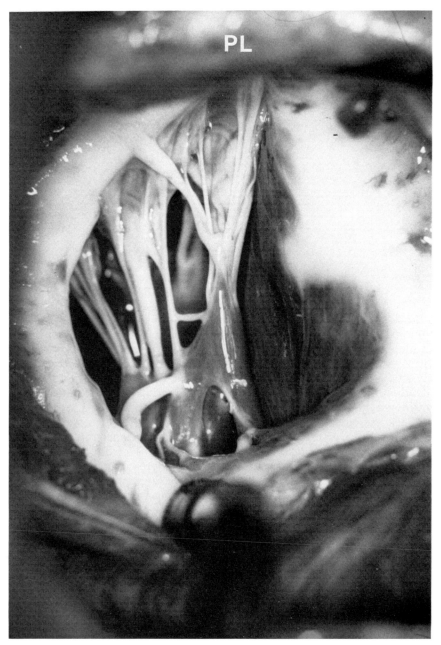

FIGURE 6-16. Intraoperative photograph through the fibrosed neck of an aneurysm, shown here as the whitish circular structure. The chordae tendineae of the posterior leaflet (PL) and its papillary muscle attachments are visible on the inner aspect of the left ventricle.

SECTION 3: HYPERTROPHIC CARDIOMYOPATHY

with WENDY A. POCOCK

Since Brock's report[1] in 1957 of "acquired aortic subvalvular stenosis" and Teare's description[2] in 1958 of the pathology of "asymmetrical hypertrophy of the heart in young adults," hypertrophic cardiomyopathy (HCM) has aroused considerable interest. HCM is not uncommon among Whites in South Africa, and by 1970 we had already studied at least 120 cases. Although four Black patients had been reported from Durban in 1973,[3] until 1982 we had not identified a Black case of HCM, and we considered the condition to be extremely rare in the South African Black. In 1983, seven Black patients with HCM, encountered during a 14-month period, were reported from this Department[4] and since then, we have encountered the condition in several others. We are uncertain whether the diagnosis was previously missed by us, whether for unknown reasons it is becoming more common in that population group, or whether the widespread use of echocardiography has enabled the diagnosis to be more easily suspected by general physicians who then refer patients to us.

In HCM there is inappropriate and sometimes considerable hypertrophy of the ventricular myocardium, predominantly affecting the left ventricle. The excessive left ventricular hypertrophy has two principal consequences: (1) ventricular relaxation and compliance are abnormal, diastolic ventricular stiffness is increased, ventricular filling is impaired and the end-diastolic pressure may be elevated; (2) myocardial contraction is more forceful, and the distorted left ventricular cavity may produce an intraventricular pressure difference during systole. The disease is often familial, inherited as a Mendelian dominant gene with variable penetrance. The symptoms of HCM include angina pectoris (due to increased myocardial oxygen demand and a diminished diastolic coronary perfusion gradient), dyspnea (the clinical manifestation of the raised left ventricular end-diastolic and left atrial pressures), and syncope (probably mainly due to arrhythmias but aggravated by the small left ventricular cavity size that limits the stroke output). Palpitations and undue fatigue are common complaints. Sudden death may supervene, especially during exercise or with emotion. Patients, including some with advanced disease, may be asymptomatic.

The pathogenesis of the inappropriate left ventricular hypertrophy is unknown. There may be an inherited malformation of muscle in different parts of the myocardium with fiber malalignment, resulting in abnormal ventricular stresses and excessive hypertrophy.[5] The distribution of the abnormal regions determines the precise geometry of the left ventricular cavity in a particular patient. When there is marked septal hypertrophy, the so-called obstructive form of the disease usually results. In most patients this "obstruction" (as seen on angiography or echocardiography) is subvalvar, but in a few instances it is midventricular (hour-glass type). Hypertrophy

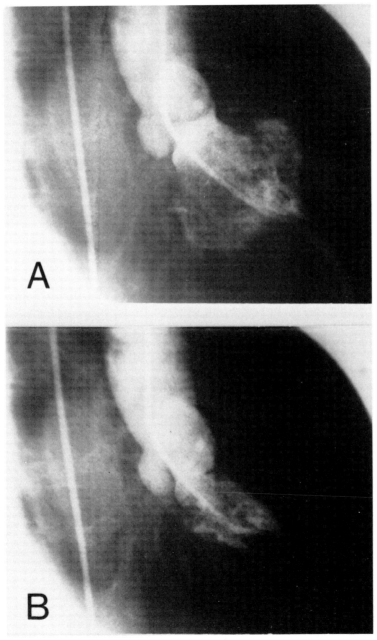

FIGURE 6-17. Left ventricular cineangiograms in the right anterior oblique projection in a 71-year-old woman with apical hypertrophic cardiomyopathy. The spadelike appearance in diastole *(A)* is typical of this condition. *B,* The systolic frame shows almost complete left ventricular emptying.

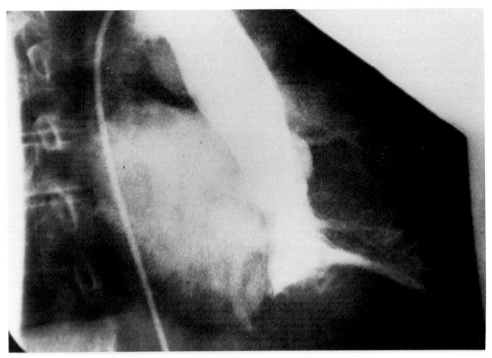

FIGURE 6-18. Left ventricular cineangiogram (right anterior oblique) demonstrates marked cavity obliteration and moderate mitral regurgitation in a patient with hypertrophic cardiomyopathy.

confined to the apical myocardium, giving a typical "spadelike" appearance on angiography (Fig. 6-17), has been emphasized by Japanese workers.[6] It has been argued, however, that the pressure difference within the left ventricular cavity does not reflect a true obstruction to ventricular emptying, but that rapid ejection during early systole and cavity obliteration (Fig. 6-18) can account for many of the homo-

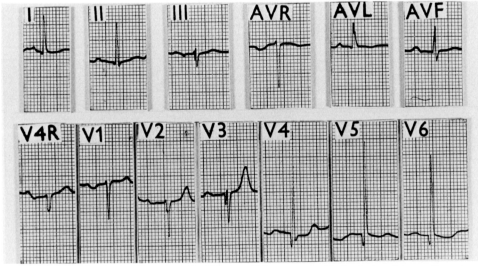

FIGURE 6-19. Electrocardiogram of a 51-year-old woman with hypertrophic cardiomyopathy, without a gradient across the left ventricular outflow tract. Prominent Q waves in V_3-V_6, left ventricular hypertrophy, left atrial enlargement, and a PR interval of 0.26 second are present.

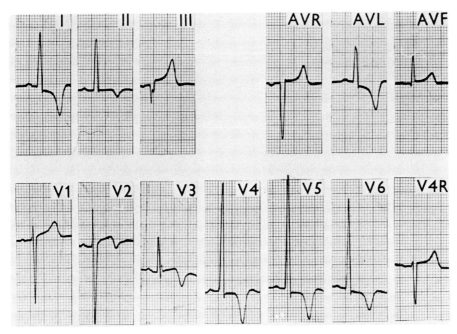

FIGURE 6-20. Giant negative T waves (10 mm in V_4) and very high QRS voltages in the precordial leads (RV5 + SV1 = 62 mm), in a 32-year-old man with apical hypertrophic cardiomyopathy. (From Steingo, L, Dansky, R, Pocock, WA, and Barlow, JB: *Apical hypertrophic non-obstructive cardiomyopathy.* Am Heart J 104:635–637, 1982, with permission.)

dynamic, echocardiographic, and angiographic features hitherto attributed to "obstruction."

The diagnosis of HCM should be suspected in any patient who has inappropriate, unexplained left ventricular hypertrophy. The arterial pulse often has a rapid upstroke, in contrast to the slow-rising pulse of aortic stenosis, since in HCM early systolic ventricular emptying is normal or increased. A second pulse wave, producing a bisferiens character, may be felt in late systole. The ECG commonly shows left ventricular hypertrophy (Fig. 6-19) but may occasionally be normal. Large septal Q waves may be present, especially in patients with excessive septal hypertrophy. Deeply inverted T waves (Fig. 6-20) are a feature of the apical form of the disease. Electrocardiographic evidence of unexplained left ventricular hypertrophy should always raise the possibility of HCM. The chest radiograph not infrequently shows only slight or even no cardiac enlargement, as assessed by the cardiothoracic ratio. However, in our experience a shelflike appearance[7] to the left heart border is characteristic of HCM (Fig. 6-21).

AUSCULTATORY FEATURES

Auscultation should remain highly important to the clinician in the diagnosis of HCM. Because of the development of echocardiography, vasoactive maneuvers that alter heart sounds and murmurs are no longer as necessary nor as frequently used. Nonetheless, these hemodynamic alterations have contributed to our understanding of HCM, and some are still useful in the clinical diagnosis of that condition. The auscultatory features of HCM, based on a study of 90 White patients, aged 5 to 62 years,[7] will be briefly described.

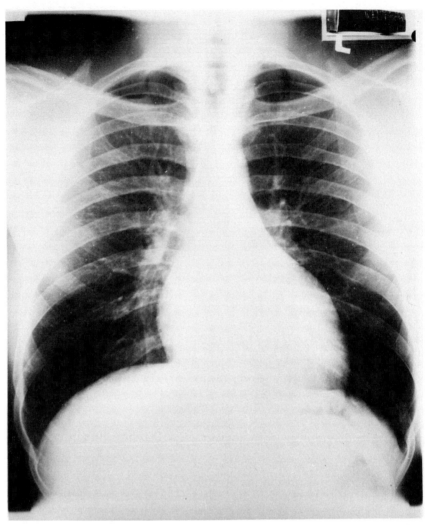

FIGURE 6-21. Posteroanterior chest radiograph of a patient with hypertrophic cardiomyopathy. The cardiothoracic ratio is 0.50, but there is a prominent shelflike appearance to the left heart border that gives the left ventricle a "bulky" appearance. (From Lewis, et al,[4] with permission.)

SYSTOLIC MURMURS

A delayed-onset crescendo-decrescendo murmur is almost invariably present in HCM, although rarely it may be absent with the patient in the supine position and only elicited by posture or vasoactive maneuvers.

The murmur is loudest at the lower left sternal border or just medial to the apex. It often has a somewhat harsh character and may resemble that of the extremely common innocent vibratory systolic murmur of childhood. In some instances, the murmur is high pitched and musical. The intensity often varies spontaneously from beat to beat, with respiration, or on different days of examination. The configuration, and thus the cadence, of the systolic murmur in 50 patients is represented diagrammatically in Figure 6-22. In all cases the onset of the murmur was delayed, and peak accentuation occurred at or near mid-systole.

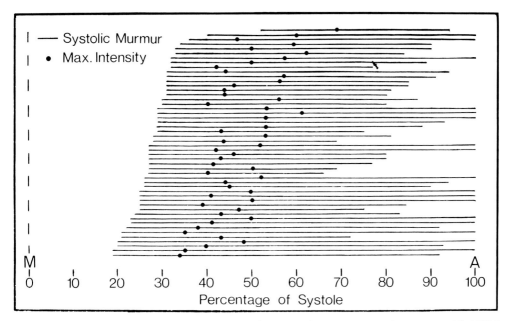

FIGURE 6-22. Diagrammatic representation of the systolic murmur in 50 patients with HCM showing the time of onset, maximal intensity, and end of each murmur, expressed as a percentage of the MA interval. M = mitral valve closure; A = aortic valve closure. (From Tucker et al,[7] with permission.)

Late vibrations extending to the aortic component of the second heart sound are usually indicative of mild mitral regurgitation. Changes in intensity of the ejection murmur in patients subjected to postural variation, amyl nitrite inhalation, and vasopressor drugs are represented in Figure 6-23. Figure 6-24 illustrates the diagnostic behavior of the ejection murmur in response to the Valsalva maneuver: during

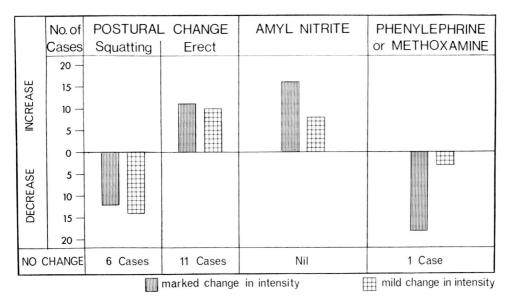

FIGURE 6-23. Histogram showing the effect on the intensity of the systolic murmur of postural change, amyl nitrite inhalation, and vasopressor drugs. The case in which there was no change after phenylephrine administration (2 mg) had a gradient of 120 mm Hg that was only reduced to 60 mm. An additional 2 mg produced equalization of left ventricular and aortic pressures, and the murmur disappeared. (From Tucker et al,[7] with permission.)

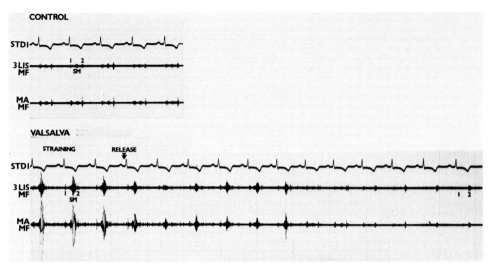

FIGURE 6-24. Phonocardiogram showing the diagnostic response of the systolic murmur (SM) of HCM during and after Valsalva maneuver. The SM is considerably louder compared to "control" during the last four cycles in the straining phase, becomes much softer, and then disappears in the late postrelease phase. (From Tucker et al,[7] with permission.)

the straining phase, there is an increase in intensity and a decrease several seconds after release. In some patients the response is that of any systolic murmur arising from the left side of the heart, in that the murmur softens during the straining phase and has a delayed return to its former intensity after release of straining. The response to the Valsalva maneuver is not infrequently equivocal.

The variable intensity of the systolic murmur at rest and with vasoactive maneuvers depends on changes in left ventricular contractility, peripheral resistance, and left ventricular end-diastolic volume. These effects of hemodynamic alterations on the systolic murmur are useful both for its clinical recognition and for distinguishing it from other murmurs with which it may be confused. In general, the murmur increases in intensity with diminished venous return, and thus decreased end-diastolic ventricular volume, or when myocardial contraction is more forceful, whereas it becomes softer if venous return and end-diastolic volume are increased and when myocardial contractility is depressed. An increased intensity can therefore be anticipated with amyl nitrite inhalation, venesection, exercise, adoption of the erect posture, and after the administration of inotropic drugs such as digoxin or isoprenaline. On the other hand, the murmur will become softer after increasing intravascular volume or after depression of myocardial contractility with beta-receptor blocking agents. It has also been observed that vasoconstrictor agents such as methoxamine and phenylephrine decrease the outflow gradient and hence soften the systolic murmur. A similar mechanism applies to squatting, but this procedure also increases venous return, so presumably both these hemodynamic changes contribute to the diminished intensity or disappearance of the murmur. In patients with severe outflow pressure differences, the response to postural and vasoactive maneuvers may be unimpressive or variable. The enhanced myocardial contractility after an ectopic beat is apparently more important than the relative overfilling of the ventricle, because the outflow gradient and the intensity of the murmur invariably increase under those circumstances. Apparent phonocardiographic confirmation of this enhanced left ventricular outflow "obstruction" during a postectopic beat, with prolongation and increased intensity of the murmur and marked reversed splitting of the second heart sound, is shown in Figure 6-25. However, Siegel and Criley[8] recently showed that left ventricular emptying was more rapid and complete during

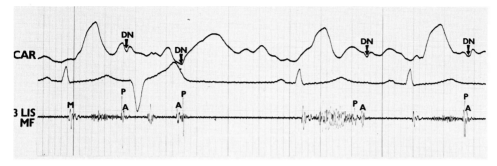

FIGURE 6-25. In the first and last cycles P (pulmonary valve closure) and A (aortic valve closure) are nearly synchronous. With the postectopic beat there is considerable increased intensity of the systolic murmur and A follows P by 0.05 second. DN marks the dicrotic notch on the indirect carotid arterial pulse tracing (CAR). (From Tucker et al,[7] with permission.)

a postectopic beat in which a gradient of at least 110 mmHg was present. Aortic valve closure and mitral valve opening were delayed despite the fact that the ventricle achieved a greater degree of emptying earlier in systole. They postulated that a more prolonged state of contraction or a reduced rate of relaxation or both are responsible for the prolonged left ventricular emptying time in patients with a pressure gradient.

It is widely accepted that HCM comprises patients with and without outflow gradients, sometimes among members of the same family. Systolic murmurs are often absent when there is no outflow pressure difference, or become softer and disappear when such pressure difference is decreased or abolished. Softening and disappearance of the murmur over time usually accompany progression of the disease and may herald sudden death.

Left ventricular cineangiography demonstrates that late systolic vibrations of the apical murmur are associated with mitral regurgitation and has shown that the regurgitation commences in mid-systole. The regurgitation is mild to moderate in degree (see Fig. 6-18), and we have not encountered patients with HCM who have mitral incompetence as a dominant feature. It is probable that mitral regurgitation is present in most patients with HCM in whom there is a significant left ventricular outflow pressure difference. The mechanism of the mitral regurgitation in HCM is probably related to abnormal traction of the hypertrophied papillary muscles on the chordae tendineae and valve leaflets.

SECOND HEART SOUND

The splitting of the second heart sound often appears abnormally narrow or reversed on clinical auscultation. The pattern of the splitting can change spontaneously, sometimes within seconds, without apparent cause. An analysis of the positions of the aortic (A) and pulmonary (P) components during natural respiration in 77 patients on whom phonocardiograms were performed, reveals five main patterns (Fig. 6-26):

Wide. P follows A by at least 0.02 second on expiration, and this interval increases to more than 0.05 second on inspiration.

Normal. Twenty-eight patients had normal splitting, in that the components merged or were no more than 0.01 second apart in expiration but were separated by 0.03 to 0.05 second during inspiration.

Narrow. Twenty-six patients had unusually narrow splitting; in these the second sound was "single" in expiration, and P followed A by not more than 0.02 second on inspiration.

	EXPIRATION	INSPIRATION	Number of Cases	
			Group A	Group B
1. Wide	M · · AP	M · A P	3	0
2. Normal	· AP	· A P	17	11
3. Narrow	· PA	· A P	19	7
4. Partially Reversed	· PA	· A P	11	1
5. Reversed	· P A	· AP	8	0

FIGURE 6-26. Diagrammatic representation of the five patterns of splitting of the second sound in HCM. Patients in Group A were referred for assessment of cardiac status, and Group B comprises subjects whose conditions were detected through examination of close relatives of individuals in Group A. (From Tucker et al,[7] with permission.)

Partially reversed. This is a stage just short of the last category in which P precedes the slightly delayed A in expiration but follows it on inspiration. The splitting of the second sound is therefore "partially reversed." Partially reversed splitting was confirmed during cardiac catheterization in some patients by recording simultaneous aortic and pulmonary artery pressures (Fig. 6-27).

Reversed. Eight patients had reversed splitting of the second sound.

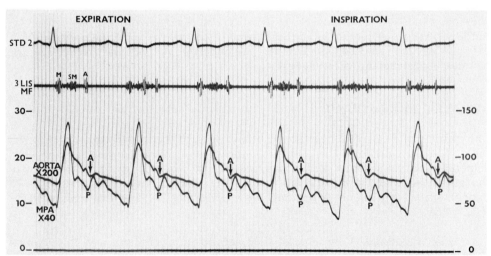

FIGURE 6-27. Simultaneous standard lead II ECG, external phonocardiogram, and aortic and main pulmonary artery (MPA) pressure tracings of an adult man with HCM. MPA pressure scale is on the left; vertical axis in millimetres of mercury; and P marks the dicrotic notch on the MPA pressure tracing. Similarly, the aortic scale is on the right vertical axis and A arrows the aortic dicrotic notch. The phonocardiogram is technically poor, but the principle of partially reversed splitting is clearly demonstrated from the pressure tracings in that P precedes A during expiration but A precedes P during inspiration. (From Tucker et al,[7] with permission.)

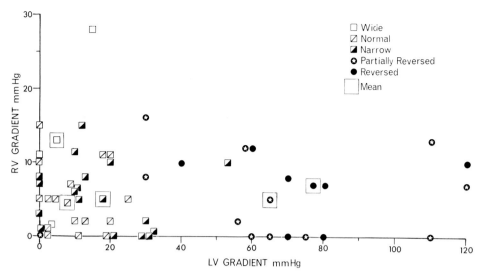

FIGURE 6-28. Correlation between the ventricular systolic pressure differences and the pattern of splitting of the second heart sound in 54 patients with HCM. Most patients with significant left ventricular (LV) outflow gradients had reversed or partially reversed splitting. (From Tucker et al,[7] with permission.)

It is well known that the ejection times of the right and left ventricles are prolonged in pulmonary and aortic stenosis, respectively, with consequent delay in closure of the relevant semilunar valves. Apparent prolongation of left ventricular ejection time in HCM has been correlated with the intraventricular systolic pressure difference. Since systolic pressure gradients may be recorded on either side of the heart, we tried to determine whether the pattern of splitting the second heart sound would correlate with these.[7] Fifty-four patients had both right and left heart catheterization and, although the phonocardiographic measurements and the intraventricular systolic pressure differences were not recorded simultaneously, some correlation was shown (Fig. 6-28). All but one of the 18 patients with reversed or partially reversed splitting had a left ventricular systolic pressure difference greater than 30 mmHg, whereas patients with narrow or normal splitting generally had small pressure differences. The largest right ventricular systolic pressure difference in our series was 26 mmHg, and this 9-year-old girl was one of the three patients with wide splitting.

FIRST HEART SOUND

The first heart sound is unremarkable in HCM, but there may be prolongation of the Q-M1 interval when measured phonocardiographically.

SYSTOLIC CLICKS

Both ejection and nonejection systolic clicks have been heard and recorded in HCM, but these are not common. The two patients with ejection clicks in Tucker's series[7] both had moderate dilatation of the ascending aorta and one had mild aortic regurgitation. Nonejection systolic clicks in HCM almost certainly arise from the mitral valve mechanism. The asymmetrical myocardial hypertrophy could well result in inequality of functional length of some chordae tendineae and thus partial billowing of the mitral leaflets. The clicks may be variable in timing and not a constant feature.

THIRD AND FOURTH HEART SOUNDS

These diastolic sounds are common in HCM and are usually left sided. Reduced compliance of the hypertrophied ventricle is probably relevant to their mechanism of production.

MID-DIASTOLIC MURMURS

Short mid-diastolic murmurs, both left- and right-sided, are a recognized feature of HCM. Cohen and associates[9] reported a 52 percent prevalence of a mitral mid-diastolic murmur in their study of HCM patients. Mid-diastolic murmurs may result from distortion of the atrioventricular valves by the asymmetrically hypertrophied myocardium or from inflow into the ventricles across hypertrophied muscle bundles. Associated disease of the mitral valve mechanism, notably anular calcification, could produce a mid-diastolic murmur in other cases.

EARLY DIASTOLIC MURMURS

Although coexistent and causally unrelated aortic leaflet disease must occur with HCM, we believe that aortic anular distortion due to asymmetrical myocardial hypertrophy causes aortic regurgitation in a few instances. The murmurs are soft and short, and the regurgitation is minimal.

ECHOCARDIOGRAPHIC FEATURES

Echocardiographic features may be diagnostic of HCM and, when unequivocal, obviate the need for cardiac catheterization in some patients. The echocardiogram, especially the real-time 2-D echocardiogram, shows the distribution and degree of left ventricular hypertrophy (Fig. 6-29), the forceful contraction of the left ventricle with cavity obliteration, and the systolic anterior motion of the mitral valve (Figs. 6-30, 6-31A), which occurs in some patients and is attributed to asymmetrical tension on the mitral apparatus by the distorted left ventricular geometry. Goodwin[10] considers that the systolic anterior movement is due to meeting the hypertrophied septum and the papillary muscles, rather than the mitral leaflet. Mid-systolic fluttering and closure of the aortic leaflets (Figs. 6-31B, and 6-32) are usually associated with a significant intraventricular pressure gradient.

ETIOLOGY

The cause of HCM is unknown, and the possible role of factors such as catecholamines remains to be clarified.[10] "Inappropriate" hypertrophy to a longstanding overload of the left ventricle may be a factor in some instances. Asymmetrical septal hypertrophy in some patients with aortic stenosis was regarded as an "adaptive mechanism" by Hess and co-workers.[11] An association between systemic hypertension and HCM is known and has recently been emphasized by Topol and colleagues.[12] It remains possible that HCM supervenes in a few cases of highly trained athletes.[13,14] Whether or not left ventricular hypertrophy is demonstrated echocardiographically to be asymmetrical, the interpretation of this finding should at present remain guarded. Shapiro and McKenna[15] emphasized the technical limitations of M-mode echocardiography in the assessment of left ventricular hypertrophy.

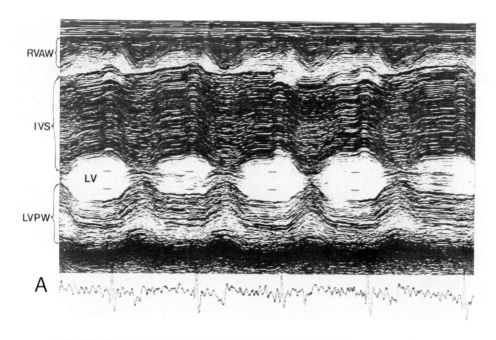

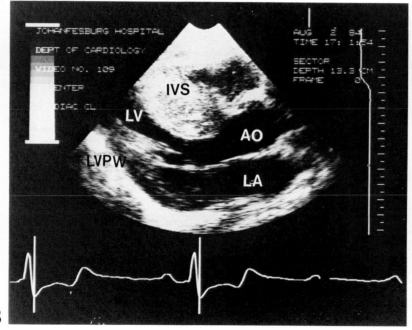

FIGURE 6-29. HCM in a 23-year-old man. *A*, M-mode echocardiogram of the left ventricle shows a markedly hypertrophied (50 mm) interventricular septum (IVS). The left ventricular posterior wall (LVPW) measures 30 mm, giving a ratio of 1.6:1. *B*, 2-D echocardiogram, long-axis view, confirms the thickened septum (IVS).

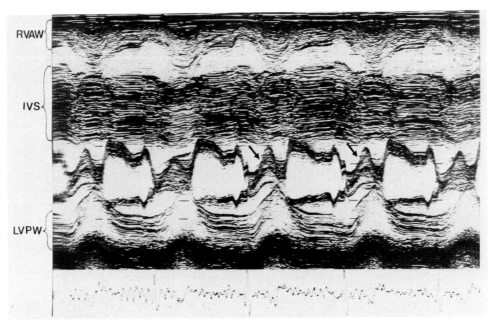

FIGURE 6-30. M-mode echocardiogram of the same patient as in Figure 6-29. Recording of mitral valve to show systolic anterior motion *(arrow)* of the anterior mitral leaflet.

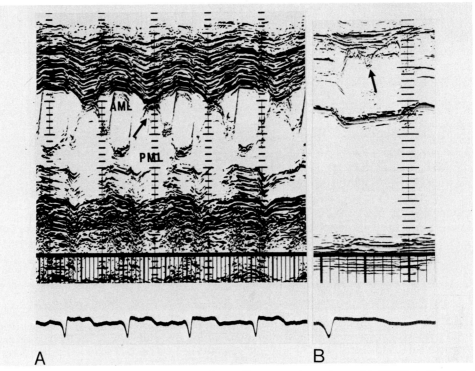

FIGURE 6-31. M-mode *(A)* and 2-D *(B)* echocardiograms of a patient with HCM. *A*, Recording of the mitral valve demonstrates systolic anterior motion (SAM) *(arrows)*. There is a reduced EF slope of the AML during diastole, with normal PML motion. *B*, Recording of the aorta shows premature aortic valve closure *(arrow)*.

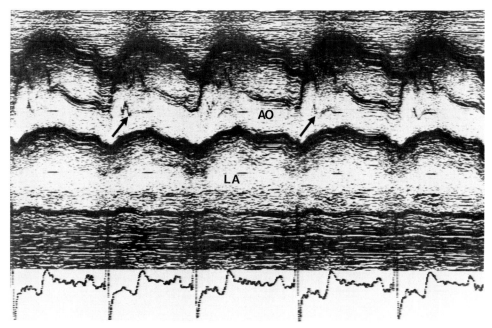

FIGURE 6-32. M-mode echocardiogram of the aortic valve in the same patient as in Figures 6-29 and 6-30. Mid-systolic closure of the aortic valve *(arrows)* is shown.

MANAGEMENT

The medical management of patients with HCM is aimed at decreasing left ventricular contractility and increasing ventricular compliance and cavity size. Beta-receptor blockade improves the hemodynamic state and is often effective in the treatment of symptoms. Through the use of large doses of propranolol in conjunction with antiarrhythmic drugs and pacemakers, Canedo and Frank[16] claimed to reduce the overall mortality rate of patients with HCM to 0.5 percent per year. The calcium antagonist verapamil also improves symptoms in some patients and, according to the observations of Kaltenbach and co-workers[17], may decrease left ventricular hypertrophy after long-term use. Since even asymptomatic patients are at risk of sudden death, all patients with HCM should undergo regular Holter monitoring in order to detect and treat potentially life-threatening arrhythmias. In 1982, Goodwin[10] expressed the strong opinion that amiodarone was the most effective antiarrhythmic drug for the management of HCM when premature ventricular extrasystoles or runs of ventricular tachycardia were detected on ambulatory monitoring. He suggested a starting dosage of 600 mg daily for one week, followed by 400 mg daily. Goodwin stated that amiodarone alone may improve dyspnea and angina but, if not, propranolol or other nonselective beta-blocking agents should be added with caution. Because of its associated Class III antiarrhythmic properties, we consider that the beta-receptor blocking agent sotalol should have a role in the treatment of some cases with HCM, and this possibility requires investigation.

In patients with large intracavitary gradients, surgical intervention (extensive left ventricular myectomy) may be indicated. Although good results have been reported, it is not established whether this alters the long-term prognosis of the disease. We have no experience of severe mitral regurgitation in HCM which in Goodwin's[10] experience occurs in "up to 5 percent of cases as a result of calcification, turbulence, or infection." We also have no experience of mitral valve replacement in order to relieve "outflow obstruction" as advocated by Cooley and colleagues.[18]

SECTION 4: ATRIAL MYXOMA

with WENDY A. POCOCK

It is always important to make a precise diagnosis in any patient with suspected heart disease but never more so than in the case of atrial myxoma. Atrial myxoma is the most common primary cardiac tumour, and the condition is invariably fatal unless surgically treated. Although most patients undergoing surgery for ischemic heart disease, valvular heart disease, and many forms of congenital heart disease can anticipate clinical improvement, the operation is usually palliative; whereas surgical removal of an atrial myxoma is curative. In patients of any age "heart failure" is never a diagnosis but merely a reflection of a state of cardiac function. The appropriate medical therapy will often vary and be influenced by the nature of the underlying heart disease. In atrial myxoma, the only meaningful treatment is surgical removal.

Before the advent of echocardiography, the clinical diagnosis was difficult, and many cases were diagnosed only by pathologists or at cardiac surgery. Constant awareness of the possibility of an atrial myxoma in any patient with an unusual presentation of heart disease was mandatory. Echocardiography, whether M-mode or 2-D, is now the easiest and most conclusive method of diagnosis. We encounter one or two cases of atrial myxoma each year. Because we have a high prevalence of rheumatic valve disease and echocardiography is readily available, many cases are now diagnosed by that investigation without having been suspected after a relatively cursory clinical examination. Echocardiography is frequently done because of recognition of unusual features in cases of "mitral valve disease." Because echocardiography is not yet readily available to all practising clinicians, it remains relevant to review briefly the clinical presentation of atrial myxoma.

CLINICAL FEATURES

Atrial myxoma has been described at all ages, and even in infants, but is most common in middle age. It is more prevalent in women and at least 80 percent are left-sided. The tumours usually arise adjacent to the foramen ovale. Following are certain features common to both left and right atrial myxoma that are of diagnostic importance.

FEATURES DEPENDENT ON INTERMITTENT OBSTRUCTION OF THE MITRAL OR TRICUSPID VALVE ORIFICE

Brief periods of complete obstruction of an atrioventricular valve, occasionally initiated by a postural change, may result in sudden breathlessness, syncope, convulsions, angina, cyanosis, and changing cardiac murmurs. Sudden death, which is not uncommon among advanced myxoma patients, probably is usually due to complete atrioventricular valve obstruction and may occasionally occur without preceding symptoms. Cardiac arrhythmias are rare, and most patients remain in sinus rhythm.

INFECTIVE ENDOCARDITIS SYNDROME

Many patients with myxoma present with anemia, intermittent pyrexia, clubbing, weight loss, increased serum globulin levels, thrombocytopenia, a raised sedimentation rate, and varying cardiac murmurs—a syndrome that mimics infective endocarditis. Blood cultures are negative. An immunologic response to the tumour tissue may be the basis for these constitutional signs, which invariably disappear after surgical removal.

Systemic emboli, sometimes causing transient or permanent neurological signs, have frequently been encountered in left atrial myxoma patients. Multiple arterial aneurysms may be the result of tumour emboli or of an autoimmune arteritis.[1] In rare instances, infection of the myxoma may occur. One such patient died after rupture of a cerebral mycotic aneurysm.[2] A systemic embolus should always raise the possibility of a left atrial myxoma. Prior to the advent of echocardiography, the occurrence of a systemic embolus created a major diagnostic problem when examination of the heart revealed no abnormality. Although a left atrial myxoma is usually large when symptoms and signs are present, the possibility of a small, completely "silent" myxoma being responsible for the systemic embolus was always present. Angiocardiography was sometimes necessary to exclude the diagnosis but has now been superseded by echocardiography. The presence of pulmonary emboli in patients with myxoma of the right atrium has also been observed.

SHORT, INTRACTABLE CLINICAL COURSE

A relatively short course, often less than two years from the onset of symptoms, with a poor response to diuretic and other medical therapy, occurs in a majority of cases. Occasionally, the course is much longer, and we have encountered two patients in whom symptoms exceeded 10 years. Intractable congestive cardiac failure with gross peripheral edema supervenes in patients with left atrial myxoma who do not die suddenly. Edema is less common when the right atrium is involved.

RADIOLOGICAL FEATURES

Radiological evidence of cardiomegaly may be absent or not as great as would be expected from the clinical state of the patient. Some left atrial enlargement (Fig. 6-33) may be detected in left atrial myxoma cases, although this is by no means invariable. Evidence of pulmonary venous hypertension such as dilated pulmonary veins

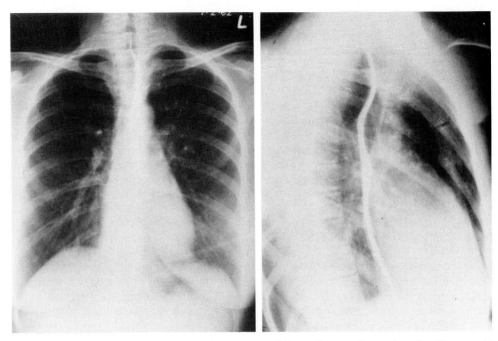

FIGURE 6-33. Posteroanterior and right anterior oblique chest radiographs of a 32-year-old woman who presented with a dense hemiplegia. The only clinical evidence of the left atrial myxoma, which was small, was a very short mid-diastolic murmur. Minimal enlargement of the left atrium is shown.

may be present, and Kerley B lines and "'miliary mottling" may result from pulmonary edema (Fig. 6-34). Dilated veins or pulmonary edema may be more pronounced unilaterally or unequally distributed in either lung field. Right atrial myxoma cases may show a dilated right atrium and some undervascularization of the lung fields (Fig. 6-35). Myxomata seldom calcify, but when this does occur they appear as large masses that on x-ray screening can be seen to swing back and forth during the cardiac cycle.

THE ELECTROCARDIOGRAM

Although P wave enlargement may be present, it is often slight and incompatible with the apparently severe "mitral or tricuspid stenosis" suggested by the clinical state. QRS voltages are usually small, especially in cases of right atrial myxoma. ST-segment depression and flattened T waves are somewhat nonspecific but may be suggestive of myocardial ischemia. There is seldom evidence of significant ventricular hypertrophy, and this feature is not in accord with the clinical state. Coronary embolism in cases of left atrial myxoma causes classic electrocardiographic features of myocardial infarction.

DIFFERENTIAL DIAGNOSES OF LEFT ATRIAL MYXOMA

MITRAL STENOSIS AND INCOMPETENCE

The almost invariable occurrence of apical systolic and diastolic murmurs—plus the commonly associated right ventricular failure; bifid P waves on the ECG; and radio-

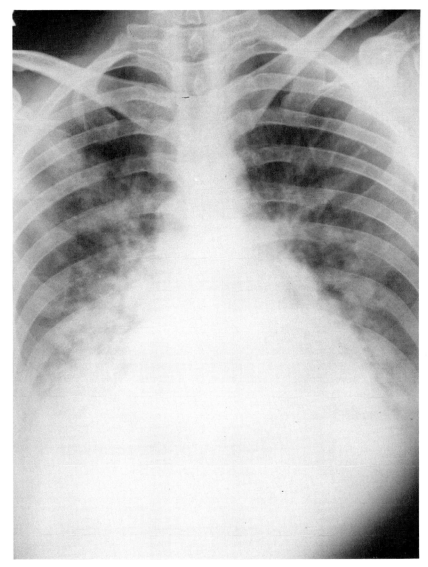

FIGURE 6-34. Posteroanterior chest radiograph showing cardiac enlargement and pulmonary edema in a 20-year-old woman with a large left atrial myxoma and intractable cardiac failure.

logical appearances of a dilated left atrium, pulmonary venous congestion, and enlarged right or left ventricle—are all suggestive of mitral valve disease, and this is the diagnosis that has usually been made. The differentiation on clinical examination of left atrial myxoma from mitral stenosis or incompetence is not easy but can be done. Although mitral murmurs are almost always detectable in left atrial myxoma, they are frequently out of accord with the symptoms and other physical signs that suggest a severe hemodynamic valve lesion. An apical systolic murmur is almost always present, and this may vary with positional changes or, more frequently in our experience, during repeated auscultation. The systolic murmur is usually Grade 1 or 2; and absence of a widely split second heart sound, a constant third heart sound, and a left atrial lift do not suggest hemodynamically significant mitral regurgitation. In rare instances, we have observed severe regurgitation from destruction of mitral leaflets by the myxoma. A true opening snap will never occur, but the so-called tumour plop can mimic an opening snap or an early third heart sound. Tumour plops are often variable in intensity, which is a clue to their identification. A mid-diastolic murmur is often heard in patients with left atrial myxoma but fre-

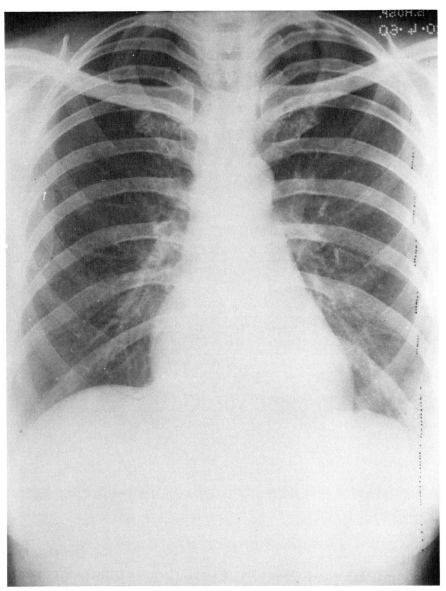

FIGURE 6-35. Posteroanterior chest radiogram of a 49-year-old woman with a right atrial myxoma. There is prominence of the right heart border compatible with an enlarged right atrium. The pulmonary vasculature is within normal limits. (From Barlow, JB: *The diagnosis of myxoma of the atrium.* Sem Hop Paris 4:51–57, 1961, with permission.)

quently has unusual features. It may be confined to presystole or be very short in early and mid-diastole. The murmur may vary with position or with repeated auscultation, and is seldom as long as would be expected in a patient with stenosis sufficiently tight to cause marked pulmonary venous hypertension or right ventricular failure. The mitral component of the first sound is often extremely loud and on phonocardiography is markedly delayed (Fig. 6-36).

Intractable right ventricular failure develops sooner or later in all patients with left atrial myxoma, except when sudden death occurs early in the course of the illness. In the absence of uncontrolled atrial fibrillation or other arrhythmia, it would

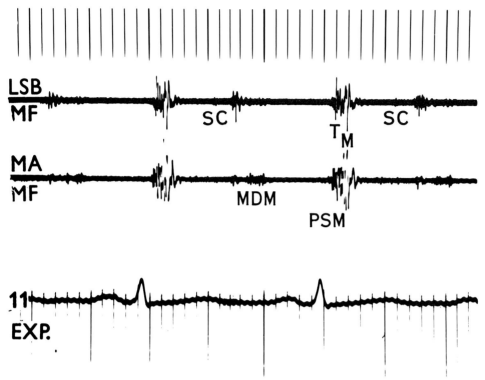

FIGURE 6-36. Phonocardiogram, recorded in expiration, of a 41-year-old man with a left atrial myxoma. The mitral component (M) of the first sound is delayed (Q–M = 0.12 second), producing reversed splitting. Left-sided mid-diastolic (MDM) and presystolic (PSM) murmurs, a soft clicking sound in systole (SC), and the tricuspid component (T) of the first sound are demonstrated. MA = mitral area; LSB = left sternal border; MF = medium frequency. Time lines 0.04 second. (From Barlow, JB and Pocock, WA: *The problem of non-ejection systolic clicks and associated mitral systolic murmurs. Emphasis on the billowing mitral leaflet syndrome.* Am Heart J 90:636–655, 1975, with permission.)

be most unusual for any case of mitral stenosis to develop right ventricular failure without a considerable increase in the pulmonary vascular resistance. This can usually be detected on the ECG by evidence of right ventricular hypertrophy. Appropriate right ventricular hypertrophy is seldom seen in myxoma cases and contrasts with the forceful and "hyperactive" right ventricular pulsation that is palpable over the lower sternum in many patients, particularly when right heart failure has supervened.

ISCHEMIC HEART DISEASE

In a patient population in which rheumatic heart disease is rare, left atrial myxoma is probably more readily suspected because of unusual features associated with mitral murmurs. Nevertheless, patients with left atrial myxoma who have attacks of constricting precordial pain (especially when associated with sweating, breathlessness, or syncope) later followed by congestive heart failure strongly mimic a clinical presentation of ischemic heart disease. Electrocardiographic evidence of myocardial ischemia may occur with myxoma, and, as previously stated, true myocardial infarction will supervene following coronary embolism. Under such circumstances, an apical systolic murmur of mitral regurgitation could well be attributed to papillary muscle dysfunction. Again, the correct diagnosis of myxoma will depend largely on any unusual aspects of the clinical presentation of "ischemic heart disease." Clues include absence of left ventricular dilatation, particularly if cardiac failure is present; mitral diastolic murmurs and an inconstant or unusual "third" heart sound; insufficient electrocardiographic evidence of ischemia or infarction; and associated systemic features.

CONGESTIVE CARDIOMYOPATHY

Symptoms of angina, fainting, and paroxysmal dyspnea, and signs of severe congestive cardiac failure, gallop rhythm, small pulse pressure, and an apical regurgitant systolic murmur are all compatible with dilated cardiomyopathy. Abnormal T waves, low-voltage QRS complexes, and Q waves, features of congestive cardiomyopathy, are also encountered in myxoma cases. Although the left ventricle is usually dilated in congestive cardiomyopathy, there are patients in whom the left ventricle has a "restrictive" pattern, and this occurs particularly in endomyocardial fibrosis. In such cases, intractable right ventricular failure, large left atrial P waves on the ECG, and radiological signs of pulmonary venous hypertension and left atrial dilatation with little or no evidence of left ventricular enlargement simulate a left atrial myxoma. Prior to echocardiography, we were often unable to make this differentiation without angiocardiography.

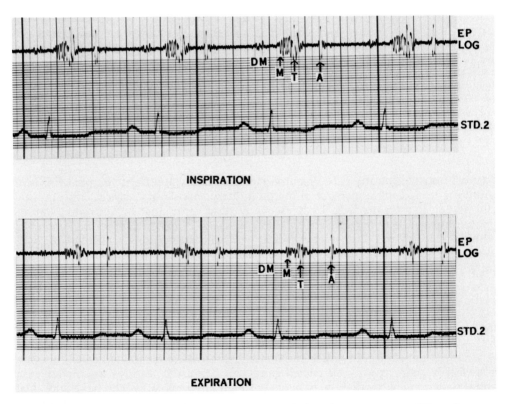

FIGURE 6-37. Logarithmic phonocardiograms recorded in the epigastrium (EP) in the same patient as in Figure 6-35. A late diastolic murmur (DM) and a "presystolic" murmur, which starts at the time of mitral valve closure (M) and ends at tricuspid valve closure (T), are shown to increase in intensity with inspiration. The loud tricuspid component of the first heart sound is delayed 0.14 second after the Q wave. Time lines 0.04 second.

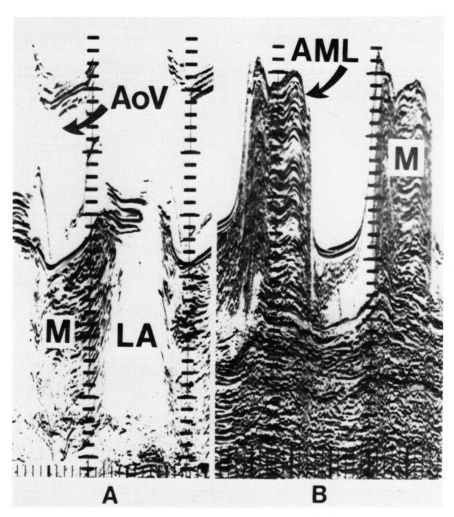

FIGURE 6-38. M-mode echocardiogram of a 14-year-old girl who presented with a right hemiplegia due to embolization from a left atrial myxoma. *A*, Echoes from the myxoma (M) in the left atrium (LA) during systole. *B*, Echocardiogram of the mitral valve shows a large mass of echoes in the mitral orifice between the mitral leaflets during diastole. AML = anterior mitral leaflet; AoV = aortic valve. (From Barlow, JB and Pocock, WA: *The importance of diagnosis in heart disease.* Cardiac Medical Journal 1:3–6, 1983, with permission.)

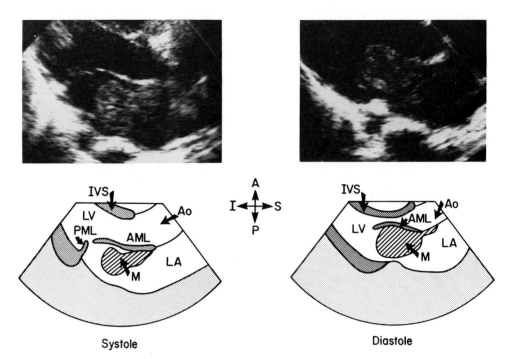

FIGURE 6-39. 2-D echocardiograms, long-axis views, of the same patient as in Figure 6-38 show the myxoma (M) within the left atrium (LA) during systole and prolapsing into the left ventricle (LV) during diastole. Each frame is accompanied by a labelled, idealized diagram. Ao = aortic root; IVS = interventricular septum; PML = posterior mitral leaflet; A = anterior; P = posterior; I = inferior; S = superior. (From Barlow, JB and Pocock, WA: *The importance of diagnosis in heart disease.* Cardiac Medical Journal 1:3–6, 1983, with permission.)

DIFFERENTIAL DIAGNOSES OF RIGHT ATRIAL MYXOMA

A total of only four patients with right atrial myxoma occurring during the last 25 years can be recalled. In one of these, the clinical presentation was clouded by severe pulmonary arterial hypertension due to thromboembolic disease, and the myxoma was diagnosed only at necropsy.

In the absence of pulmonary hypertension and severe pulmonary embolic disease, right atrial myxoma presents with systemic venous congestion and "tricuspid" murmurs, principally diastolic (Fig. 6-37). These clinical signs with recent onset of symptoms, often including upper abdominal pain due to hepatic congestion, make right atrial myxoma easier to suspect than left atrial myxoma. Ebstein's anomaly, constrictive pericarditis, and carcinoid syndrome have all been considered in the differential diagnoses of reported cases of right atrial myxoma but should be able to be distinguished by their characteristic physical and other features.

Probably because of lower pressures on the right side of the heart, tricuspid regurgitation in right atrial myxoma is not as prevalent as is mitral regurgitation in cases of left atrial myxoma. Right atrial myxoma most closely mimics severe isolated tricuspid stenosis. Congenital tricuspid stenosis is extremely rare as an isolated lesion. The most common cause of tricuspid stenosis is rheumatic heart disease, but this is seldom encountered in the absence of associated mitral or aortic valve involvement. Diagnosis of a right atrial myxoma should always be considered in a patient with a hemodynamically significant isolated tricuspid "stenosis."

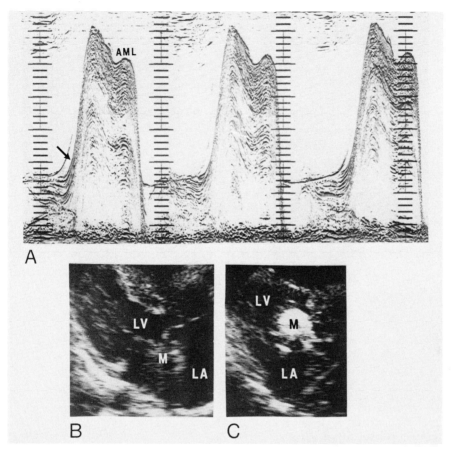

FIGURE 6-40. Echocardiograms in a patient with a left atrial myxoma. *A*, M-mode shows dense echoes on the atrial surface of the anterior mitral leaflet (AML) with a small echo-free space *(arrow)* in early diastole. *B, C*, 2-D, long-axis view, in systole *(B)* and diastole *(C)*. The myxoma (M) moves from the left atrium (LA) into the ventricle (LV) during diastole.

ECHOCARDIOGRAPHY OF ATRIAL MYXOMA

Both M-mode (Fig. 6-38) and 2-D echocardiography (Fig. 6-39) have superseded angiography in the diagnosis and definition of atrial myxomata. Cardiac catheterization is unnecessary and possibly hazardous in these cases. Surgery can be recommended on the basis of the echocardiogram alone, provided the image is of high quality and the diagnosis established beyond doubt (Fig. 6-40). The subxiphoid view (Fig. 6-41) is especially useful for visualizing the interatrial septum, to which most atrial myxomas are attached.

Differential diagnoses of atrial tumour on echocardiography include a ball-valve thrombus and vegetations due to infective endocarditis. Atrial thrombi are not always shown echocardiographically, but de Pace and associates[3] demonstrated that 2-D echocardiography is an effective technique for diagnosing laminated adherent clot in the left atrium. Ball-valve thrombi may be indistinguishable electrocardiographically from atrial myxomata. A ball-valve thrombus in the left atrium is invariably associated with some mitral valve stenosis and is much rarer than left atrial myxomata.[4]

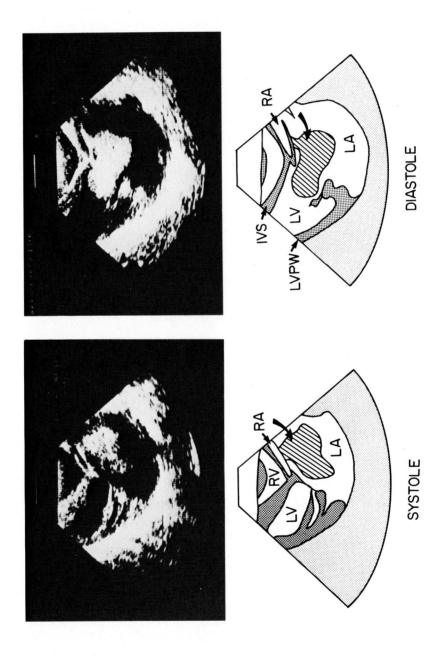

FIGURE 6-41. Cross-sectional echocardiograms (subxiphoid view) in systole (*left*) and diastole (*right*) of a left atrial myxoma in a 60-year-old woman. A large mass (*arrow*) is present in the left atrium (LA) attached to the lower interatrial septum. In late diastole the mass has prolapsed into the mitral orifice. RA = right atrium; RV = right ventricle; LV = left ventricle. (From Lewis, BS, Stein, MG, Agathangelou, NE, and Barlow, JB: *High-quality imaging of a left atrial tumour using real-time two-dimensional echocardiography.* S Afr Med J 61:165–167, 1982, with permission.)

REFERENCES

SECTION 1

1. ROBERTS, WC: *Morphologic features of the normal and abnormal mitral valve.* Am J Cardiol 51:1005–1028, 1983.
2. NESTICO, PF, DE PACE, NL, MORGANROTH, J, KOTLER, MN, AND ROSS, J: *Mitral annular calcification: Clinical pathophysiology, and echocardiographic review.* Am Heart J 107:989–996, 1984.
3. TAKAMOTO, T AND POPP, RL: *Conduction disturbances related to the site and severity of mitral anular calcification: A 2-dimensional echocardiographic and electrocardiographic correlative study.* Am J Cardiol 51:1644–1649, 1983.
4. RYTAND, DA: *An auricular diastolic murmur with heart block in elderly patients.* Am Heart J 32:579–598, 1946.
5. LABOVITZ, AJ, NELSON, JG, WINDHORST, DM, KENNEDY, HL, AND WILLIAMS, GA: *Frequency of mitral valve dysfunction from mitral anular calcium as detected by Doppler echocardiography.* Am J Cardiol 55:133–137, 1985.
6. OSTERBERGER, LE, GOLDSTEIN, S, KHAJA, F, AND LAKIER, JB: *Functional mitral stenosis in patients with massive mitral annular calcification.* Circulation 64:472–476, 1981.

SECTION 2

1. ABRAHAMS, DG, BARTON, CJ, COCKSHOTT, WP, EDINGTON, GM, AND WEAVER, EJM: *Annular subvalvular left ventricular aneurysms.* Q J Med 31:345–360, 1962.
2. COCKSHOTT, WP, ANTIA, A, IKEME, HA, AND UZODIKE, VO: *Annular subvalvar left ventricular aneurysms.* Br J Radiol 40:424–435, 1967.
3. CHESLER, E: *Aneurysms of the left ventricle.* M.D. Thesis, University of Witwatersrand, Johannesburg, South Africa, 1968.
4. KANAREK, KS, BLOOM, KR, LAKIER, JB, POCOCK, WA, AND BARLOW, JB: Clinical aspects of submitral left ventricular aneurysms. S Afr Med J 47:1225–1229, 1973.
5. DAVIS, MD, CASPI, A, LEWIS, BS, MILNER, S, COLSEN, PR, AND BARLOW, JB: *Two-dimensional echocardiographic features of submitral left ventricular aneurysm.* Am Heart J 103:289–290, 1982.

SECTION 3

1. BROCK, R: *Functional obstruction of the left ventricle: Acquired aortic subvalvular stenosis.* Guy's Hospital Reports 106:221–238, 1957.
2. TEARE, D: *Asymmetrical hypertrophy of the heart in young adults.* Br Heart J 20:1–8, 1958.
3. LEWIS, BS, ARMSTRONG, TG, MITHA, AS, AND GOTSMAN, MS: *Hypertrophic obstructive cardiomyopathy in the South African Bantu.* S Afr Med J 47:599–604, 1973.
4. LEWIS, BS, AGATHANGELOU, NE, FLAX, H, TAAMS, MA, AND BARLOW, JB: *Hypertrophic cardiomyopathy in South African Blacks.* S Afr Med J 63:266–270, 1983.
5. MARON, BJ: *Myocardial disorganisation in hypertrophic cardiomyopathy. Another point of view.* Br Heart J 50:1–3, 1983.
6. YAMAGUCHI, H, ISHIMURA, T, NISHIYAMA, S, NAGASAKI, F, NAKANISHI, S, TAKATSU, F, NISHIJO, T, UMEDA, T, AND MACHII, K. *Hypertrophic nonobstructive cardiomyopathy with giant negative T waves (apical hypertrophy): Ventriculographic and echocardiographic features in 30 patients.* Am J Cardiol 44:401–412, 1979.
7. TUCKER, RBK, ZION, MM, POCOCK, WA, AND BARLOW, JB: *Auscultatory features of hypertrophic obstructive cardiomyopathy. A study of 90 patients.* S Afr Med J 49:179–186, 1975.
8. SIEGEL, RJ AND CRILEY, JM: *Comparison of ventricular emptying with and without a pressure gradient in patients with hypertrophic cardiomyopathy.* Br Heart J 53:283–291, 1985.
9. COHEN, J, EFFAT, H, GOODWIN, JF, OAKLEY, CM, AND STEINER, RE: *Hypertrophic obstructive cardiomyopathy.* Br Heart J 26:16–32, 1964.

10. GOODWIN, JF: *The frontiers of cardiomyopathy.* Br Heart J 48:1–18, 1982.

11. HESS, OM, SCHNEIDER, J, TURINA, M, CARROLL, JD, ROTHLIN, M, AND KRAYENBUEHL, HP: *Asymmetric septal hypertrophy in patients with aortic stenosis: An adaptive mechanism, or a coexistence of hypertrophic cardiomyopathy.* J Am Coll Cardiol 3:783–789, 1983.

12. TOPOL, EJ, TRAILL, TA, AND FORTUIN, NJ: *Hypertensive hypertrophic cardiomyopathy of the elderly.* N Engl J Med 312:277–283, 1985.

13. OAKLEY, DG AND OAKLEY, CM: *Significance of abnormal electrocardiograms in highly trained athletes.* Am J Cardiol 50:985–989, 1982.

14. BARLOW, JB AND POCOCK, WA: *Mitral valve prolapse, the athletes heart, physical activity and sudden death.* J Sports Cardiol 1:9–24, 1984.

15. SHAPIRO, LM AND MCKENNA, WJ: *Distribution of left ventricular hypertrophy in hypertrophic cardiomyopathy: A two-dimensional echocardiographic study.* J Am Coll Cardiol 2:437–444, 1983.

16. CANEDO, MI AND FRANK, MJ: *Therapy of hypertrophic cardiomyopathy: Medical or surgical? Clinical and pathophysiologic considerations.* Am J Cardiol 48:383–388, 1981.

17. KALTENBACH, M, HOPF, R, KOBER, G, BUSSMAN, WD, KELLER, M, AND PETERSEN, Y: *Treatment of hypertrophic obstructive cardiomyopathy with verapamil.* Br Heart J 42:35–42, 1979.

18. COOLEY, DA, LEACHMAN, RD, AND WAKASCH, DC: *Diffuse muscular subaortic stenosis: Surgical management.* Am J Cardiol 31:1–6, 1973.

SECTION 4

1. LEONHARDT, ETG AND KULLENBERG, KPG: *Bilateral atrial myxomas with multiple arterial aneurysms—a syndrome mimicking polyarteritis nodosa.* Am J Med 62:792–794, 1977.

2. GRAHAM, HV, VON HARTITZSCH, B, AND MEDINA, JR: *Infected atrial myxoma.* Am J Cardiol 38:658–661, 1976.

3. DE PACE, N, SOULEN, R, KOTLER, M, AND MINTZ, GS: *Two dimensional echocardiographic detection of intraatrial masses.* Am J Cardiol 48:954–960, 1981.

4. GILMER, D AND CAMPANELLA, C: *Echocardiographic diagnosis of left atrial ball-valve thrombus. A case report.* S Afr Med J 65:662, 1984.

BIBLIOGRAPHY

SECTION 1

NAIR, CK, SUDHAKARAN, C, ARONOW, WS, THOMSON, W, WOODRUFF, MP, AND SKETCH, MH: *Clinical characteristics of patients younger than 60 years with mitral anular calcium: Comparison with age- and sex-matched control subjects.* Am J Cardiol 54:1286–1287, 1984.

WALLER, BF AND ROBERTS, WC: *Cardiovascular disease in the very elderly. Analysis of 40 necropsy patients aged 90 years or over.* Am J Cardiol 51:403–421, 1983.

SECTION 2

SZARNICKI, RJ, DE LEVAL, MR, AND STARK, J: *Calcified left ventricular aneurysm in a 6-year-old Caucasian boy.* Br Heart J 45:464–466, 1981.

WOLPOWITZ, A, ARMAN, B, BARNARD, MS, AND BARNARD, CN: *Annular subvalvular idiopathic left ventricular aneurysms in the Black African.* Ann Thorac Surg 27:350–355, 1979.

SECTION 3

BERTRAND, ME, TILMANT, PY, LABLANCHE, JM, AND THIEULEUX, FA: *Apical hypertrophic cardiomyopathy: Clinical and metabolic studies.* Eur Heart J 4:127–133, 1983.

BOROGGREFE, M, KUHN, H, KÖNIGER, HH, STÖTER, H, BREITHARDT, G, LOOGEN, F, SCHULTE, HD, AND BIRCKS, W: *Arrhythmias in hypertrophic obstructive and non-obstructive cardiomyopathy.* Eur Heart J 4:245–451, 1983.

GOODWIN, JF: *Hypertrophic cardiomyopathy: A disease in search of its own identity.* Am J Cardiol 45:177–180, 1980.

GOODWIN, JF: *An appreciation of hypertrophic cardiomyopathy.* Am J Med 68:797–800, 1980.

KEREN, G, BELHASSEN, B, SHEREZ, J, MILLER, HI, MEGIDISH, R, BERENFELD, D, AND LANIADO, S: *Apical hypertrophic cardiomyopathy: Evaluation by noninvasive and invasive techniques in 23 patients.* Circulation 71:45–56, 1985.

KOGA, Y, ITAYA, K-I, AND TOSHIMA, H: *Prognosis in hypertrophic cardiomyopathy.* Am Heart J 108:351–359, 1984.

MCKENNA, WJ, HARRIS, L, ROWLAND, E, KLEINEBENNE, A, KRIKLER, DM, OAKLEY, CM, AND GOODWIN, JF: *Amiodarone for long-term management of patients with hypertrophic cardiomyopathy.* Am J Cardiol 54:802–810, 1984.

MARON, BJ, EPSTEIN, SE, AND ROBERTS, WC: *Hypertrophic cardiomyopathy: A common cause of sudden death in the young competitive athlete.* Eur Heart J 4:135–144, 1983.

SECTION 4

BULKLEY, BH AND HUTCHINS, GM: *Atrial myxomas: A fifty year review.* Am Heart J 97:639–643, 1979.

GERSHLICK, AH, LEECH, G, MILLS, PG, AND LEATHAM, A: *The loud first heart sound in left atrial myxoma.* Br Heart J 52:403–407, 1984.

GOODWIN, JF: *Diagnosis of left atrial myxoma.* Lancet 1:464–468, 1963.

7

RHEUMATIC FEVER AND RHEUMATIC HEART DISEASE

with ROBIN H. KINSLEY and WENDY A. POCOCK

EPIDEMIOLOGY

There is almost universal agreement that for rheumatic fever and rheumatic heart disease to occur, there must have been previous infection with Group A betahemolytic streptococcus. Other important factors related to a higher risk of rheumatic fever developing after infection with Group A streptococcus are significant antibody responses, the presence of an exudative as opposed to a nonexudative pharyngitis, and the persistence of the Group A streptococcus in the pharynx for at least 21 days during convalescence.

In most developed countries, the reported incidence of both rheumatic fever and rheumatic heart disease has declined drastically. Because the onset of this decline preceded the advent of antibiotics, other factors must have played a role. Despite worldwide research, the factors causing a high prevalence of rheumatic heart disease in any community remain uncertain. It is favored that socioeconomic factors are important; hence, the continued high prevalence of rheumatic heart disease in Third World countries. Unlike our experience 15 to 20 years ago, it is now rare to encounter White patients under the age of 20 years with rheumatic heart disease. The clinical experience of those involved with the diagnosis and treatment of Black patients in this country is that rheumatic heart disease remains prevalent and continues to affect young children. Approximately 300 Black patients with rheumatic heart disease are operated on annually in our institution, and about 35 percent of these are subjects under 20 years of age. In 1972, we conducted a survey of 12,050 Black schoolchildren in the Johannesburg area[1] and detected an overall prevalence rate of rheumatic heart disease of 6.9/1000, with a peak rate of 19.2/1000 in children aged about 15 to 18 years. A more recent survey by Bundred and Kitchiner[2] in South West Africa, showed results similar to those of our 1972 study. Rheumatic heart disease remains a major challenge to cardiologists in the Asian-Pacific area. In 1978, Padmavati[3] concluded that "prophylaxis was hardly worthwhile" in patients encountered for the first time with a late stage of rheumatic heart disease. Such cases comprised 75 percent of those considered for a secondary prophylaxis programme in India between 1968 and 1974.

The exact nature of the relevant "co-factor" (or "co-factors") that predispose to rheumatic fever or rheumatic heart disease remains uncertain. In 1930, Glover[4] stated that "no disease has a clearer-cut 'social incidence' than acute rheumatism which falls perhaps thirty times as frequently upon the poorer children of the industrial town as upon the children of the well-to-do . . . the incidence of acute rheumatism increases directly with poverty, malnutrition, overcrowding and bad housing." Since Glover's comments, the socioeconomic factors that have received the most attention are poor nutrition and overcrowding. Hereditary, racial, geographical, and blood group factors have also been studied but are probably of minor or no importance. From the data obtained in our survey, we concluded that overcrowding was of great importance but that it alone was not the sole factor. All schools are "overcrowded" in that the pupils are in close contact with one another, and this will facilitate spread of the betahemolytic streptococcus. As many as 9 percent of pupils at an exclusive Johannesburg preparatory school in 1975[5] had throat swabs that tested positive for the betahemolytic streptococcus, yet rheumatic fever or rheumatic heart disease has not, to our knowledge, been encountered in a pupil at that school during the last 20 years. A recent survey,[6] in which the throats of Coloured and of Indian schoolchildren were swab-tested, revealed Group A betahemolytic streptococci in 24 and 21 percent, respectively, during the summer months. The total number of 226 children examined was relatively small, but none had rheumatic heart disease. We did not detect significant malnutrition in the Black schoolchildren who we examined in 1972, but it is possible that poor nutrition during the first year of life renders a child susceptible to rheumatic fever and rheumatic heart disease. Aryanpur-Kashani[7] made this assumption in 1980, and it requires further investigation.

RHEUMATIC FEVER PROPHYLAXIS

PRIMARY

Eradication of the betahemolytic streptococcus from the pharynx by treatment with penicillin in adequate doses will prevent subsequent rheumatic fever. One intramuscular injection of benzathine penicillin G (1,200,000 units for adults and 600,000 units for children) or oral penicillin 250,000 units (250 mg) four times daily for 10 days is recommended. Under ideal circumstances, treatment of acute pharyngitis due to betahemolytic streptococcus should be based on a positive throat swab test result. Failing those ideal circumstances, all cases of acute pharyngitis in a potentially susceptible population should be so treated. This would require teaching medical practitioners and the general population that such treatment of sore throats is both necessary and practicable, a formidable and often impossible undertaking in Third World countries because of a shortage of medical practitioners and of funds. Furthermore, about one third of the cases of rheumatic fever occur without a previous symptomatic streptococcal throat infection. Thus, for primary prophylaxis to be effective, the streptococcal infection must be actively sought or prevented, which would entail frequent routine throat cultures on schoolchildren. An alternative policy is for antibiotics to be given prophylactically to the entire school population at times of increased risk, such as during the winter months; this also would have considerable practical problems. Parenteral benzathine penicillin is the most reliable form of treatment and prevention, but its use in an apparently normal school population would be limited by local discomfort and the risk, however small, of fatal anaphylaxis. The use of oral penicillin or sulphonamides is more practicable, although it has disadvantages owing to the erratic compliance of schoolchildren. The development of an effective antistreptococcal vaccine that could be given to all children would clearly obviate these disadvantages and provide an immediate and simple means of primary prophylaxis. Such a vaccine is not yet available for general use. We remain pessimistic about decreasing significantly the incidence of rheumatic heart disease amongst South African Blacks until their socioeconomic conditions improve. If the relevance of malnutrition in infancy is valid, then improvement in nutrition and possibly also in the treatment of infections should produce beneficial results. In our view, the institution of such measures would be a meaningful and practicable attempt to achieve primary prophylaxis against rheumatic heart disease in Third World countries, including South Africa. Irrespective of whether the co-factor to the hemolytic streptococcus relates to malnutrition and sickness during infancy, this approach would have great overall benefit to public health.

SECONDARY

All subjects who have had a definite attack of rheumatic fever or who have established rheumatic heart disease require prophylaxis against recurrent rheumatic activity. Preferably, this should be administered in the form of intramuscular benzathine penicillin G 1,200,000 units every three or four weeks (600,000 units for children weighing less than 30 kg) or as oral penicillin V 250,000 units (250 mg) twice a day. It is mandatory that patients understand the importance of this treatment, whether or not they are symptomatic. Secondary prophylaxis should be continued until at least the age of 21 years, and we currently favor 25 years. Many patients, and certainly the majority of South African Blacks, are reluctant to continue medication in the absence of symptoms. Even when the rationale and importance of the therapy is understood, economic factors contribute to the lack of compliance. It is regrettable that a large proportion of the operations for rheumatic heart disease is doomed to fail in the long term because of ongoing rheumatic activity. It is not unusual for a patient to require aortic valve replacement two to three years after successful mitral valve replacement as the result of persistent or recurrent rheumatic activity. In some instances, the patient returns with organic tricuspid valve disease and further myocardial damage several years after successful aortic and mitral valve replacement. Our experience is very different from that of John and co-workers[8] in Vellore, India, who apparently seldom encounter rheumatic activity after mitral valve replacement.

ACUTE RHEUMATIC FEVER AND RELATIVELY MILD RHEUMATIC ENDOCARDITIS

"Classic" rheumatic fever is no longer common, even in the South African Black population. Approximately 45 cases of rheumatic fever are encountered annually in the pediatric wards (children aged 10 years or under) at Baragwanath Hospital. The clinical features are the most reliable in making the diagnosis of active rheumatic carditis. Patients are usually young, aged 10 to 14 years, and are in sinus rhythm. The ECG reveals a relatively prolonged PR interval in about 60 percent of cases. We have seldom assessed the QT intervals, but QRS and T-wave changes are unremarkable. Laboratory investigations invariably confirm a raised erythrocyte sedimentation rate; a mild normochromic anemia is not infrequent;[9] and the antistreptolysin titre is raised in more than 50 percent of patients. C-reactive protein and mucoprotein are also increased. The laboratory findings are nonspecific and unhelpful in differentiating rheumatic activity from other pyrexial illnesses, most importantly infective endocarditis. It is customary to administer intramuscular benzathine penicillin G in a dose of 1,200,000 units (600,000 for children <30 kg). This is repeated thereafter at three- to four-week intervals; or oral penicillin 250 mg twice daily is given as secondary prophylaxis. Strict bed rest is necessary until evidence of rheumatic activity has disappeared. No evidence exists that steroids will prevent valve lesions or decrease their severity, and they are rarely indicated for symptomatic relief. Arthralgia and arthritis invariably respond to salicylate therapy. In our experience, symptomatic acute pericarditis is rare in the absence of virulent carditis and hemodynamically severe valve involvement.

It is well known that mild mitral regurgitation may occur with active rheumatic carditis and be reversible. We have observed apical pansystolic murmurs to become late systolic and then disappear entirely. We postulated that "anular dysfunction" is the probable mechanism for transient mitral regurgitation.[10] Bundred and Kitchiner[2] have observed 66 patients with mitral regurgitation lose their systolic murmurs after adequate penicillin and other therapy extending over a nine-year period. The murmurs of the majority of their patients disappeared within 24 months after the commencement of treatment.

Our survey[1] of 12,050 "normal" Black schoolchildren revealed 80 with rheumatic heart disease. In 39 (49 percent) there was no history to suggest previous rheumatic activity. A definite history of rheumatic fever was elicited from only nine children, while the remaining 32 had had symptoms compatible with previous rheumatic activity such as repeated sore throats, arthralgia, and arthritis. Clinical features suggestive of rheumatic activity were detected in only four children at the time of examination. Mitral regurgitation was the most common valvular lesion, occurring in 76 (95 percent) of the affected children and was an isolated lesion in 38. Thirty-eight children (47.5 percent) had some mitral stenosis, but pure stenosis was present in two children only. Aortic incompetence was diagnosed in nine children, three of whom had associated aortic stenosis. Eight of the nine had clinical evidence of mitral valve involvement. Ninety-two percent of the children with rheumatic heart disease denied cardiac symptoms.

ACTIVE, SEVERE RHEUMATIC CARDITIS

A fulminating form of active rheumatic carditis continues to be encountered by us. Such cases have been observed by one of us (JBB) for more than three decades, and the pattern of presentation remains unchanged. It is difficult to assess the incidence, but there is no evidence to suggest that it is decreasing. In fact, because of an expanding cardiac surgical service, the number of patients with severe heart disease seen annually is increasing. During 1983, 359 open heart operations for valve disease were performed on Black patients in our institution. Nearly all were on the basis of rheumatic heart disease, and approximately 35 percent were performed on subjects under 20 years of age. In many of the younger patients, active rheumatic carditis was present at the time of surgery.

From July 1974 to July 1979, 80 patients underwent valve replacement or repair, or both, while in the active phase of rheumatic carditis.[9] On the basis of an analysis of those patients, the clinical picture can be described.

CLINICAL FEATURES

All but four of the 80 patients were under the age of 21 years. Eighteen patients (23 percent) were less than 10 years old, and the youngest patient was 5 years old (Fig. 7-1). The children or their parents commonly claimed that symptoms such as tiredness, breathlessness, cough, and arthralgia had been present for a few weeks only. Tachycardia of more than 100 beats per minute and pyrexia greater than 38°C (Table 7-1) are almost invariable features and were present in 96 percent of patients. The clinical picture is often compatible with infective endocarditis, but the differentiation

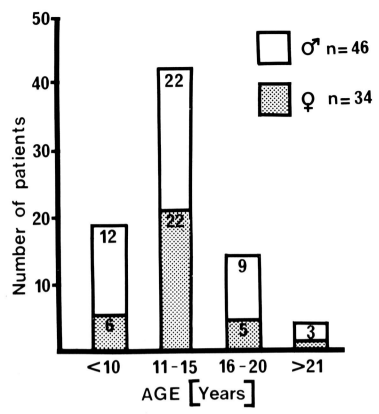

FIGURE 7-1. Age and sex of 80 patients who underwent valve replacement, repair, or both while in the active phase of rheumatic carditis. (From Kinsley et al,[9] with permission.)

TABLE 7-1. Clinical Features of Active Severe Rheumatic Carditis

	NUMBER OF PATIENTS	PERCENT
Age (yr)		
<10	18	23
10–20	58	72
>20	4	5
Tachycardia (>100/min)	77	96
Pyrexia	77	96
Chest pain	31	39
Arthralgia	13	16
Epistaxis	10	13
Cardiothoracic ratio		
(57 patients) >0.6	53	93
<0.6	4	7
PR interval (55 patients)		
>0.2	30	55
<0.2	25	45
Cachexia	34	49
Emergency operation	52	65

can usually be made. Relevant distinguishing features are negative blood cultures and lack of splinter hemorrhages (or other evidence of systemic embolism), lack of vegetations on echocardiography, and lack of response to a trial of antibiotic therapy. Definite clubbing of the fingernails was present in about 15 percent of patients. This is a little-recognized feature of active rheumatic carditis and may mislead clinicians into diagnosing infective endocarditis. Splenomegaly was present in about 15 percent of patients. It is uncertain whether this is causally related to the rheumatic activity or a coincidental feature in a population with a high prevalence of parasitic infestation. A notable symptom was severe anterior chest pain (in 31 patients), which is typically aggravated by pressure of the palm of the examiner's hand on the sternum. A pericardial rub may be detected in such cases, and acute fibrinous pericarditis was confirmed at surgery in 24 of these patients. Significant cachexia was present in 34 patients, and this may be extremely marked in some instances (Fig. 7-2). Arthralgia or arthritis is uncommon and occurred in only 16 percent. Rheumatic nodules and erythema marginatum were rarely encountered.

Considerable cardiomegaly is readily apparent on clinical examination and confirmed by a cardiothoracic ratio on chest roentgenogram of at least 60 percent in nearly all cases. Regurgitation is invariably the predominant valvular lesion (Table 7-2), and this almost always involves the mitral valve. A left atrial lift is an easily elicited and highly contributory physical sign, especially if the apical systolic murmur is only Grade 2 or less in intensity.

Although the apex beat is sustained throughout systole and heaving, it is sometimes suggestive of associated myocardial dysfunction in that the apical heave is less forceful than would be expected with the severe valvular lesion. Concomitant aortic regurgitation was present in 47 of our 80 patients, but marked aortic regurgitation as an isolated lesion (that is, without detectable associated mitral valve involvement) was encountered in only six subjects. Dominant mitral stenosis occurred in only one patient in this series, and there was no case of significant aortic stenosis. Associated tricuspid regurgitation is common and usually due to dilatation of the tricuspid anulus. This was confirmed at operation in 22 patients. The systolic murmur of tricuspid regurgitation is often unimpressive or absent, but the entity may be clinically recognized by prominent "CV" waves in the jugular venous pressure and systolic pulsation of the enlarged liver. Unlike Stollerman,[11] we have never observed rheumatic involvement of the pulmonary valve.

Although left ventricular myocardial dysfunction is frequently present, it is important to emphasize that, contrary to previous reports, left or right ventricular failure does *not* result from active rheumatic carditis without a hemodynamically severe valvular lesion. The entity of "toxic rheumatic myocarditis" discussed by Stollerman[11] is indeed an important component of the cardiac involvement by the active rheumatic process, but, unlike viral myocarditis, it alone does not cause ventricular dilatation or heart failure. The contribution of medical therapy to these patients is therefore limited, and heart failure and rheumatic activity seldom resolve on medical therapy only. We want to emphasize strongly that steroids are never a "lifesaving measure" in these patients who always have a severe valvular lesion. The only contributory therapy is cardiac surgery. Steroids are likely to make the tissues more friable and the task of the surgeon more difficult. Although we have encountered many patients with fulminating rheumatic carditis and severe regurgitant valve lesions treated by pediatricians and others with steroid therapy, we have yet to observe improvement with such therapy.

So-called rheumatic pneumonitis has provoked discussion as to whether the condition is a rheumatic manifestation or a complication of heart failure. The histological findings are unusual for pulmonary edema in that the lungs are grossly hemorrhagic and resemble pulmonary infarction. Nonetheless, we have not observed this entity in the absence of fulminating carditis and a hemodynamically significant valvular, invariably mitral regurgitant, lesion. It subsides if valvular surgery is successful, but the surgical risk is greater because of postoperative pulmonary compli-

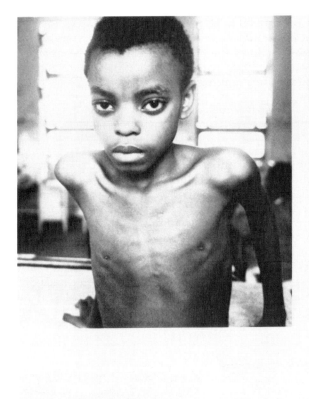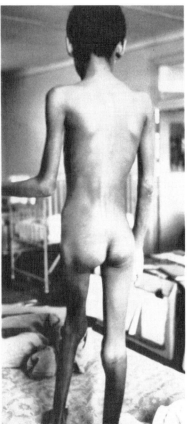

FIGURE 7-2. An 8-year-old cachectic girl with severe rheumatic mitral regurgitation and acute carditis.

cations. We believe treatment of so-called rheumatic pneumonitis with steroid therapy is meaningless and contraindicated. The condition is presumably an unusual manifestation of pulmonary venous hypertension and appropriate surgical therapy is indicated.

Another interesting observation in these patients has been the persistence of signs of active rheumatic carditis, most notably pyrexia and tachycardia, despite all medical therapy until surgery improves or "cures" the valvular lesions. The decrease of the temperature and of the tachycardia several days postoperatively is often dramatic. Other signs of improvement after surgery are equally impressive. Patients develop large appetites and gain weight; chest pain and arthralgia subside. We are

TABLE 7-2. Hemodynamic Lesions

	NUMBER OF PATIENTS		PERCENT
Mitral regurgitation	72		90
Pure		58	
Predominant		14	
Aortic regurgitation	53		66
Isolated		6	
Associated with mitral regurgitation		47	
Tricuspid regurgitation (functional)	22		28
Mitral stenosis	1		1

not aware that this remarkable improvement in all parameters after surgery has been reported previously. The relevant factor may be removal of the cardiac workload by correction of the valve lesion, which allows the carditis to subside. The excessive workload on the heart is analogous to a child with active rheumatic carditis and a *mild* valve lesion being forced to exercise strenuously.

OPERATIVE FINDINGS

Although most patients are young, mitral anular dilatation invariably allows the insertion of an adult-sized prosthesis. Despite friability of tissues during the active phase, we have attempted mitral anuloplasties or valvuloplasties in some patients.[12] Long-term results of these conservative procedures have not been satisfactory in the past, but we have seldom been certain whether penicillin was taken regularly by these patients. As a general principle, we have considered it advisable to insert a prosthesis rather than try to conserve the valve when severe active rheumatic carditis is evident, and particularly when subsequent patient compliance is in doubt. More recent experience in our unit, however, which is summarized under the "Concluding Remarks" of this chapter, reflect our reservations on this policy. A successful valvuloplasty, especially in a young subject, is clearly preferable to the insertion of any prosthetic valve.

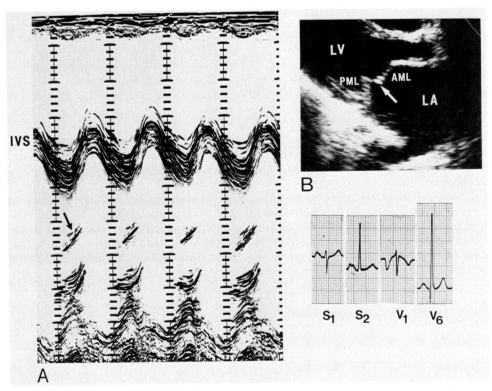

FIGURE 7-3. M-mode (*A*) and 2-D (*B*) echocardiograms in a 10-year-old patient with severe rheumatic carditis and acute mitral regurgitation due to ruptured chordae tendineae and a flail anterior leaflet (AML). *A*, Increased excursion of the septum (IVS) in a volume overloaded left ventricle. Echoes (*arrows*) in the left ventricular cavity owing to ruptured chordae. *B*, Long-axis view shows the flail AML (*arrow*). Selected ECG leads show left atrial enlargement and the typical pattern of left ventricular hypertrophy in mitral regurgitation. PML = posterior mitral leaflet.

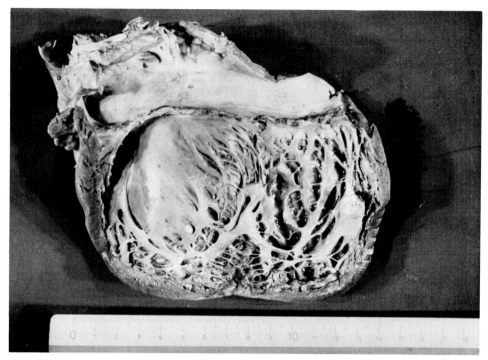

FIGURE 7-4. Necropsy specimen showing marked dilatation of the mitral anulus and left ventricular cavity with relative thinning of the left ventricular wall. (From Kinsley et al,[9] with permission.)

At least two thirds of patients suspected clinically of having active rheumatic carditis will have obvious macroscopic evidence at surgery to confirm this.[9] Features include acute fibrinous pericarditis, an aortitis characterized by macroscopic edema of the aortic adventitia, fibrin vegetations on valves, and edema of valve leaflets. The fibrinous vegetations occur on the atrial surface of the mitral leaflets, which themselves are friable, inflamed, and less transparent. The vegetations may extend along the chordae tendineae. In some patients, no morphologic alteration of the mitral leaflets is apparent, but mitral regurgitation results from a combination of dilatation of the anulus and elongation or rupture of the chordae tendineae, principally to the anterior leaflet (Fig. 7-3). The left atrium is invariably markedly dilated.

In at least half the patients, there is obvious left ventricular dilatation together with an apparent thinness of the left ventricular wall (Fig. 7-4). In some instances, pericardial adhesions over the left side of the heart make assessment of the size of the left ventricle at operation unreliable.

HISTOLOGICAL FINDINGS

In this series of 80 patients, tissues from valves, pericardium, atria, and aortic wall were removed when practicable for histological diagnosis. Three histological stages of the disease were recognized. In three patients the specimen was inadequate for histological examination.

Stage I: Alterative (Exudative-Degenerative) Phase

The 35 patients with this stage had an acute inflammatory cell infiltration, including polymorphonuclear leukocytes, lymphocytes, histiocytes, and eosinophils, into leaflet tissue. Mucoid edema of the ground substance was present, with fragmentation of collagen fibers. In several patients, the inflammatory process extended into the region of insertion of the posterior leaflet of the mitral valve and into the basal myocardium. Thirty-four patients with morphologic evidence of aortitis showed an acute, inflammatory cell infiltration on histology.

Stage II: Granulomatous Phase

Twenty-eight patients had disease in this stage. Twenty-one of these had Aschoff bodies in valve tissue, four had Aschoff bodies in the left atrial wall, three in the left ventricular myocardium at necropsy examination, and two in the right atrial appendage. Some patients had Aschoff bodies in several sites. The criteria used for recognizing Aschoff bodies were those proposed by Saphir[13] and modified by Roberts and Virmani.[14]

Stage III: Chronic (Healing) Phase

The 15 patients in this group had considerable fibrosis of leaflet tissue without histological evidence of acute inflammatory or granulomatous changes.

PATHOGENESIS OF RHEUMATIC MITRAL VALVULAR DISEASE

The *primary* effects of active rheumatic carditis are anular dilatation and an inflammatory valvulitis (Fig. 7-5). Dilatation of atrioventricular and semilunar valve anuli is common and usually enables the insertion of an adult-sized prosthesis even in children younger than 10 years. Dilatation of the mitral anulus may be extremely marked and measure as much as twice the normal area. Why do the mitral and aortic

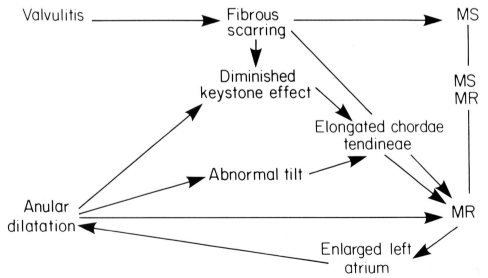

FIGURE 7-5. Pathogenesis of functional abnormality of rheumatic mitral valve disease. MR = mitral regurgitation; MS = mitral stenosis.

anuli dilate in active fulminant rheumatic carditis? The dimensions of the mitral and aortic orifices are controlled by muscular and fibrous tissue factors. The muscular component is the left ventricular basal myocardium, which incorporates the mitral and aortic anuli. Separating the anuli is the anterior leaflet of the mitral valve, situated between the two dense left and right fibrous trigones and suspended from the thickened triscalloped fibrous anulus of the aortic valve (see Fig. 1-7). The mitral leaflets themselves form a fibrous ring because of the 5 to 8 mm union in the commissural regions. Posteriorly, the mitral valve does not have a distinct anulus; rather, the posterior leaflet merges almost imperceptibly with the basal myocardium, which itself forms the posterior "anulus." Not surprisingly, mitral anular dilatation is maximal posteriorly. It would appear that fibrous rather than muscular factors are of greater importance in resisting anular dilatation. Thus, significant mitral anular dilatation does not occur with the ventricular dilatation associated with congestive cardiomyopathy, ischemic heart disease, and longstanding aortic regurgitation.[15,16] On the other hand, massive dilatation of the mitral or aortic anuli is common with Marfan's syndrome, a disease of connective tissue. The rheumatic process damages collagen fibres and the ground substance of connective tissue in the heart. We have confirmed the observations of Sacks[17] that the area of maximum infiltration of left ventricular myocardium with Aschoff bodies is close to the atrioventricular and semilunar valve rings. Concentration of acute inflammatory cells to the region of insertion of the posterior leaflet of the mitral valve into the basal left ventricular myocardium has also been noted. Thus, the failing, diffusely diseased myocardium affected by acute rheumatic carditis has a tendency to dilate. This tendency is not resisted by the weakened connective tissue of the mitral and aortic valve rings.

Secondary changes supervene following mitral anular dilatation. In the normal mitral valve, chordae tendineae are subjected to minimal tension during systole because of the keystone mechanism of leaflet coaptation (Fig. 7-6A). The directional velocity of blood is normally through the aortic valve, with mitral and aortic anuli being at an angle of approximately 130° to each other. When the mitral anulus dilates, the supportive keystone mechanism is lost and the angle between the aortic and mitral anuli is increased so that their relationship approximates the horizontal (Fig. 7-6B). The mitral leaflets (and hence the chordopapillary mechanism) are thus subjected to greater pressure and are under more tension during left ventricular ejection. Moreover, and as discussed in Chapter 1, left ventricular dilatation also causes an inefficient lateral, rather than vertical, pull of the papillary muscles. All these factors contribute to increased tension on the chordae tendineae and leaflets, themselves weakened by the rheumatic process, and result in elongated or ruptured chordae tendineae and flail leaflets. Another consequence of mitral anular dilatation is the stretching of the posterior leaflet so that it may become functionally retracted (Fig. 7-6B). This process in turn may be further aggravated by left atrial dilatation and by true retraction of the posterior leaflet owing to its fibrosis or thickened, shortened chordae tendineae.

Whereas the effects of active rheumatic carditis in the young tend to be concentrated on anular changes with secondary involvement of other structures, valvulitis may also result in considerable scarring of the valve with commissural fusion, thickened leaflets, and fused chordae tendineae (Fig. 7-7). These features are of a more chronic nature and account for the relative rarity of isolated mitral stenosis in the very young. Similarly, rheumatic aortic stenosis, especially in isolation, is exceptional. However, we have seen a small number of patients with active rheumatic carditis and moderately severe mitral regurgitation, presumably owing to anular dilatation, who present years later with mitral stenosis as the chronic effects of valvulitis prevail. This mode of progression probably accounts for the observation that some patients with chronic mitral stenosis have a dilated anulus at surgery. It would also explain the dilatation of the left ventricular cavity (see Chapter 5) that we occasionally encounter in adult patients with pure mitral stenosis.

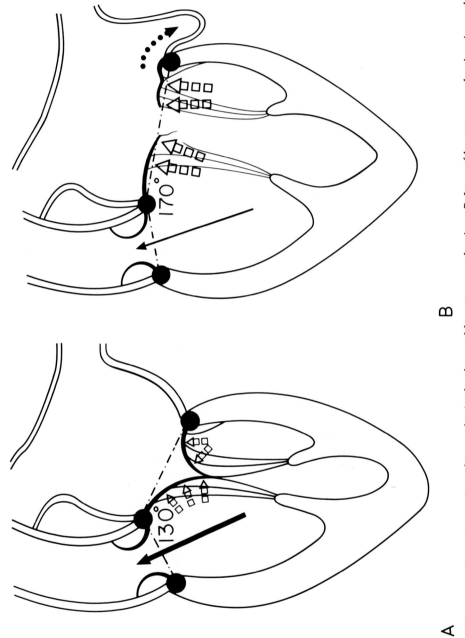

FIGURE 7-6. *A,* Diagrammatic representation of normal mitral valve and keystone mechanism. *B,* Loss of keystone mechanism in anular dilatation produces increased chordal tension and rupture. (For details, see text.)

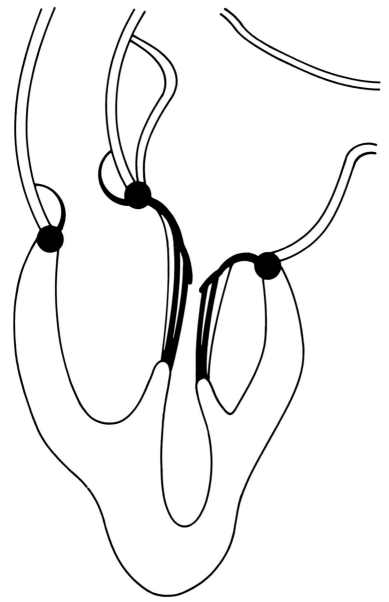

FIGURE 7-7. Diagrammatic representation of chronic rheumatic valvulitis showing thickened leaflets, fused thick chordae tendineae, and narrowed orifice of the mitral valve.

PATHOGENESIS OF RHEUMATIC AORTIC VALVULAR DISEASE

Similar changes may occur in the morphology of the aortic valve as in the rest of the heart in active rheumatic carditis (Fig. 7-8). Dilatation of the aortic anulus is a salient feature. Areas of greater dilatation have not been identified in the aortic anulus, possibly because the thick triscalloped fibrous anulus is of equal density throughout its circumference. Anular dilatation and a lateral displacement of commissures both contribute to a failure of cusp coaptation and thus to prolapse of the cusps.

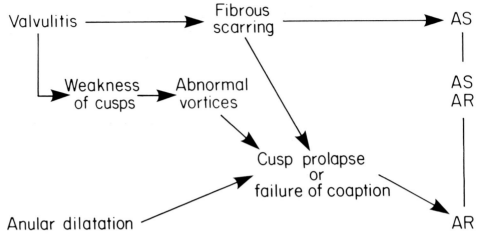

FIGURE 7-8. Pathogenesis of functional abnormality of rheumatic aortic valve disease. AR = aortic regurgitation; AS = aortic stenosis.

Not infrequently, especially in young patients with rheumatic aortic regurgitation, only very mild anatomical abnormalities of the aortic valve are detected at surgery despite the presence of free aortic regurgitation. We postulate that there are subtle changes in cusp geometry, owing to an acquired weakness of cusp tissue resulting from the rheumatic process. These changes, together with anular dilatation, may modify the aortic root vortices necessary for proper valve closure. Prolapse of the aortic cusps with gross regurgitation may result when the cusps fail to coapt.

When aortic valvulitis predominates, the chronic sequelae of cusp thickening, retraction, and commissural fusion ensue with variable degrees of aortic regurgitation and aortic stenosis.

MYOCARDIAL DYSFUNCTION IN ACUTE RHEUMATIC CARDITIS

Although there is little doubt that the myocardium is always affected in patients with active fulminant rheumatic carditis, the extent of the involvement is variable. The nature of the rheumatic myocardial dysfunction remains ill-defined. Histological changes such as Aschoff nodes, inflammatory cell infiltrates, and "coronary arteritis" are insufficient to explain the myocardial dysfunction; and Stollerman has postulated that there is a "toxic" effect. It cannot be emphasized too strongly, however, that left or right ventricular failure will not occur in the absence of a hemodynamically severe valvular, usually mitral regurgitant, lesion. Similarly, although relatively small pericardial effusions are not infrequent with active rheumatic carditis, we have rarely encountered a significant hemodynamic alteration from such an effusion with only a mild valvular lesion (Fig. 7-9).

There are two main causes of left ventricular dysfunction during or after active fulminating rheumatic carditis. The first, and probably more important, is the rheumatic myocarditis regarded by Stollerman as a "toxic" myocarditis. The second is related to the work overload produced by the severe mitral regurgitation similar to the left ventricular dysfunction, which supervenes in severe nonrheumatic mitral regurgitation and which reputedly may progress after repair or replacement of the valve. Because of the severe mitral regurgitation that is invariably present, echocardiographic assessment of myocardial function is usually misleading. It is common to find good, even supernormal, left ventricular contraction on echocardiography in

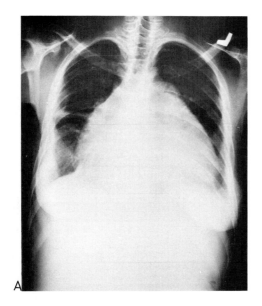

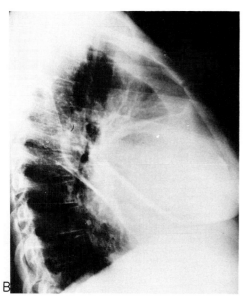

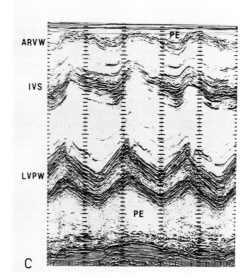

FIGURE 7-9. Posteroanterior (*A*) and lateral (*B*) chest radiographs of a patient with acute rheumatic carditis, mitral regurgitation, and a pericardial effusion. There is marked diffuse cardiomegaly. Interlobar effusions are visible in the lateral projection. *C*, M-mode echocardiogram shows echo-free spaces of the pericardial effusion (PE) surrounding the heart. There is paradoxical motion of the interventricular septum (IVS). ARVW = anterior right ventricular wall; LVPW = left ventricular posterior wall.

patients who were assessed on clinical examination as having dilated and poorly contracting left ventricles. Shortly after mitral valve replacement or repair, left ventricular contractile indices as assessed echocardiographically are invariably depressed. We have found it impossible to predict the long-term prognosis in the individual patient. Whereas some do well for many years, others do not improve and die of progressive myocardial dysfunction after two or three years. However, the long-term postoperative medical management in our experience has often been unsatisfactory. Many of these young patients attempt to exercise too early and fail to take adequate diuretic or vasodilator therapy or penicillin prophylaxis. We suspect

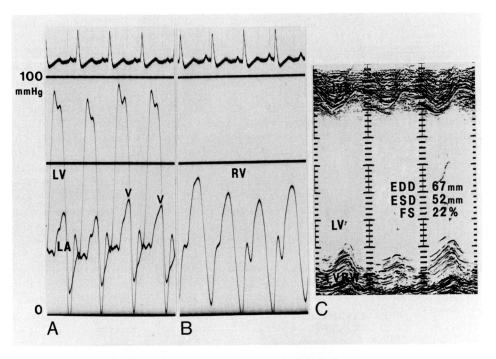

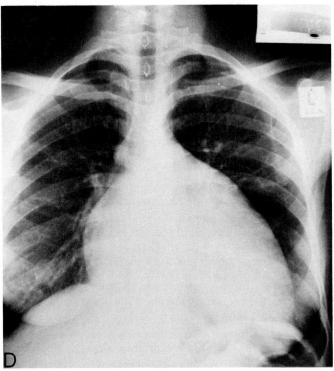

FIGURE 7-10. Severe mitral regurgitation with poor left ventricular function in a patient who refused surgery. *A,* Simultaneous left ventricular (LV) and left atrial (LA) pressures showing raised end-diastolic pressures and prominent V wave. *B,* Raised right ventricular (RV) systolic and end-diastolic pressures. *C,* M-mode echocardiogram demonstrates the dilated left ventricular cavity with poor contraction. *D,* Marked cardiomegaly depicted on the posteroanterior chest radiograph. EDD = end-diastolic diameter; ESD = end-systolic diameter; FS = fractional shortening.

that the long-term prognosis could be improved with ideal medical management. A few patients have such poor left ventricular function preoperatively that, despite significant mitral regurgitation, left ventricular contraction is depressed on echocardiography (Fig. 7-10). Even in those patients, the operative mortality is low, although the long-term prognosis is commonly but not invariably poor. It is very seldom that left ventricular dysfunction precludes cardiac surgery.

Although we favor that progressive myocardial dysfunction after valve replacement and the breakdown of some mitral valvuloplasties are important reflections of ongoing rheumatic activity due to recurrent streptococcal infections, there are three other factors that may contribute to progressive myocardial damage despite excellent patient compliance with prophylactic penicillin therapy. Two of these are recognized throughout the world following open heart surgery for nonrheumatic as well as rheumatic valve disease and are not entirely understood. Both are discussed in more detail in Chapter 8. The first has already been mentioned as a factor causing myocardial damage in patients with active rheumatic carditis and relates to the irreversible, and reputedly sometimes progressive, myocardial dysfunction, which may manifest or persist after successful surgical treatment of hemodynamically severe valve lesions. The second is the so-called postperfusion cardiomyopathy. It is the third factor that is of much interest to us and that relates to the possibility of ongoing rheumatic activity despite good secondary prophylaxis and thus eradication of recurrent streptococcal throat infections. We are convinced that active rheumatic carditis is considerably aggravated by the increased workload of an associated hemodynamically significant valve lesion; and we have already mentioned our frequent observation that pyrexia, cachexia, pericarditis, arthralgia, laboratory findings, and other parameters of severe rheumatic activity subside dramatically after successful valve surgery. In addition, we have observed the acute onset of active rheumatic carditis, despite definite penicillin prophylaxis, in several patients with chronic and presumably slowly progressive hemodynamically significant valve disease. There is therefore also a possibility that a dilated left ventricle, which is necessarily at a mechanical disadvantage, predisposes to some ongoing rheumatic activity following valve replacement despite virtually normal valve function.

CONCLUDING REMARKS

Active fulminant rheumatic carditis remains common in undeveloped populations including South African Blacks. For a number of reasons, we and others have to date failed to organize effective primary or secondary prophylactic programmes. We are pessimistic about anticipating a significant reduction in the high prevalence of rheumatic carditis in our Black population until socioeconomic factors improve. We are uncertain of the most pertinent socioeconomic factors but favor that malnutrition and infection during the first year of life may be important and that this possibility requires investigation.

Active rheumatic myocarditis never causes intractable heart failure in the absence of a hemodynamically significant valve lesion, most commonly mitral regurgitation. The regurgitant valve lesion results predominantly from anular dilatation, and leaflet pathology may be mild or absent. The treatment of such heart failure is essentially valvular surgery. We believe steroid therapy is not indicated and is never "lifesaving." "Rheumatic pneumonitis" is probably an unusual manifestation of severe pulmonary venous hypertension. It does not respond to steroid therapy but to improvement in the heart failure.

Active severe rheumatic carditis, with a hemodynamically significant valve lesion but without heart failure, will also often not respond to medical therapy. The hemodynamic lesion seems to perpetuate or aggravate the rheumatic carditis, and in such instances the patient should be treated surgically. Furthermore, a chronic and presumably progressive valve lesion may initiate acute rheumatic activity despite secondary prophylactic treatment.

Because of the importance of restoring normal or near-normal valve function and of problems with patient compliance relating to long-term secondary prophylaxis, we have favored the general principle of mitral valve replacement rather than valvuloplasty in patients with severe active rheumatic carditis that required surgical management. To date, however, all patients in whom we have implanted tissue and prosthetic valves have had significantly high valve-related morbidity or mortality. Conservation of the native mitral valve has obvious advantages, especially in children, young adults, and patients in whom tightly controlled anticoagulation is rarely practicable and valve failure may be catastrophic. During a two-year period, from 1983 to 1985, cardiac surgical colleagues in our unit operated on 70 patients with severe active rheumatic carditis. Early mortality (within 30 days of operation) was 4 percent. In 27 percent, operations were undertaken as emergency procedures. Mitral valvuloplasty was attempted in 30 patients (by MJ Antunes or PR Colsen) and was successful in 21 of these, with marked clinical improvement at the time of discharge from hospital. We plan a long-term follow-up but currently conclude that mitral valve repair is technically feasible during severe active carditis and that it is justifiable to persist with this policy.

During a two-year period ending in July 1985, members of our department analyzed the data on an additional 61 Black patients with active rheumatic carditis who were subjected to correction of severe mitral regurgitation. The active rheumatic carditis was confirmed at operation in all 61 patients. There were 40 females and 21 males, with a mean age of 13 ± 4 years. Mitral valve replacement was performed in 34 and mitral valvuloplasty in 27 patients. Histological corroboration of the diagnosis was available in 48 patients. In 13, all of whom underwent valvuloplasty, insufficient tissue was submitted for histological evaluation. Sixteen patients also required aortic valve replacement. All patients were classified as NYHA Class III (36 patients) or Class IV (25 patients). Cardiomegaly was confirmed radiologically by a mean cardiothoracic ratio of 66 ± 7 percent. Intraoperative pressures confirmed the severity of the mitral regurgitation and showed the following: mean left atrial pressure 26 ± 9 mmHg; mean left atrial V wave 49 ± 18 mmHg; mean left ventricular end-diastolic pressure 16 ± 6 mmHg. Preoperative 2-D and M-mode echocardiography demonstrated a markedly prolapsing or flail anterior leaflet in 57 patients, which was confirmed in all at operation. Mitral anular dilatation was present in 54 (95 percent), chordal elongation in 50 (88 percent), and chordal rupture in 4 (7 percent). Of the total 61 patients, some fibrosis and retraction of mitral leaflet tissue was noted in eight. This study confirmed that a severely prolapsing or flail anterior mitral leaflet is an extremely prevalent abnormality in severe mitral regurgitation caused by active rheumatic valvulitis. Flail or severely prolapsing anterior leaflets result from chordal elongation, which is almost always accompanied by anular dilatation. Chordal rupture was uncommon in this study, and this is in accord with our previous experience.

REFERENCES

1. McLaren, MJ, Hawkins, DM, Koornhof, HJ, Bloom, KR, Bramwell-Jones, DM, Cohen, E, Gale, GE, Kanarek, K, Lachman, AS, Lakier, JB, Pocock, WA, and Barlow, JB: *Epidemiology of rheumatic heart disease in Black schoolchildren of Soweto, Johannesburg.* Br Med J 3:474–478, 1975.
2. Bundred, P and Kitchiner, D: Personal communication, 1985.
3. Padmavati, S: *Rheumatic fever and rheumatic heart disease in developing countries.* Bull WHO 56(4):543–550, 1978.
4. Glover, JA: *Incidence of rheumatic diseases.* Lancet 1:499–505, 1930.
5. Devaux, P: *Some aspects of rheumatic fever in Soweto.* The Leech 49:67–68, 1979.

6. RANSOME, OJ, ROODE, H, SPECTOR, I, AND REINACH, SG: *Pharyngeal carriage of group A beta-haemolytic streptococci in Coloured and Indian schoolchildren.* S Afr Med J 64:779–781, 1983.

7. ARYANPUR-KASHANI, I: *On rheumatic fever in children.* (Letter to Editor.) Am Heart J 100:942–943, 1980.

8. JOHN, S, JAIRAJ, PS, RAVIKUMAR, E, KRISHNASWAMY, S, CHERIAN, G, AND SUKUMAR, IP: *Mitral valve replacement in the young patient with rheumatic heart disease. Early and late results in 118 subjects.* J Thorac Cardiovasc Surg 86:209–216, 1983.

9. KINSLEY, RH, GIRDWOOD, RW, AND MILNER, S: *Surgical treatment during the acute phase of rheumatic carditis.* In NYHUS, LM (ED): *Surgery Annual,* Vol. 13. Appleton-Century-Crofts, East Norwalk, CT, 1981, pp 299–323.

10. BARLOW, JB AND POCOCK, WA: *The problem of nonejection systolic clicks and associated mitral systolic murmurs: Emphasis on the billowing mitral leaflet syndrome.* Am Heart J 90:636–655, 1975.

11. STOLLERMAN, GH: *Rheumatic Fever and Streptococcal Infection.* Grune & Stratton, New York, 1975, pp 127–131, 139.

12. ANTUNES, MJ, COLSEN, PR, AND KINSLEY, RH: *Mitral valvuloplasty: A learning curve.* Circulation 68 (Suppl II):70–75, 1983.

13. SAPHIR, O: *The Aschoff nodule.* Am J Clin Pathol 31:534–539, 1959.

14. ROBERTS, WC AND VIRMANI, R: *Aschoff bodies at necropsy in valvular heart disease. Evidence from an analysis of 543 patients over 14 years of age that rheumatic heart disease, at least anatomically, is a disease of the mitral valve.* Circulation 57:803–807, 1978.

15. PERLOFF, JK AND ROBERTS, WC: *The mitral apparatus: Functional anatomy of mitral regurgitation.* Circulation 46:227–239, 1972.

16. BULKLEY, BH AND ROBERTS, WC: *Dilatation of the mitral anulus. A rare cause of mitral regurgitation.* Am J Med 59:457–463, 1975.

17. SACKS, B: *The pathology of rheumatic fever: A critical review.* Am Heart J 1:750–772, 1926.

BIBLIOGRAPHY

ATTIE, F, KURI, J, ZANONIANI, C, RENTERIA, V, BUENDIA, A, OVSEYEVITZ, J, LOPEZ-SORIANO, F, GARCIA-CORNEJO, M, AND MARTINEZ-RIOS, MA: *Mitral valve replacement in children with rheumatic heart disease.* Circulation 64:812–817, 1981.

AYOUB, EM: *The search for host determinants of susceptibility to rheumatic fever: The missing link.* Circulation 69:197–201, 1984.

BORMAN, JB AND GOTSMAN, MS: *Rheumatic valvular disease in children.* Springer-Verlag, Berlin, West Germany, 1980.

CHESLER, E, LEVIN, S, DU PLESSIS, L, FREIMAN, I, ROGERS, M, AND JOFFE, N: *The pattern of rheumatic heart disease in the urbanized Bantu of Johannesburg.* S Afr Med J 40:899–904, 1966.

DISCIASCIO, G AND TARANTA, A: *Rheumatic fever in children.* Am Heart J 99:635–658, 1980.

SUBRAMANYAN, R, KARTHA, CC, AND BALAKRISHNAN, KG: *Intramyocardial coronary arterial changes in rheumatic mitral valve disease. Relation to left ventricular function.* Cardiology 71:233–238, 1984.

TARANTA, A AND MARKOWITZ, M: *Rheumatic Fever. A guide to its recognition, prevention and cure. With special reference to developing countries.* MTP Press Ltd, Boston, 1981.

ZABRISKIE, JB: *Rheumatic fever: The interplay between host, genetics, and microbe.* Circulation 71:1077–1086, 1985.

8

SURGICAL ASPECTS OF MITRAL VALVE DISEASE

SECTION 1: PREOPERATIVE, PERIOPERATIVE, AND POSTOPERATIVE FACTORS

with MANUEL J. ANTUNES and WENDY A. POCOCK

Ideally, the diseased mitral valve, whether stenosed, incompetent, or both, should be repaired or replaced before damage to the myocardium is irreversible or the patient significantly symptomatic and disabled. However, the decision to subject a patient to valve surgery is made more difficult by the lack of a perfect prosthesis and by the fact that a large number of diseased mitral valves cannot be repaired. In this section, we discuss aspects of this complex problem that reflect some of our past and current experiences.

MITRAL STENOSIS

Stenosed mitral valves are often amenable to conservative surgery in the form of either open or closed mitral commissurotomy, both of which are currently associated with an extremely low mortality, provided patients with severe pulmonary arterial hypertension or marked tricuspid regurgitation are excluded. A mobile anterior leaflet is a prerequisite for a nonrestrictive and competent valve after commissurotomy. A rigid valve structure and the presence of heavy calcification usually preclude a good result, and valve replacement is required.

It has been suggested[1] that early operation might arrest the progressive fibrosis and distortion of the valve. Hence, we suggest surgery to many patients classified as NYHA Grade II, who are assessed as having conservable mitral valves. If mitral valve replacement is considered likely, patients are treated medically at least until Grade III symptoms ensue. Although the indication for operation in severely symptomatic patients (Grade IV) is seldom in question, the timing of surgery remains a problem and it is difficult to generalize.

In our experience, patients with tight mitral stenosis who present with pulmonary edema, with or without evidence of hepatic or renal failure, carry a high surgical mortality and "emergency" surgery is contraindicated. Aggressive medical therapy, which includes diuretics, inotropic drugs, and mechanical ventilation, achieves a dramatic improvement in most patients. After several days, rarely more than two weeks, patients can then be subjected to mitral valve surgery with little more than standard operative risk. We find it important, when possible, not to operate on patients until frank pulmonary edema has cleared and cardiac jaundice is subsiding. Moreover, we prefer to manage medically severe peripheral edema and ascites prior to undertaking surgery. In the exceptional cases when therapy fails to improve pulmonary edema or jaundice, we experience a perioperative hospital mortality of at least 25 percent.

CLOSED VERSUS OPEN MITRAL COMMISSUROTOMY

In the early days of cardiac surgery, closed mitral commissurotomy was the only method available for the treatment of mitral stenosis. With the advent of cardiopulmonary bypass, relief of the stenosis under direct vision became feasible, with the likelihood of improved results. Consequently, closed commissurotomy became increasingly uncommon and has been abandoned in many units. In our view, the closed operation still has a definite place in the treatment of certain types of stenosed mitral valves. Adequate leaflet pliability and normal subvalvar anatomy are essential for a good result. Absence of calcification must be demonstrated echocardiographically and fluoroscopically. These favorable characteristics are encountered in many of our young patients in the second to fourth decades of life. An ideal candidate for closed mitral commissurotomy is a patient aged 15 to 45 years, in sinus rhythm, without previous history of systemic embolization and with a pliable and noncalcified valve. The procedure is particularly useful during late pregnancy and in the presence of mild aortic valve disease. Relative contraindications to closed operation include atrial fibrillation, previous embolic episodes, and old age. The presence of only one relative contraindication does not preclude closed commissurotomy. Intraatrial clot and marked calcification of the valve are absolute contraindications. In our experience, most children with tight mitral stenosis have rigid valves, and open commissurotomy or valvuloplasty is preferable.

Immediate mitral valve replacement has been required in less than 2 percent of our patients referred for closed commissurotomy. In these rare cases, valve replacement has been possible through the same left thoracotomy incision that is extended posteriorly. An advantage of closed commissurotomy, often disregarded, is the relatively low cost. With the soaring costs of cardiac surgery, this is a distinct benefit provided that a good result can be anticipated and the patient's safety is not jeopardized. Practical experience with the operation is important, especially in units that are not equipped for open heart surgery. A problem with the closed technique is that it is difficult to teach. In inexperienced hands, good results are less certain with the closed than with the open procedure. Precise assessment of the characteristics of the valve, especially of commissures and subvalvar structures, is more difficult than when an open approach is used. However, this difficulty should be offset by an accurate preoperative assessment which, in our experience, proves correct in over 90 percent of the cases.

A detailed description of the technique of commissurotomy, open or closed, is outside the scope of this book. However, we consider that a brief account of some of the technical aspects, as practiced in our unit, is warranted.

Technique of Closed Commissurotomy

Closed commissurotomy is performed through a small left anterior thoracotomy and the orientation of the skin incision, in a submammary position in the female, is such that it may be extended posteriorly should the need for a valve replacement arise. Access to the pleural cavity is through the sixth intercostal space. The pericardium is opened longitudinally, anterior to the phrenic nerve and its posterior edge retracted posteriorly towards the edges of the thoracotomy wound, simultaneously retracting the left lung. A double-pledgeted horizontal mattress suture is placed in the apex of the left ventricle, and a purse string suture is inserted on the lateral wall of the left atrial appendage. After simultaneous measurement of the left atrial and left ventricular pressures (Fig. 8-1A), a clamp is applied over the base of the left atrial appendage and an incision, large enough to admit an exploratory index finger, made into the left atrium (Fig. 8-2). The anatomical characteristics of the valve and the degree of regurgitation, if any, are assessed by palpation. The Tubb's dilator is introduced through a small stab wound in the apex of the left ventricle and guided through the mitral valve orifice into the left atrium. The opening of the dilator is preset according to the size of the patient. In most cases it should be opened to 3.6 to 3.8 cm for an adult female and 3.9 to 4.1 cm for a male. The dilator is then opened fully in a slow but forceful movement. Frequently, there is an incomplete split of one of the commissures, which should then be opened further by digital dissection. With experience and practice, fused chordae tendineae and papillary muscles can be separated by this method. After final assessment of the valve, both the dilator and the finger are removed and the sutures tightly snared. Transvalvular pressures are measured again (see Fig. 8-1B). It has been our clinical experience that a residual transvalvular gradient predisposes to an increased rate of restenosis. This contrasts with the excellent long-term results of a completely unrestricted valve.

Rarely, immediate valve replacement is required owing to severe regurgitation produced by the tearing of a leaflet or rupture of chordae. In these cases, we prefer to use the same left thoracotomy incision that is extended posteriorly. Cardiopulmonary bypass is instituted by retrograde cannulation of the right ventricle through the main pulmonary artery and valve for venous drainage, and of the ascending or descending aorta for arterial return. A longitudinal incision of the left atrial appendage extended almost into the orifice of the left superior pulmonary vein usually provides adequate exposure of the mitral valve. The technique of implantation of the

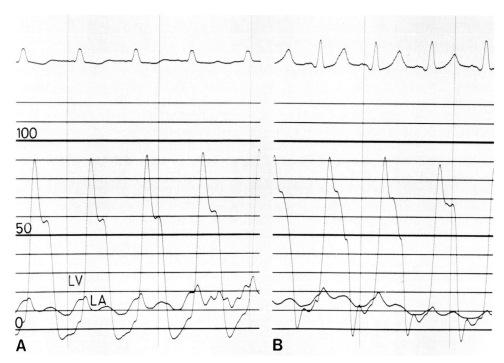

FIGURE 8-1. Intraoperative simultaneous left ventricular (LV) and left atrial (LA) pressures (mmHg) measured before (A) and after (B) closed mitral commissurotomy demonstrate a marked reduction in the diastolic gradient between the two cavities.

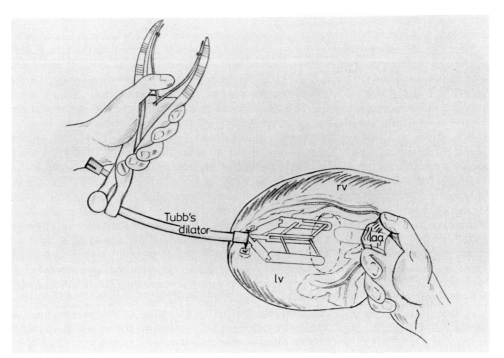

FIGURE 8-2. Technique of closed commissurotomy. An index finger is introduced through the left atrial appendage (laa) into the left atrium and helps guide the Tubb's dilator, which is introduced via the apex of the left ventricle (lv), through the mitral valve. rv = right ventricle.

prosthesis is similar to that used in elective valve replacement, which will be discussed later.

Technique of Open Commissurotomy

Open commissurotomy is performed through a median sternotomy, under standard cardiopulmonary bypass conditions, with moderate hypothermia and cardioplegic myocardial protection. Good exposure of the valve is essential. The line of commissural fusion is often difficult to identify. Vertical traction on the free edge of both leaflets with nerve hooks creates a wrinkle furrow that identifies that line. Alternatively, gentle distension of the left ventricle with cold cardioplegic solution or saline makes the relatively more pliable leaflet bodies bulge, thereby delineating the commissural furrow.

The scalpel incision is commenced in the central orifice and follows a gentle upward curve towards the anulus (Fig. 8-3a). This method facilitates the identification of the commissural chordae. The incision of the commissures must stop 5 to 8 mm short of the anulus in order to preserve the normal continuity of the leaflets at commissural level. Fused chordae are split longitudinally into the apex of the relevant papillary muscle (Fig. 8-3b). If the free movement of the posterior leaflet is impaired by thickening of secondary and basal chordae at the site of insertion, these are thoroughly resected (Fig. 8-3c). In order to achieve unrestricted flow through the mitral orifice, it is mandatory to relieve the chordal system of any obstructive component. In the central area of the orifice, fused chordae, which extend down to their insertion into the papillary muscles, often form a partial or complete curtain. This causes a severe obstruction to blood flow and impairs free movement of the leaflets, even in the absence of commissural fusion. Fenestration of this curtain, with excision of triangular windows of fibrous tissue, creates several "new" marginal chordae (Fig. 8-3d).

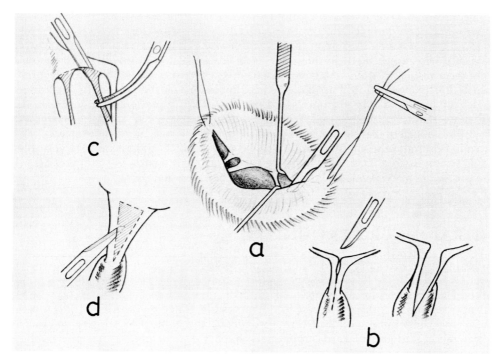

FIGURE 8-3. Technique of open commissurotomy. *a*, Sharp division of the commissures helped by retraction of the free edges of the two leaflets. *b*, When the chordae tendineae and the papillary muscle heads are fused at commissural level these are incised longitudinally. *c*, Thickened secondary and basal chordae contribute to the thickening and immobility of the posterior leaflet and are resected thoroughly. *d*, Fused chordae tendineae obstructing the flow of the blood are fenestrated by the removal of triangular portions of the fibrosed tissue.

Localised areas of fibrosis or calcification may be excised from the leaflet substance. However, large calcium masses are preferably treated by leaflet resection, provided enough tissue remains for reconstruction of the leaflet, which limits this method to the commissural areas of the posterior leaflet.

A good result is evidenced in the arrested heart by the "fall" of the two leaflets into the ventricular cavity, leaving a large mitral orifice. The valve is then tested for regurgitation by injecting cold cardioplegic solution or saline through an apical ventricular vent. In most cases, a water-tight valve is achieved. Small localised jets of incompetence at commissural level usually indicate that the incision was extended too far into the anulus. More centrally situated jets of incompetence are invariably caused by residual traction on the leaflets by abnormal shortened chordae tendineae, which must then be corrected. The intraoperative assessment of the adequacy of the operation is more difficult after open procedures than after closed procedures. All methods of valve testing during open heart surgery are nonphysiological, whereas direct palpation of the valve and assessment of incompetence jets are easier after closed commissurotomy.

RESULTS OF COMMISSUROTOMY

The mortality for open commissurotomy is approximately 1 percent, whereas that for closed procedures is slightly higher, at 2 to 3 percent.[2,3] The difference is probably related to a lower incidence of embolization of clot and calcium with the open procedure. It is important to note, however, that most reports are based on consecutive rather than concomitant series, closed procedures having been performed much earlier. Furthermore, mortality and morbidity rates do not include cases in which the procedures had to be followed by immediate valve replacement, which is more frequent after open commissurotomy (11 percent)[4] than after closed (2 percent)[5] commissurotomy. Claims that open mitral valvotomy is curative rather than palliative have not been confirmed. In our view, open commissurotomy will give improved long-term results in valves with significant involvement of the subvalvar structures, which, in any event, would not have been suitable for a closed procedure. We remain to be convinced that closed commissurotomy is not the operation of choice when the valve mechanism is pliable.

The long-term results for both methods are influenced by patient selection and most importantly, the variable rigidity of the valve, which makes comparisons unreliable or impossible. The assessment by the surgeon as regards the completeness of the procedure also correlates with the long-term functional result.[6]

MITRAL REGURGITATION

Again, there is difficulty in deciding on the timing of surgery. Despite gross regurgitation and marked cardiomegaly, patients may remain asymptomatic for many years. Deterioration of left ventricular function may not be evident clinically or on echocardiography until it is severe and irreversible. Since myocardial function is an important determinant of long-term prognosis, the timing of surgery is crucial. Improved techniques of cardiopulmonary bypass and of myocardial preservation have resulted in markedly decreased mortality and morbidity. Elective replacement of the mitral valve is now achieved with a mortality lower than 2 to 3 percent in most institutions.[7] Conversely, mortality will be higher for patients with cardiac cachexia, just as long-term results are also less likely to be satisfactory in these patients. However, the risk of a poor long-term result must be weighed against the potential valve-related morbidity and mortality risks of a mechanical or tissue mitral prosthesis or the likelihood of a failed valvuloplasty. Premature surgery should be avoided, and many surgeons are reluctant to operate on asymptomatic patients. On the other hand, we have had a number of patients with severe chronic mitral regurgitation who deny symptoms. Our policy is to operate on Class II patients if they have large hearts (cardiothoracic ratio of about 60 percent on roentgenogram) or left ventricular hypertrophy with "strain" on the ECG. Patients with Class III symptoms and good left ventricular function stand to benefit the most from surgery. However, it must be remembered that left ventricular dysfunction may be masked by mitral regurgitation and may only be evident after correction of the valve lesion. We remain uncertain of or unconvinced by any echocardiographic criteria that purport to indicate or preclude surgery. Poor left ventricular function preoperatively (Fig. 8-4) is usually a sign of severe myocardial damage and probably has grave prognostic significance, yet we cannot regard this as a definite contraindication to surgery in an individual patient. Patients with mitral regurgitation presenting with pulmonary edema also respond to medical therapy, but surgery should not be unduly delayed after the lungs have improved if the regurgitation is severe.

Patients with mixed mitral valve disease (stenosis and regurgitation) are treated on similar principles. In our experience, less than 25 percent of these valves are amenable to valvuloplasty procedures. We usually operate only on patients with at least Class III symptoms.

There is to date no ideal substitute mitral valve. Mechanical valves have a high incidence of thromboembolic complications; tight anticoagulation control is difficult to attain and has its own risks. Bioprosthetic valves have a high failure rate after five years in adults and much sooner in children. Consequently, operative techniques that aim at conservation of the patient's native mitral valve remain attractive. Techniques of reconstructive surgery, however, are not as reproducible nor are the results as predictable as with valve replacement.

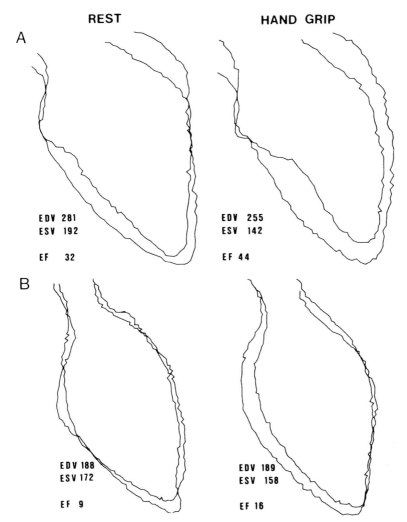

REST   HAND GRIP

A

EDV 281   EDV 255
ESV 192   ESV 142

EF 32   EF 44

B

EDV 188   EDV 189
ESV 172   ESV 158

EF 9   EF 16

FIGURE 8-4. Diagrammatic representation of frames from the left ventricular cineangiogram of a 20-year-old patient with severe mitral regurgitation. Systolic and diastolic frames at rest and during hand-grip exercise preoperatively (*A*) and after valve replacement (*B*). The ejection fraction (EF) is reduced at rest (32 percent) but improves with exercise to 44 percent. Postoperatively, the extremely low ejection fraction of 9 percent, increasing to only 16 percent with exercise, reflects the marked left ventricular dysfunction, which is unmasked by correction of the regurgitation. EDV = end-diastolic volume; ESV = end-systolic volume.

RECONSTRUCTIVE SURGERY FOR MITRAL REGURGITATION

Motivated by the inadequacies of mitral valve replacement, we have adopted a policy of mitral valve conservation whenever possible. More than 40 percent of about 750 patients who were subjected to isolated open mitral valve surgery for pure or predominant regurgitation during the last five years had conservative procedures. In the last year, the number has been 65 to 70 percent. Initially, this consisted of conventional mitral anuloplasty, but late results of this procedure have been disappointing. After eight years, the actuarial survival, free from reoperation, was only 42 percent; and only 27 percent of the survivors had normal or near normal valve function.[8] Why should mitral anuloplasty have such a high failure rate in underdeveloped populations? Certainly, continued rheumatic activity must contribute, but it cannot be the only factor. Carpentier[9] has emphasized that rheumatic carditis affects all the components of the mitral valve apparatus: the anulus, leaflets, papillary muscles, and chordae tendineae. Correction of only one abnormal component is an incomplete repair. Logically, therefore, surgical correction should be directed at repair of all affected components of the mitral valve. This concept of comprehensive valvuloplasty has not yet had universal acceptance, although enthusiasm appears to be increasing, and its sound functional and anatomical basis cannot be denied. The operation is more difficult to perform, especially by an inexperienced surgeon.

One of the most difficult problems facing surgeons who perform conservative mitral valve surgery is the "complex of guilt." The weight of a failed valvuloplasty is borne largely by the surgeon, as opposed to his or her "immunity" in relation to the complications of prosthetic valve replacement. This "complex" may be intensified by the attitudes of others, especially the cardiologist and the patient. Increasing litigation, which has almost philosophically become a consequence of medical practice, has also had a dampening effect on the surgeon's will to preserve the mitral valve. Hence, it is essential that surgeons be technically prepared and psychologically motivated when undertaking these conservative procedures. A larger number of failures early in their experience is inevitable. Moral support of the policy by the cardiologists is crucial, and the patient should be informed of the possibility of technical failure. When cardiac surgery is indicated and potentially lifesaving, however, we do not consider that is is necessarily to the patient's advantage to be involved in discussions on problems or possible complications of which he or she has little knowledge. The bona fides of surgeon and cardiologist have to be accepted, but peer review, always practicable in an academic department, is mandatory.

The Technique of Valvuloplasty

The basic concept on which valvuloplasty is based is that mitral valve disease, especially of rheumatic etiology, may involve all components of the mitral valve mechanism.[9] Hence, the mitral valve is seen as a functional unit and reconstructed as such (Fig. 8-5). Because of its complexity, the procedure requires longer cardiopulmonary bypass and aortic cross-clamp times, thus myocardial protection assumes special importance. In our opinion, the use of cardioplegia is essential, although the assessment of the valve anatomy may be more accurate when performed under ischemic arrest. Such assessment requires experience and sound knowledge of the functional anatomy of the mitral valve. Good exposure is required, and all components of the mitral valve, including the leaflets, anulus, chordae tendineae, and papillary muscles, must be examined meticulously in a sequential manner.

Isolated rheumatic mitral valve regurgitation often results from a combination of leaflet prolapse, leaflet retraction, and anular dilatation. Leaflet prolapse occurs in 75 percent of the cases and is caused by elongated or ruptured chordae tendineae. The former is corrected by shortening the elongated chordae (Fig. 8-5a). Ruptured chordae to the posterior leaflet are treated by quadrangular resection of the leaflet (Fig. 8-5b), which can be reduced to about half its length. Similar techniques applied to the anterior leaflet are usually unsuccessful, owing to the critical relationship between its surface area and closure of the valve. While some surgeons[10,11] favor the construction of new chordae tendineae, fashioned from either artificial or natural materials, transposition of chordae from the posterior to the anterior leaflet appears to give the better results (Fig. 8-5c). The presence of ruptured strut chordae to the anterior leaflet is probably a contraindication to valvuloplasty.

Diminished leaflet mobility, owing to retraction by fused chordae or scarring of the leaflet itself, is a cause of mitral regurgitation and is usually associated with a degree of stenosis. The posterior leaflet is often markedly retracted by the thickened triangular base of implantation of secondary and basal chordae, which must then be resected. An occasional secondary chorda that prevents full mobility of the anterior leaflet should also be resected. Masses of fused marginal chordae are divided or

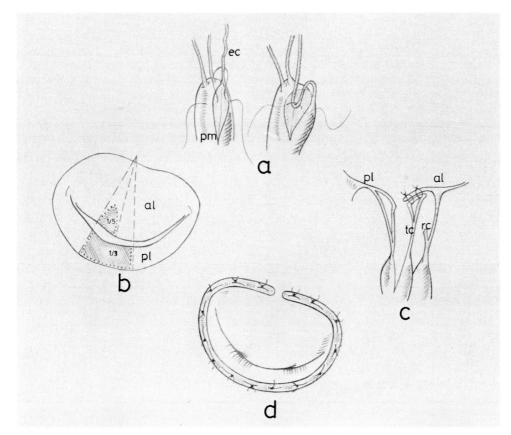

FIGURE 8-5. Technique of valvuloplasty for correction of mitral regurgitation. *a,* Shortening of elongated chordae tendineae (ec) by burying the excessive length into a trench created in the papillary muscle (pm). *b,* Leaflet resection; the two leaflets are resected following the triangular outline indicated. The anterior leaflet (al) can only tolerate small resections of up to one fifth of its free edge, while the posterior leaflet (pl) is amenable to a much wider resection, of up to one third of its substance. *c,* Transposition of chordae tendineae (tc) from the posterior leaflet (pl) to the anterior leaflet (al) to replace ruptured chordae (rc). *d,* Final result after implantation of Carpentier ring to consolidate the repair and to reshape the anulus.

fenestrated in order to restore near normal function. A mitral valve can only be repaired if the leaflets are made sufficiently pliable to open passively during diastole. Localised areas of thickening, including calcium deposits, should be "shaved" from the leaflet substance.

Dilatation of the anulus occurs in about 80 percent of cases of rheumatic mitral valve regurgitation. The anulus is not only dilated but also deformed. Hence, the implantation of a semirigid Carpentier ring is a most important part of the technique of valvuloplasty (Fig. 8-6). A main function of the ring is to reshape the anulus, but it is also important in securing the integrity of the anulus in cases of posterior leaflet resection. In order to avoid excessive narrowing and to allow unrestricted blood flow during diastole, a ring of appropriate size must be selected and placed in a position that conforms to the normal anatomy of the anulus.

After completion of the valvuloplasty, the valve is tested. In testing under cardioplegic conditions, the surgeon encounters the same problems as in the initial assessment of the functional anatomy of the valve. We observe for normal valve configuration, a good line of leaflet edge apposition, and absence of leaflet prolapse (Fig. 8-7). Simultaneous left atrial and left ventricular pressures are measured at the end of the procedure (Fig. 8-8).

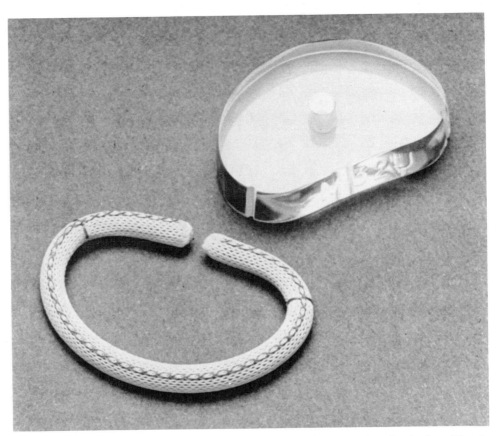

FIGURE 8-6. Carpentier ring for mitral anuloplasty and the respective plastic sizer. The size of the ring is chosen to match that of the surface area of the anterior leaflet.

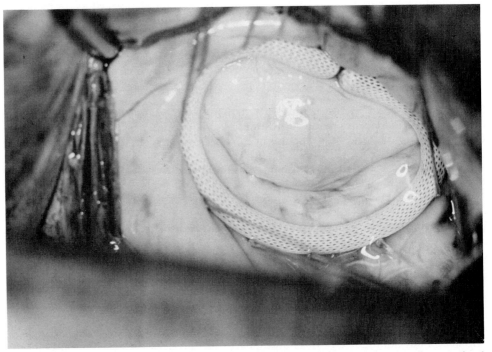

FIGURE 8-7. Intraoperative photograph of mitral valve after successful completion of valvuloplasty. Note that the apposition line between the anterior and posterior leaflets is regular and parallel to the posterior anulus of the mitral valve.

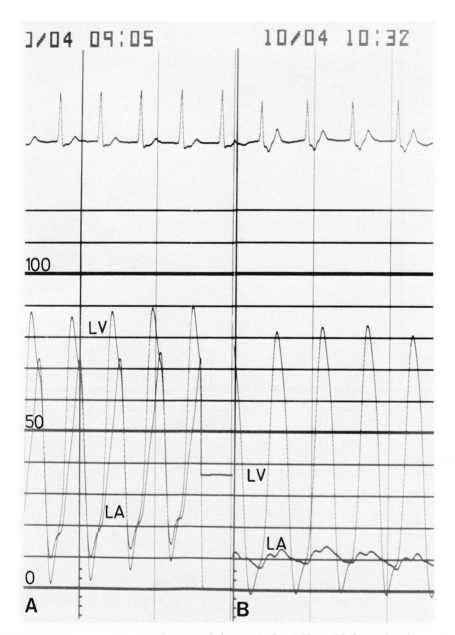

FIGURE 8-8. Intraoperative simultaneous left ventricular (LV) and left atrial (LA) pressures (mmHg) before (*A*) and after (*B*) mitral valvuloplasty for correction of severe acute mitral regurgitation. Note the amplitude of the V wave in the preoperative tracing.

RESULTS. The best results of mitral valvuloplasty are obtained in valves whose pathologies are of a degenerative etiology. Rheumatic valves are more difficult to repair and the results, especially in children, are not as good. In young rheumatic patients, ongoing rheumatic carditis further scars and distorts the valve mechanism, rendering the repair unstable. Even in the absence of clinically evident active carditis, it is probable that the healing process has not yet stabilised. In the past four years, one of us (MJA) and our colleague PR Colsen have performed mitral valve reconstruction on over 300 rheumatic patients, the majority for isolated or predominant mitral regurgitation, with an operative mortality of 2 percent. The late mortality was 3.1 percent per patient-year and was valve related in 40 percent of the cases. Ten

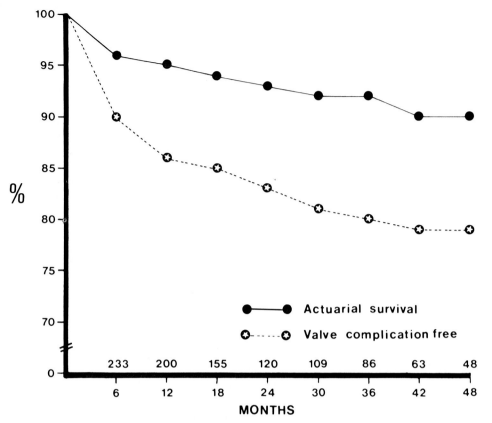

FIGURE 8-9. Actuarial global survival and survival complication-free of a group of 241 patients subjected to mitral valvuloplasty. After four years the global survival was 90 percent, and 78 percent of the patients were free from valve-related complications.

percent of the patients (4.9 percent per patient-year) have required reoperation, mainly for persistent or recurrent valve regurgitation. The incidence of valve failure was 6.1 percent per patient-year and was two times higher in patients younger than 12 years (7.8 percent per patient year) than in those older than 12 years (3.9 percent per patient-year), which probably reflects the influence of recurrent rheumatic activity in the younger age group. After four years, the actuarial survival was 90 percent, and 78 percent of the patients were free from valve complications (Fig. 8-9). These figures compare favorably with those of Carpentier and associates,[12] considering the differences in the population characteristics. They also compare very favorably with the actuarial survival of 78 percent and the valve-free complication of 63 percent in a similar population in which Medtronic-Hall mitral prostheses were inserted (Fig. 8-10). One of us (JBB) has assessed clinically the results of mitral valvuloplasty within 2 to 3 weeks of surgery in 125 patients from February 1984 to September 1985, without knowing the preoperative diagnosis. The results are shown in Figure 8-11.

Other complications were extremely rare after valvuloplasty. Systemic embolism or infective endocarditis occurred in less than 0.6 percent per patient-year in our patients. Only patients with atrial fibrillation were treated with anticoagulants.

PROSTHETIC MITRAL VALVE REPLACEMENT

The valve prosthesis is regarded as one of the major advances in the management of heart disease. Since the introduction of the caged ball valve by Starr in 1960,

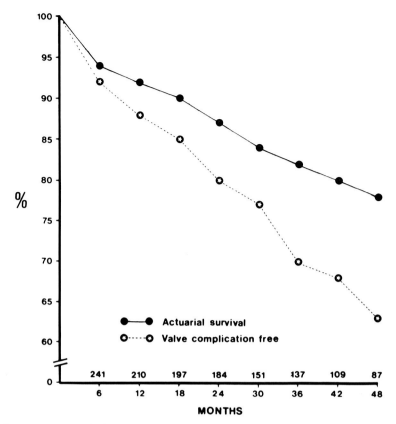

FIGURE 8-10. Actuarial global survival and survival complication-free of a group of 269 patients subjected to mitral valve replacement with a Medtronic-Hall prosthesis during the same period. After four years the global survival was 78 percent, and the survival free from complication was 63 percent.

nearly a million prostheses have been implanted in patients throughout the world. The characteristics of an ideal valve substitute include good hemodynamics, freedom from thrombogenicity, availability, and lifelong durability.[13] Other important features are ease of implantation, silent function, and low cost. Despite the progress made in the past two decades with evolution in design and materials, the ideal valve substitute has not been found. The variety of prostheses available for implantation testifies to the inadequacies of all existing designs.

Prostheses currently available for use as a mitral valve substitute fall into two categories: tissue valves and mechanical valves.

Tissue Valves

This type of valve was developed as a response to the thromboembolic complications that plagued the original mechanical valves. However, optimistic anticipation of complete freedom from thrombogenicity has not materialized, and thromboembolic rates of 2 to 5 percent per patient-year have been reported[14,15] for mitral valve replacement and in our experience is 1.3 percent per patient-year. These rates are much lower than those of mechanical prostheses, especially when it is considered that the patients are often not treated with anticoagulants. Absence of the necessity for anticoagulation remains the major advantage of these valves. Porcine and bovine (pericardial) xenografts are the most commonly used tissue valves.

The most popular porcine xenografts are the Hancock and the Carpentier-Edwards (Fig. 8-12, *top*) prostheses; and these are the tissue valves with which we

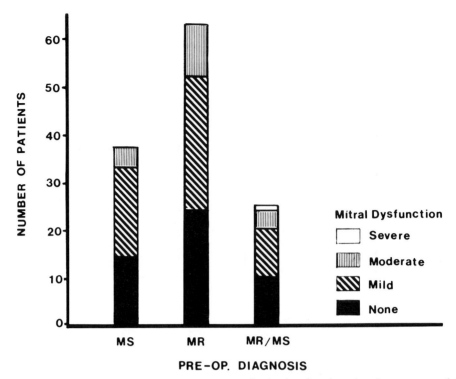

FIGURE 8-11. Early postoperative assessment of mitral valve function in a group of 125 patients subjected to mitral valvuloplasty showing that no or only mild mitral valve dysfunction was present in over 85 percent of the patients. MS = mitral stenosis; MR = mitral regurgitation; MR/MS = mixed mitral valve disease with significant mitral regurgitation.

have had most experience. Their original designs were modified, resulting in significant reductions of transvalvular gradients, which now compare favorably with those observed in some of the commonly used mechanical prostheses. One of the valves that evolved from the quest for a better hemodynamic performance was the bovine pericardial valve, developed by Ionescu and perfected and marketed by the Shiley laboratories. The popularity of the pericardial valve has increased, and both the Edwards and Hancock laboratories produce and market their own models. The mean transvalvular diastolic gradients of mitral pericardial prostheses are similar to those of the porcine xenografts. One of the disadvantages of the Ionescu-Shiley valve was its high profile, which sometimes encroached on the ventricular wall and left ventricular outflow tract. A lower-profiled design was used by the Edwards laboratory with their pericardial valve (Carpentier-Edwards) (Fig. 8-12, *bottom*); and this concept is also used in a new Ionescu-Shiley model.

The major disadvantage of tissue valves is lack of durability. Early degeneration and calcification are particularly evident in children (Fig. 8-13). In our experience,[16] only 19 percent of 135 patients under 20 years of age remained with a valve free from degeneration after a mean follow-up of 5.5 years, with a linearized valve failure rate of 22.5 percent per patient-year. The rate of failure was much lower in an adult population, but current evidence points to a mean duration of 8 to 12 years in the original glutaraldehyde-preserved models.[17] There is to date no confirmation that the durability of the pericardial valve is better than that of porcine xenografts. Moreover, modifications of the stent, of the fixation process (low pressure) and of chemical treatment (Hancock T6) have not yet demonstrated improved long-term durability of porcine bioprostheses. Amongst the new valves incorporating some of these advances is the Xenotech prosthesis, currently undergoing clinical testing.

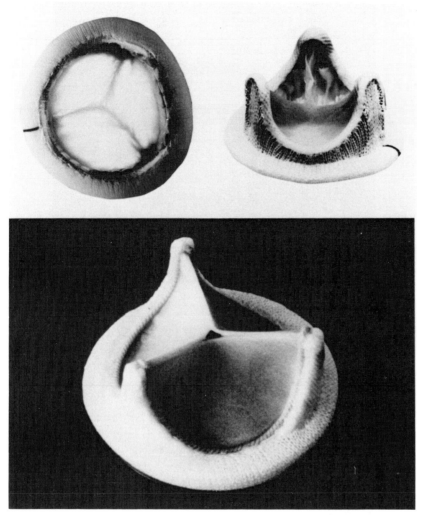

FIGURE 8-12. Bioprostheses used for mitral valve replacement. *Top,* Glutaraldehyde-preserved porcine Carpentier-Edwards bioprosthesis. *Bottom,* Carpentier-Edwards bovine pericardial valve.

Mechanical Valves

Of the many types of mechanical valves, some of which had little or no practical impact, two have stood the test of time and remain as the yardstick against which other prostheses are usually judged. These are the caged ball (Starr-Edwards) and the tilting disc prostheses.

The Starr-Edwards valve has been the most widely used but has had many modifications of the original design. These include the curation of the silicone rubber poppet (1965), cloth-covered struts (1967), a hollow stellite ball (1967), a composite seat (1972), and extended cloth cover of the ring. Only a slight improvement was achieved in the thromboembolic rate, which is reported between 2 percent and 9 percent per patient-year for all the models in the mitral position. Ironically, some of these modifications introduced other complications, such as hemolysis and thrombotic obstruction; and there has been a return to the old non–cloth-covered Silastic ball (model 6120), which is the only model currently available (Fig. 8-14). A problem

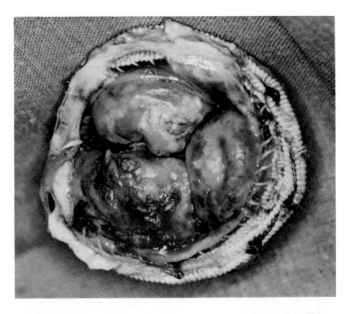

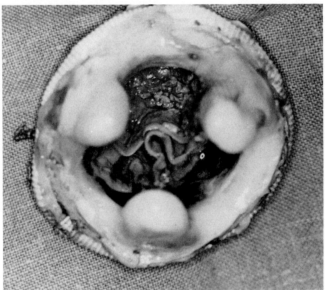

FIGURE 8-13. Degenerated bioprosthesis removed surgically, after two and a half years of implantation in the mitral position. *Top*, Atrial surface with partial tear of one of the cusps and some fibrin clot. *Bottom*, Ventricular aspect showing calcification of one of the cusps and the "creep" of the struts.

with the caged ball prosthesis is the small "third orifice" (represented by the space for blood flow between the ball and the ventricular wall), which may occur in patients with previous mitral stenosis and a small cavity of the left ventricle. In extreme cases, the ventricular wall impinges on the cage and impairs movement of the poppet. Hence, it is probably appropriate to limit the use of this prosthesis to patients with large ventricular cavities owing to volume overload by pure or predominant mitral regurgitation.

The tilting disc prosthesis was for a long period best exemplified by the Björk-Shiley valve, which has good hemodynamic properties and a central flow pattern. However, it has a high rate of thromboembolism and thrombotic obstruction (Fig. 8-15), which in our experience has reached 8 percent per patient-year. Some modifi-

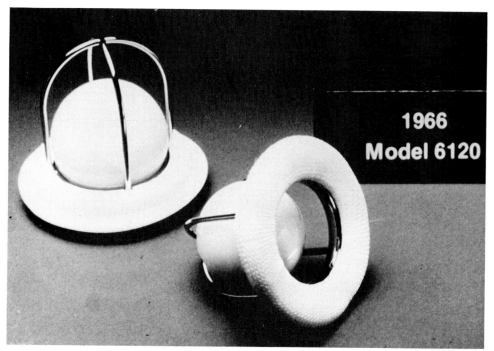

FIGURE 8-14. Starr-Edwards mitral prosthesis model 6120. This model, which was one of the earliest produced, is now the only one commercially available.

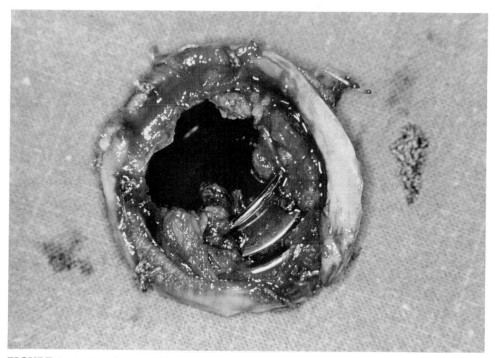

FIGURE 8-15. Atrial view of a thrombosed Björk-Shiley prosthesis removed surgically after three years of implantation. The large mass of blood clot obstructs the orifice and immobilises the disc.

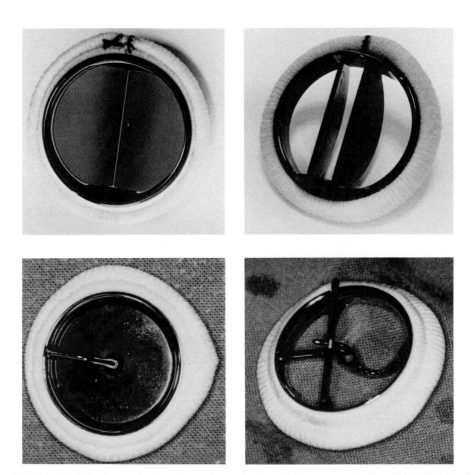

FIGURE 8-16. Mitral prosthetic valves currently inserted by our unit. *Top,* St. Jude bileaflet valve in closed *(left)* and open *(right)* position. *Bottom,* Medtronic-Hall valve, closed *(left)* and open *(right).*

cations were introduced, including the concave-convex disc and more recently, the monostrut valve. The former has had catastrophic structural failures, and the latter requires more clinical experience for accurate assessment.

Recently, a new generation of mechanical valves has been introduced, ostensibly with better hemodynamic and antithrombotic properties. These are the St. Jude Medical bileaflet and the Medtronic-Hall valves (Fig. 8-16). In our unit, these two valves have been implanted in over 2500 patients, who have been followed for nearly 5000 patient-years. Relatively low thromboembolic and thrombotic obstruction rates, varying with the population group, were observed. Both valves have negligible transvalvular gradients, other than in very early diastole, which is inevitable for all mechanical and tissue prostheses and which presumably relates to the absence of the "active" opening mechanism of a native mitral valve. Although slightly higher increased hemolysis was noticed with the Medtronic-Hall valve, this had little clinical significance.[18]

Choice of Prostheses

With the many types of prostheses available, the choice is difficult. The type of pathology and age of the patient are pertinent. A policy should be adopted to insert a limited variety of prostheses. A mechanical prosthesis is our choice for our relatively young Black population, most of whom have rheumatic heart disease. In this population group, we have had poor experience with tissue prostheses. The St. Jude Medical and the Medtronic-Hall valves have yielded the best results of mechanical prostheses used in our unit, and we currently favor their use in all population groups. The question of the advisability of using bioprostheses in older patients is as yet unanswered. Although the biodegradation rate is much slower in this age group, currently available models have a limited durability, and reoperation is required after several years in a number of patients, with increased risk in the aged patient. On the other hand, bioprostheses are probably indicated in women who may become pregnant. They should also be chosen for insertion in patients in whom anticoagulation is contraindicated or undesirable. Anticoagulation with coumarin derivatives has significant hemorrhagic complications and is not used by us in patients with peptic ulceration or coagulation disorders. We would prefer to avoid their use, but this is often not possible, in the large number of patients in whom tight anticoagulant control is impracticable.

Technique of Mitral Valve Replacement

Mitral valve replacement is performed through a median sternotomy, under standard cardiopulmonary bypass conditions, moderate hypothermia (25 to 28°C), and cardioplegic preservation of the myocardium. The same technique is used for the first valve replacement and for subsequent procedures, using cannulation of the descending aorta and of both vena cavae, through the right atrium. A second cannula placed in the aortic root is initially used for the perfusion of cardioplegia and later for the evacuation of air. The left atrium is opened longitudinally just posteriorly to the interatrial groove. The diseased valve is excised, leaving a 2 to 3 mm rim of leaflet in order to avoid disruption of the anulus. It is currently preferred to use a continuous suture technique. The sutures are passed through a firm fibrous area of the anulus. Using a continuous suture technique, a mitral valve can be replaced within a 12- to 20-minute aortic clamping time. An interrupted suture technique is preferred, however, in second and subsequent valve replacements. Depending on the size of the valve, 12 to 15 "figure-of-eight" or U stitches are placed at regular intervals. The use of Teflon pledgets is avoided, especially in the case of infected patients.

After implantation, the valve is made temporarily incompetent with a Foley catheter, in order to vent the left ventricle. Any thrombus is evacuated from the left atrial appendage. The left atrial wall suture line is left loose until the Foley catheter is removed near the end of bypass. Cardiopulmonary bypass is discontinued on reaching normothermia and after adequate de-airing of the left heart. Inotropes are not used routinely, although 1 g of calcium chloride is frequently added to the perfusate in the pump towards the end of the procedure.

In a repeat operation, only the right side of the pericardium is freed from adhesions. More extensive dissection is not necessary to achieve adequate exposure of the valve and is hazardous because of increased bleeding and the risk of left atrial or ventricular rupture. De-airing is facilitated by vigorously shaking the chest wall and by tilting the operating table sideways several times.

RESULTS. The operative mortality for isolated mitral valve replacement depends largely on the functional class of the patient at the time of surgery. From 1980 to 1983, a total of 689 patients of all racial groups had mechanical mitral valve prostheses inserted in our department. This includes all grades of disability, including emergency operations, and the early mortality was 5.6 percent. However, considering only Class III patients, the mortality rate was less than 3 percent. Patients with isolated mitral stenosis have a higher mortality than those with mitral regurgitation. Other factors that increase operative mortality include the presence of severe tricuspid regurgitation (10 percent) and hepatic or renal dysfunction (25 percent). The most prevalent causes of early death were myocardial failure with low cardiac output

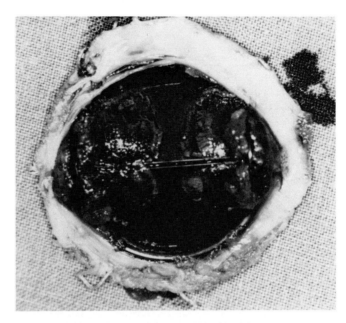

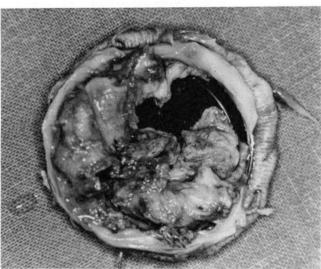

FIGURE 8-17. Thrombosed mechanical prostheses. *Top*, Atrial surface of a St. Jude prosthesis with leaflets immobilised by large clots that appear to originate from the hinge areas. *Bottom*, Thrombosed Medtronic-Hall prosthesis with the disc almost completely covered by a mass of organized blood clot.

(42.9 percent) and technical problems during surgery (35.7 percent). Late mortality averaged 4 percent to 7 percent per patient-year. With mechanical prostheses, late mortality was valve related in 25 percent to 39 percent of the cases, depending on the patient population (the initial percentage refers to developed country populations and the latter to Third World populations). Thromboembolic events (systemic emboli and thrombotic obstruction), anticoagulation-related hemorrhage, and prosthetic infective endocarditis were the cause in 39 percent, 36 percent, and 25 percent, respectively, of the developed country populations and in 45 percent, 6 percent, and 26 percent, respectively, of the Third World populations. In 16 percent of the latter group, bland periprosthetic leaks were the cause of the valve-related mortality. Systemic thromboembolism occurred at a linearized rate of 2.74 percent to 4.16 percent per patient-year, of which as many as 2.14 percent per patient-year were fatal or left neurological sequelae. The incidence of systemic thromboembolism was 4 to 5 times greater in patients with atrial fibrillation than in those with sinus rhythm. Thrombotic obstruction (Fig. 8-17) occurred in 0.65 percent to 0.80 percent per patient-year, and two thirds of the episodes were fatal. Overall actuarial survival was 78 percent to 87 percent at five years, but only 63 percent to 75 percent of the survivors were free of valve-related complications during the same period.

EARLY POSTOPERATIVE COMPLICATIONS AND MANAGEMENT

HEMORRHAGE

Excessive hemorrhage in the immediate postoperative period occurs in 5 percent to 10 percent of the patients and may be technically related (inadequate intraoperative hemostasis) or due to a deficiency in the coagulation system.

Clotting abnormalities that exist before surgery are most commonly related to low prothrombin levels, either from coumarin derivatives or from chronic hepatic distention due to prolonged tricuspid regurgitation. Patients with low prothrombin levels are given vitamin K preoperatively. Fresh frozen plasma is included in the pump prime or administered immediately after cardiopulmonary bypass. Other bleeding problems may relate to cardiopulmonary bypass, to the use of platelet-depleted stored blood, and to heparin. Fresh blood should be used in the pump whenever possible. Alternatively, the retransfusion of autologous blood, collected from the patient prior to the institution of cardiopulmonary bypass, or the use of a bloodless prime, has been shown by some[9] to decrease the amount of blood loss in the immediate postoperative period. The control of heparinization during and immediately after discontinuation of cardiopulmonary bypass is greatly facilitated by monitoring the activated clotting time. The aim is to return it to preoperative values. Small doses of protamine sulphate should be administered in the intensive care unit (ICU) to counteract the phenomenon of heparin rebound.

The definition of excessive bleeding varies widely. In our unit, amounts of less than 350 cc in the first hour and 250 cc in each of the next four hours in an adult (correspondingly less for children and teenagers) are considered acceptable. Quantities larger than these or signs of cardiac tamponade constitute an indication for surgical re-exploration, provided that deficiencies in coagulation have been excluded and corrected.

We have found positive end-expiratory pressure (PEEP) to be useful when the source of hemorrhage is within the anterior mediastinum, rather than within the pericardium. The approximation of the two mediastinal pleura presumably contributes to hemostasis in low-grade venous oozing resulting from the surgical dissection. The accumulation of large amounts of thrombus in the pericardial sac or anterior mediastinum appears to delay hemostasis by impeding the approximation of tissues. We recommend removal of these clots with a tracheal suction catheter introduced under strict aseptic conditions via the drainage tubes. This is often followed by a dramatic fall in the bleeding rate.

Following this policy, re-exploration of the mediastinum has been required in less than 1 percent of our cases subjected to open heart procedures. At such surgery there is often a significant amount of fresh thrombus, but no major bleeding point is usually identified. The pericardial space and anterior mediastinum are evacuated of clots and thoroughly irrigated with an antibiotic saline solution.

PERICARDIAL EFFUSION

Pericardial fluid probably occurs in at least 50 percent of patients following cardiac surgery and is unrelated to the type of operation. Clinical suspicion may be confirmed by 2-D echocardiography, which also gives an indication of the amount and location of the fluid. Low-grade pyrexia may be present. Most patients are asymptomatic and have a normal or a mildly raised systemic venous pressure. The majority of effusions occur in the first postoperative week but reabsorb spontaneously within a few days. Complete resolution may take several weeks. We are not convinced that the rate of resolution is hastened by medication, but symptomatic therapy includes salicylates and other nonsteroidal anti-inflammatory drugs. Significant hemodynamic alteration must be carefully sought, and, in the case of cardiac tamponade, pericardiocentesis is lifesaving. We have experienced a few patients in whom drainage had to be established as an extreme emergency by reopening the lower extremity of the fresh mediastinal wound while the patient was in the ward. Dramatic clinical improvement followed the drainage. In some instances, the effusion recurs after removal of the drain, or the fluid collection may be loculated making drainage difficult. The establishment, through a small left thoracotomy, of a pericardial window for free drainage into the pleural cavity is occasionally indicated.

POSTOPERATIVE INFECTION

All our patients subjected to cardiac surgery are treated prophylactically with antibiotics. We administer 2 g cephradine (Cefril) intravenously before cardiopulmonary bypass and continue with 1 g every six hours for 48 hours or until the chest drainage tubes are removed. Alternatively, cefazolin sodium (Kefzol), 1 g initially and 500 mg every eight hours intravenously, is used. Early prosthetic infective endocarditis is now rare in our experience. Superficial wound infection usually occurring 5 to 10 days postoperatively is easily recognized and treated by simple drainage procedures by breaking through the thin layer of epithelium covering the small cutaneous abscesses. Antibiotics are seldom required, and the septic focus is usually eliminated immediately after drainage. Deep mediastinal infection is rare and develops mainly in patients with a complicated immediate postoperative period, especially those who required external cardiac massage or who are very obese. The infection is often diagnosed or confirmed only after dehiscence of the sternum occurs. This serious complication requires surgical intervention involving reopening the skin and subcutaneous tissues, removing the sternal wires, clearing the mediastinum of all septic material, and irrigating the mediastinum with an antibiotic or antiseptic solution. Irrigation of the mediastinum is continued for 5 to 10 days, and the drainage catheter is then withdrawn progressively. Occasionally, contrast sinography is performed to exclude the presence of residual infected cavities. Adequate antibiotic cover is mandatory.

ANTIFAILURE THERAPY

Patients with mitral valve disease who have had a cardiopulmonary bypass may be fluid overloaded in the early postoperative period. We prescribe antifailure therapy (Table 8-1) to most patients subjected to mitral valve surgery as soon as possible and invariably continue this for at least six weeks and usually longer. Antifailure therapy is particularly important in patients who have had reconstructive mitral valve surgery, those with poor left ventricular function, and those with preoperative tricuspid regurgitation. Furosemide is routinely started in doses of 40 to 240 mg daily, and the dosage is later adjusted according to the response and the requirements. We have found good potentiation of the effect of furosemide by metolazone and use this com-

TABLE 8-1. Oral Antifailure Therapy After Mitral Valve Surgery

DRUG	USUAL DAILY DOSAGE
DIURETICS	
Furosemide	40–240 mg
Spironolactone	50–200 mg
Metolazone	2.5–10 mg
VASODILATORS	
Hydralazine	60–150 mg
Prazosin	1.5–3 mg
Captopril	25–75 mg

bination in patients with intractable cardiac failure. We frequently prescribe vasodilators (Table 8-1) including hydralazine, prazosin, and captopril in cases of previous pure or dominant mitral regurgitation, especially when associated left ventricular dysfunction is apparent.

SECTION 2: LATE POSTOPERATIVE COURSE AND COMPLICATIONS: EMPHASIS ON THE "RESTRICTIVE-DILATATION" SYNDROME

with WENDY A. POCOCK, MANUEL J. ANTUNES, PINHAS SARELI, and THEO E. MEYER

PERICARDIAL TAMPONADE

Although pericardial hemorrhage or effusion causing significant hemodynamic alteration most commonly occurs within two weeks of cardiac surgery and therefore before the patient is discharged from hospital, cardiac tamponade has been observed several months later. This complication is particularly dangerous, may occur without warning, and should be suspected in any patient with postoperative hemodynamic deterioration. There are often no associated symptoms or clinical features of the postcardiotomy syndrome.

Patients may complain of recent onset of breathlessness, swelling of the ankles, and tiredness. An important symptom, which may mislead the unwary medical advisor, is severe upper abdominal pain due to acute hepatic distension. The clinical signs include pulsus paradoxus, marked elevation of the jugular venous pulse, stony dullness to cardiac percussion, tender nonpulsatile hepatomegaly, faint heart sounds, small QRS voltages, and often an "electrical alternans." Echocardiography will confirm the pericardial effusion. Immediate pericardiocentesis, either by needle aspiration or surgical drainage, is mandatory. The fluid may be straw colored or bloodstained. In the latter instance, we suspect that anticoagulant therapy has caused or contributed to the pericardial effusion. Patients are treated with anti-inflammatory drugs and monitored by echocardiography. Drainage may need to be repeated, and in resistant cases a pericardial window is indicated.

Although some pericardial fluid can be demonstrated echocardiographically after cardiac surgery in many patients, this is usually not hemodynamically important and therapy with anti-inflammatory drugs may suffice. Pericardial effusion causing significant hemodynamic alteration, especially after discharge from hospital, is a life-threatening complication, and medical therapy alone should not be attempted.

VALVE DYSFUNCTION

Our clinical experience of Björk-Shiley, porcine, St. Jude, and Medtronic-Hall valves is large, and clinical aspects of their dysfunction will now be discussed.

PARAVALVULAR REGURGITATION

Ring leaks may be present immediately after valve replacement or may develop at any time thereafter. Late onset of paravalvular regurgitation should always arouse suspicion of infection, but this is not invariably responsible. Hancock and Carpentier-Edwards porcine valves in the mitral position frequently produce an apical systolic murmur that may be difficult to differentiate from mitral regurgitation. This "normal" murmur is somewhat harsh, often Grade 2 or 3 in intensity, and probably arises from the struts. A recent alteration of its character, particularly if it becomes musical or honking, is diagnostic of mitral regurgitation. When regurgitation supervenes several years after insertion, it may be difficult on auscultation to distinguish a ring leak from valve degeneration and consequent prolapse of one the leaflets. If the systolic murmur is musical, leaflet prolapse is the more likely.

Paravalvular regurgitation of any prosthetic valve in the mitral position should be suspected when the postoperative course is unsatisfactory or the patient's condition deteriorates at any time during the postoperative period. Recent onset of left or right ventricular failure, a left atrial lift, and appropriate auscultatory features should be carefully sought. In our experience, a ring leak of a Björk-Shiley, St. Jude, or Medtronic-Hall valve has never been completely silent, although, even with a severe ring leak, the pansystolic murmur may be localised and only Grade 1 in inten-

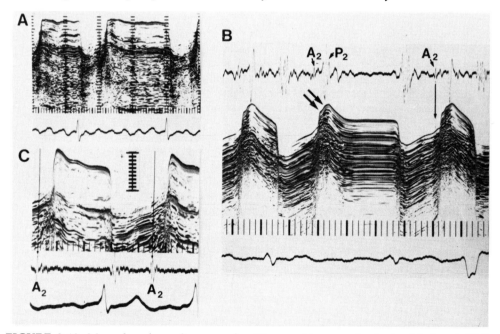

FIGURE 8-18. M-mode echocardiogram of a 45-year-old man who had a Medtronic-Hall valve inserted for mixed mitral valve disease (A) and who three weeks later developed a paravalvular leak (B). A, normal pattern of Medtronic-Hall valve opening. B, Rounded opening movement ("hump") of the disc (*double arrow*) with a very short interval between A2 (*long arrow*) and mitral valve opening. C, After correction of the paravalvular regurgitation, the valve opening movement is normal and the "hump" has disappeared. The time interval from A2 (*long arrow*) to opening of the mitral valve is normal. A2 = aortic valve closure; P2 = pulmonary valve closure.

sity. Radiation of the murmur is variable, depending on the site of the leak and therefore of the direction of flow of the regurgitant jet. It may radiate to the sternum, towards the base, or over the back. Such sites of radiation of a soft systolic murmur due to native mitral valve regurgitation would be unusual. A second highly contributory sign of a Björk-Shiley, St. Jude, or Medtronic-Hall valve ring leak is a long mid-diastolic murmur. In the absence of associated aortic regurgitation, these prosthetic valves do not normally produce a long mid-diastolic murmur. The murmur is presumably caused by the large volume of blood returning rapidly, through both the prosthetic valve orifice and the ring leak itself, to the left ventricle and resulting in turbulence around the open disc or discs. Similarly, the short mid-diastolic murmur occurring with a normal porcine valve may become much louder and longer in the presence of a ring leak. Associated tricuspid stenosis as a cause of a long mid-diastolic murmur is a diagnostic pitfall for the unwary.

Increased hemolysis may ensue with a ring leak of any prosthetic valve and assists in confirming the diagnosis.

Echocardiographic features of significant paravalvular regurgitation are loss of paradoxical movement of the interventricular septum, systolic expansion of the left atrium, and a relatively "hyperactive" left ventricle. An early diastolic "hump" has proved a reliable echocardiographic sign of a mitral ring leak in Björk-Shiley and Medtronic-Hall valves (Fig. 8-18). The sign is reliable when detected, but we have not always been able to demonstrate it, even in the presence of severe paravalvular regurgitation.

VALVE DEGENERATION OR OBSTRUCTION

Björk-Shiley Mitral Prosthesis

The normal opening and closing clicks of this prosthesis in the mitral position are easily audible; the opening click is softer than the closing click. The clicks are usually best heard near the apex but may be loudest or only audible in a localised area near the sternal border or at the base of the heart. The normally functioning prosthesis may produce a soft, short mid-diastolic murmur; but this is unusual. Recent onset of a mid-diastolic murmur should arouse suspicion of endothelial ingrowth or early thrombus formation.

Patients with thrombosis of a Björk-Shiley mitral valve commonly present with acute, progressive dyspnea occurring over several days or even over a few hours. The most reliable auscultatory sign is disappearance of the opening click, but the continued presence of the opening click does not exclude the possibility of early thrombus formation. With thrombosis of this valve, a mid-diastolic murmur is often inaudible, or it may be short and soft. The closing click may become muffled but is frequently still audible even when the valve orifice is almost completely occluded. Clinical features of acute occlusion include right ventricular failure, a hyperdynamic right ventricle with a loud pulmonary closure sound, and radiological signs of pulmonary edema. Dense echos (Fig. 8-19) on M-mode echocardiography, diminution of the amplitude of valve disc excursion, and slowing of the opening and closing rates confirm the diagnosis. Cinefluoroscopy may confirm limitation of disc movement (less than 60°) in the newer models, in which a thin radio-opaque wire encircles the disc. The cinefluoroscopic findings should be interpreted with caution. We have experienced severely thrombosed mitral Björk-Shiley prostheses when cinefluoroscopic evidence of disc movement had appeared nearly normal.

From the rapid progression of symptoms and clinical deterioration, it is apparent that once thrombosis commences on a mitral Björk-Shiley prosthesis, critical obstruction to forward flow quickly ensues. Delay necessitated by cardiac catheterization is dangerous and should be avoided. The clinical features alone are almost always sufficiently characteristic for obstruction of a mitral Björk-Shiley prosthesis

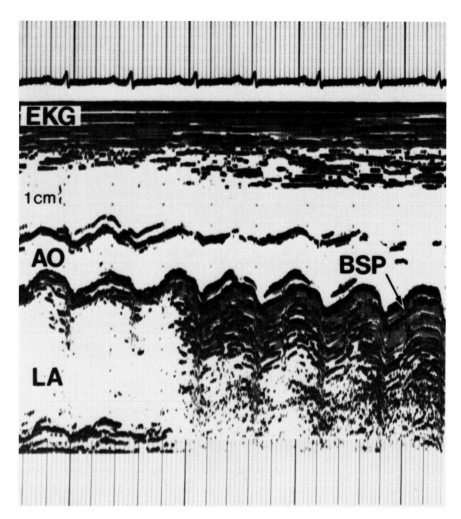

FIGURE 8-19. M-mode echocardiogram of a thrombosed Björk-Shiley mitral prosthesis (BSP). The amplitude of valve excursion is diminished, the opening and closing rates are reduced, and dense echoes posterior to the prosthesis reflect the thrombus. (From Copans, M, Lakier, JB, Kinsley, RH, Colsen, PR, Fritz, VU, and Barlow, JB: *Thrombosed Bjork-Shiley mitral prostheses.* Circulation 61:169–174, 1980, with permission.)

to be diagnosed but should if possible be confirmed by echocardiography and cinefluoroscopy. As soon as obstruction of the prosthesis is recognized, it is mandatory that the patient be referred for immediate surgery. This is lifesaving surgery, and the operative results are excellent.

Porcine Bioprostheses

We have experience of the Hancock and the Carpentier-Edwards porcine bioprosthetic valves. Within two or three years the valves calcify in children and young adults, and within about seven years in the older patient there is a high incidence of torn leaflets owing to valve fatigue. For these reasons, we have virtually abandoned the use of porcine bioprostheses in the mitral position.

The closing click of the normal porcine bioprosthesis is similar to a loud normal left-sided component of the first heart sound. The opening click is seldom heard. A short mid-diastolic murmur may occur normally. Onset of mitral regurgitation may be detected by the presence of high-frequency pansystolic vibrations and by other clinical evidence of regurgitation. A long mid-diastolic murmur is compatible with a ring leak, increased rigidity of leaflets, or significant regurgitation due to a flail leaflet. We have not encountered retraction or shortening of porcine valve leaflets as a result of degeneration. A musical systolic murmur is diagnostic of a partially torn, prolapsed, or flail leaflet despite hemodynamically mild mitral regurgitation. More severe regurgitation is inevitable after days or weeks, and a musical systolic murmur arising in a mitral tissue valve is an indication for early valve replacement.

Apart from the detection of calcification, cinefluoroscopy has been of limited assistance in the assessment of dysfunction of porcine bioprostheses in the mitral position. Thickening of severely degenerated leaflets may be detected echocardiographically. Echocardiography will confirm other features of severe regurgitation, such as left atrial systolic expansion; but we have seldom been able to demonstrate a flail leaflet.

Although there is usually a more gradual progression of symptoms resulting from a degenerating porcine bioprosthesis compared with that of thrombotic occlusion on disc prosthetic valves, we have experienced notable exceptions. Development of a flail leaflet may produce sudden-onset severe mitral regurgitation. Alternatively, we encounter extremely severe stenosis of degenerated porcine leaflets, especially in young Black patients who have denied symptoms until a few weeks or even days before admission to hospital. Our current policy is to perform regular echocardiographic studies at six-month intervals in patients with porcine prostheses to detect calcification and degeneration.

Medtronic-Hall Disc Prosthesis

Previously known as the Hall-Kaster prosthesis, this prosthesis is mechanically sound and easily assessed clinically, and we continue to use it. The opening click is always audible but may be confined to a fairly small area on the chest at the sternal border, apex, or base of the heart. Although disappearance of the opening click indicates abnormal disc movement, it is important to appreciate that an opening click may be heard despite considerable limitation of disc opening. Systolic and long mid-diastolic murmurs arising at the Medtronic-Hall prosthesis in the mitral position have similar significance to those murmurs occurring with mitral Björk-Shiley and St. Jude prostheses.

An early diastolic "hump" on echocardiography is a reliable sign of a ring leak with this prosthesis. To date, we have encountered false-negative but not false-positive results of this sign. Incomplete opening of the disc, owing to tissue ingrowth or thrombus, may be confirmed both echocardiographically and cinefluoroscopically (Fig. 8-20).

St. Jude Bileaflet Prosthesis

Although we favor and continue to use this prosthesis, we find it more difficult to assess clinically than the Medtronic-Hall prosthesis. The normal mitral opening click is usually soft or even inaudible in a large number of patients. Conversely, we have encountered patients in whom the opening click remained audible because only one of the two leaflets was immobilised by thrombosis. The closing click is clearly audible, except when advanced thrombotic occlusion has supervened. As with the Medtronic-Hall and Björk-Shiley prostheses, a long mid-diastolic murmur is abnormal and requires explanation.

The St. Jude prosthesis is not seen on a plain chest radiograph, but movement of the leaflets can be assessed accurately on cinefluoroscopy and by echocardiography.

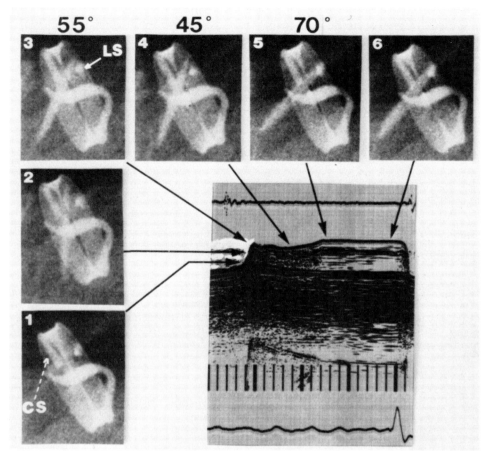

FIGURE 8-20. M-mode echocardiogram of a 24-year-old man with atrial fibrillation who had a Medtronic-Hall mitral prosthesis inserted two years previously. He presented with a transient hemiparesis and was hemodynamically stable with an intermittent soft opening click but no mid-diastolic murmur. Movement of the disc on echocardiography has been correlated with cinefluoroscopy *(arrow)* and demonstrates that complete opening of the disc (70°) only occurred late in diastole (frames 5 and 6). At surgery tissue ingrowth was confirmed. LS = lateral strut; CS = central strut.

LATE-ONSET LEFT OR RIGHT HEART FAILURE

This discourse relates to the evaluation and treatment of a patient who has been subjected to mitral valve surgery but who then presents weeks, months, or years later with symptoms and signs of left or right heart failure. There are five principal causes for this, which, in our view, may interact with and aggravate each other, producing a *vicious cycle.* We suggest that it is appropriate to call this entity the "restrictive-dilatation" syndrome (Fig. 8-21). Although the manifestations of this syndrome have been recognized by one of us (JBB) for several years, the interactions of the five main factors have not hitherto been clarified or reported by us or by others. The potential roles of all five factors should be borne in mind when considering the assessment and management of such a patient. Successful treatment of one or more of the factors will delay the progression or interrupt the cycle. The five factors are:

1. Mitral valve dysfunction
2. Myocardial dysfunction or other reason for left ventricular dilatation

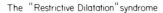

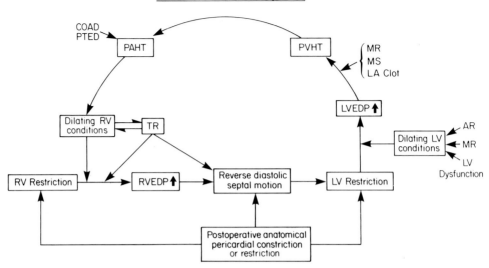

FIGURE 8-21. Diagrammatic representation of interrelated factors causing cardiac failure after cardiac surgery. (See text for details.) AR = aortic regurgitation; COAD = chronic obstructive airways disease; LA = left atrial; LV = left ventricular; LVEDP = left ventricular end-diastolic pressure; MR = mitral regurgitation; MS = mitral stenosis; PAHT = pulmonary arterial hypertension; PTED = pulmonary thromboembolic disease; PVHT = pulmonary venous hypertension; RV = right ventricular; RVEDP = right ventricular end-diastolic pressure; TR = tricuspid regurgitation.

3. Pulmonary thromboembolic disease and chronic obstructive airways disease
4. Functional or organic tricuspid regurgitation
5. Pericardial restriction or constriction

Before discussing these five factors and their respective contributions to the "vicious cycle" (Fig. 8-21), the interrelationship of ventricular function requires consideration. Pulmonary hypertension, tricuspid regurgitation, and pericardial constriction or restriction independently or, more significantly, in combination, will

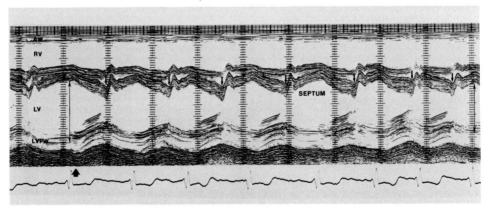

FIGURE 8-22. M-mode echocardiographic recording in a patient with pulmonary hypertension and a dilated right ventricle (RV), before and during abdominal compression. Paper speed 100 mm/sec. With compression *(bottom arrow to end of tracing)* blood is displaced from the inferior vena cava to the RV, which dilates at the expense of the left ventricular (LV) cavity, an effect seen in conditions of right ventricular overload. Diastolic septal motion is indicated by the *small arrows. Bidirectional arrows* measure LV cavity size before (52 mm) and at the end of abdominal compression (44 mm). AW = anterior wall of RV; LVPW = left ventricular posterior wall.

result in left ventricular restriction. The pathophysiological common denominator underlying the development of such left ventricular restriction is dilatation of the right ventricle at the expense of the left ventricular cavity, especially in the context of postoperative pericardial adhesions (Fig. 8-22).

Right ventricular filling commences marginally before left ventricular filling in normal patients. It starts even sooner in patients with right ventricular volume overload and pericardial restriction, because the higher the right atrial pressure, the earlier will be the diastolic pressure crossover between the right atrium and ventricle. In right ventricular volume overload, the rapid right ventricular early diastolic filling with consequent elevation of right ventricular diastolic pressure, in conjunction with the relatively delayed left ventricular filling, creates a trans-septal gradient that displaces the interventricular septum during early diastole (Fig. 8-23) towards the left ventricular cavity. If the right ventricular free wall is restricted by pericardial adhesions when right ventricular volume overload conditions coexist, the right ventricular diastolic pressure will be further elevated, causing even more marked left ventricular cavity restriction (Fig. 8-24).

The "vicious cycle" may be initiated when any pathology affecting the left side of the heart causes raised pulmonary venous and hence pulmonary arterial pressure. Conditions that usually dilate the left ventricle, such as left ventricular dysfunction and mitral or aortic valve regurgitation, may thus cause significant elevation of the left ventricular end-diastolic pressure when the left ventricular cavity size is limited by pericardial adhesions and diastolic septal shift. Other conditions causing pulmonary venous hypertension, notably mitral stenosis and mitral regurgitation, may initiate or enhance the cycle. Similarly, pulmonary arterial hypertension caused or aggravated by pulmonary thromboembolism or by obstructive airways disease may also participate in the process.

The five important factors responsible for creating and perpetuating this "vicious cycle" will be hereafter briefly considered.

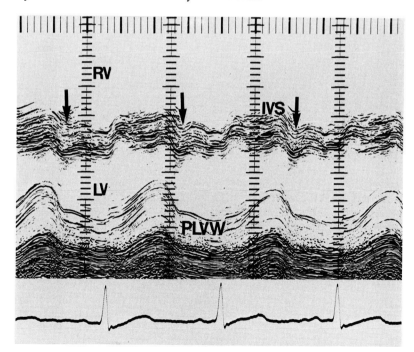

FIGURE 8-23. M-mode echocardiographic recording (paper speed 100 mm/sec) of right ventricular (RV) cavity, interventricular septum (IVS), left ventricular (LV) cavity, and the posterior left ventricular wall (PLVW) in a 28-year-old man with isolated tricuspid regurgitation and pericardial restriction following a stab wound to the chest and emergency thoracotomy nine years previously. Note the marked posterior septal motion in early diastole (arrows).

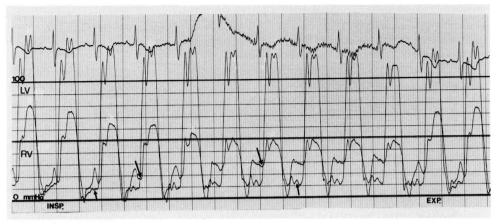

FIGURE 8-24. Simultaneous left (LV) and right (RV) ventricular pressures in a patient with pulmonary hypertension due to pulmonary thromboembolic disease. During inspiration (INSP) the RV systolic pressure drops, owing to increased right ventricular transmural pressure (afterload), with a concomitant rise in right ventricular end-diastolic pressure *(long arrows)*. With the progressive rise in RVEDP, the LV diastolic pressure tracing becomes more restricted, exhibiting a dip and plateau pattern *(short arrows)*.

MITRAL VALVE DYSFUNCTION

A principal cause of a patient's deterioration late after cardiac surgery is mitral valve dysfunction. This cause is particularly likely to be relevant if the deterioration has been sudden. Infective endocarditis must always be sought as a cause of regurgitation or stenosis of a native or prosthetic valve. In the absence of infection, investigation should exclude restenosis after mitral commissurotomy, obstruction or regurgitation of a prosthetic valve, or increasing regurgitation after commissurotomy or valvuloplasty. Relatively mild mitral regurgitation following cardiac surgery may have increased hemodynamic significance months or years later, when restriction due to adhesions increases. In other words, relatively mild regurgitationwill be functionally more significant if the left ventricular end-diastolic pressure rises because the ventricle is unable to dilate or is actively constricted by tightening adhesions or right ventricular dilatation. In such instances, correction of the mitral lesion, usually involving valve replacement, will be helpful.

LEFT VENTRICULAR DYSFUNCTION OR DILATATION

There are several possible causes of left ventricular dysfunction that occurs months or years after surgery (Fig. 8-25), but it is not always possible to establish which cause is applicable or whether a combination of factors is relevant. Occlusive coronary artery disease must be excluded, because, although bypass surgery may improve left ventricular function, occlusive coronary artery disease is seldom the cause, especially in our Black patients, of the deteriorating left ventricular function. The respective roles of myocardial dysfunction following prolonged severe mitral regurgitation, ongoing rheumatic activity in young patients who fail to comply with antibiotic prophylaxis, or myocardial dysfunction as a result of cardiopulmonary bypass are often uncertain. In addition, the development of hemodynamically significant aortic valve disease may contribute to the left ventricular dilatation. The essential result of any of these causes is a rise of left ventricular end-diastolic pressure, and the contribution of this to the "vicious cycle" is readily apparent.

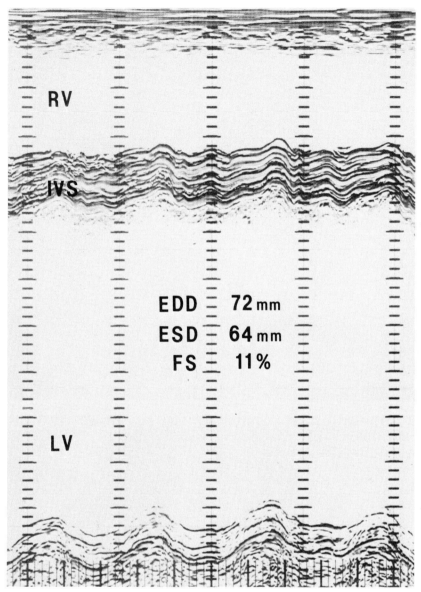

FIGURE 8-25. M-mode echocardiographic recording in a patient after aortic and mitral valve replacement showing a dilated left ventricle with poor contraction. EDD = end-diastolic diameter; ESD = end-systolic diameter. FS = fractional shortening (normal, 25 percent).

PULMONARY THROMBOEMBOLIC DISEASE AND CHRONIC OBSTRUCTIVE AIRWAYS DISEASE

Chronic obstructive airways disease may be an associated condition in patients (particularly the middle-aged and elderly) who have been subjected to previous mitral valve surgery. When this condition is severe, resultant pulmonary hypertension will predispose to right ventricular dilatation.

   In our experience, chronic pulmonary thromboembolic disease is the principal cause of persistence of a raised pulmonary vascular resistance in patients who have undergone mitral valve surgery (Fig. 8-26). The pulmonary arterial hypertension caused by hemodynamically significant mitral stenosis, regurgitation, or both,

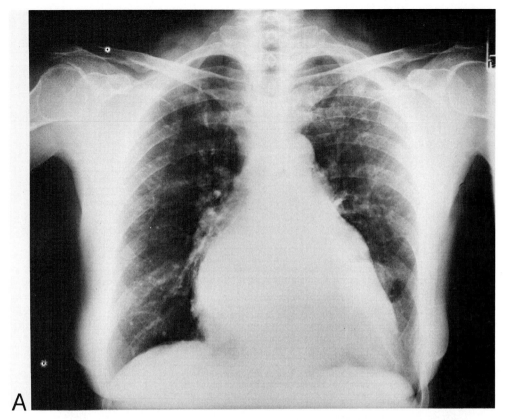

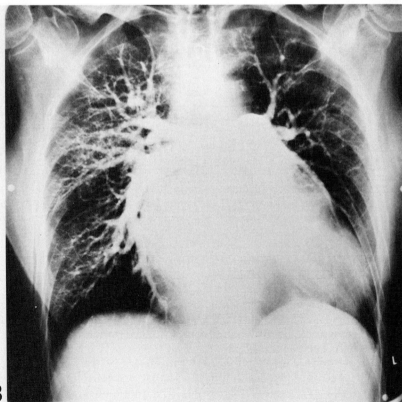

FIGURE 8-26. Posteroanterior chest radiograph (*A*) and pulmonary angiogram (*B*) in a 61-year-old woman with pulmonary thromboembolic and chronic obstructive airways disease. Pulmonary hypertension persisted after mitral valve replacement 10 years earlier.

should return to normal when the valve lesion is corrected. If the left-sided hemo-dynamics are normal and there is no chronic obstructive airways disease or other parenchymatous lung pathology, then the cause of a sustained increased pulmonary vascular resistance is invariably pulmonary thromboembolic disease. This common condition is underdiagnosed by many clinicians. It frequently occurs without previous history of an acute pulmonary embolus, and we postulate that the pulmonary arterial occlusions are often primarily thrombotic. Once started, further thrombosis will supervene because of stasis and propagation of thrombus. Treatment comprises long-term anticoagulation with warfarin, which most patients with mitral valve disease will be receiving already for other reasons.

FUNCTIONAL OR ORGANIC TRICUSPID REGURGITATION

Tricuspid regurgitation resulting from dilatation of the anulus is prevalent in patients with rheumatic heart disease and, in the absence of leaflet scarring, is usually

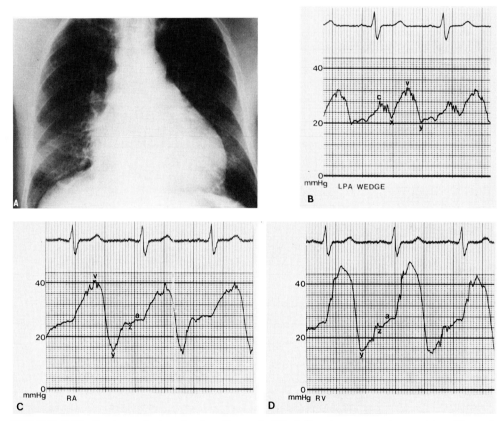

FIGURE 8-27. Posteroanterior chest radiograph (A), left pulmonary artery wedge (B), and right atrial (C) and right ventricular (D) pressures in a 62-year-old man with the "restrictive dilatation" syndrome. Mitral valvotomy was performed 12 years previously and a Björk-Shiley aortic valve inserted seven years later. Marked tricuspid regurgitation with a restrictive diastolic pattern is demonstrated in C and D. Clinical examination, echocardiography, and cinefluoroscopy indicated mild mitral valve disease, suggesting that the elevated left pulmonary artery (LPA) wedge pressure (B) reflected the left ventricular end-diastolic pressure. Tricuspid valve surgery was recommended. Prior to operation, the patient became uremic and died. At necropsy, the tricuspid anulus was grossly dilated with virtually normal leaflets; the mitral valve showed only mild abnormality, and the prosthetic aortic valve was perfect. Dense adhesions encased the heart, attaching it to the chest wall.

regarded as "functional." It is probable that this lesion is often partly or mainly organic and that there is anular disease analogous to the anular dilatation affecting the mitral valve. When the tricuspid leaflets are involved, the regurgitant murmur is more prominent and a mid-diastolic murmur may also be detected. If commissures are fused, some tricuspid stenosis will be present. Closed tricuspid commissurotomy, a disastrous operation that should no longer ever be performed, was another cause of severe tricuspid regurgitation with or without residual stenosis.

Any cause of raised pulmonary arterial pressure, principally left-sided abnormalities or pulmonary thromboembolic disease, may initiate or will aggravate tricuspid regurgitation. We have observed patients after mitral valve surgery with normal or near-normal left ventricular systolic function and with minimal or mild mitral valve disease but in whom gross tricuspid regurgitation remained or developed (Fig. 8-27). Such patients may be very symptomatic because of peripheral edema, ascites, and hepatomegaly. Cardiac catheterization confirms a raised left ventricular end-diastolic pressure with a "restrictive" pattern (Fig. 8-28). Surgery confined to the tricuspid valve (whether anuloplasty, valvuloplasty, or valve replacement with a tissue valve) has resulted in marked reduction of symptoms and disappearance of signs of tricuspid regurgitation. It is difficult to generalize as to when such surgery is indicated. We operate only when patients are symptomatic, with marked hepatomegaly or peripheral edema despite large doses of diuretics, and provided that neither pulmonary thromboembolic disease nor an inoperable left heart hemodynamic abnormality is the dominant manifestation.

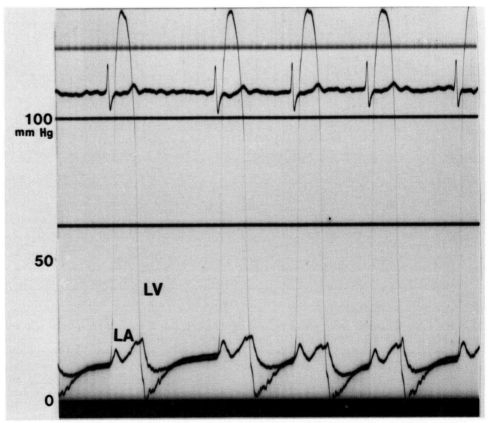

FIGURE 8-28. Raised left ventricular end-diastolic pressure with a dip and plateau pattern in a patient with severe tricuspid regurgitation after double valve replacement (aortic, Björk-Shiley; and mitral, Carpentier-Edwards).

In view of our conviction that rheumatic anular disease is an important factor in initiating or aggravating so-called functional tricuspid regurgitation, an aggressive policy towards tricuspid anuloplasty is justified at the time of initial surgery for rheumatic mitral valve disease. We consider that this should prevent or retard the later development of the "restrictive-dilatation" syndrome. It is better to create, in fact, some tricuspid stenosis than to leave tricuspid regurgitation. The former will not be detrimental, whereas the latter may progress to play a profound role in the vicious cycle of the syndrome.

PERICARDIAL RESTRICTION OR CONSTRICTION

Ribeiro and colleagues[1] summarized relevant literature and concluded that true constrictive pericarditis is a rare complication of cardiac surgery. This has been our experience also in patients undergoing surgery for congenital cardiac abnormalities or coronary artery disease. However, we have found that cardiac restriction is common in patients subjected to surgery for rheumatic valvular heart disease. Such "restriction" may become a functional "constriction" when either ventricle must dilate. Many patients have had two or more operations, often a left thoracotomy for closed mitral commissurotomy followed later by a midsternal incision for valve replacement. In most of these patients, there are factors that contribute to the functional constriction (Fig. 8-29) by the pericardial or mediastinal adhesions. Surgical relief of

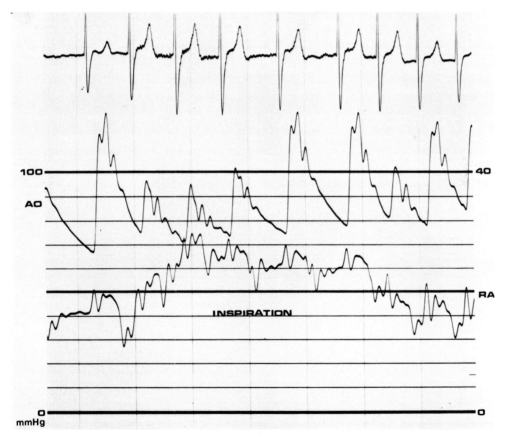

FIGURE 8-29. Pulsus paradoxus and a positive Kussmaul's sign in a 33-year-old man with the "restrictive-dilatation" syndrome and marked tricuspid regurgitation due to anular dilatation. He had had a previous mitral commissurotomy. AO = aorta; RA = right atrium.

this restriction has been attempted but has usually been unsuccessful because of numerous dense adhesions outside the pericardium that are difficult to remove and are a major cause of the functional constriction. Even in cases in which the pericardium itself is thickened and therefore constricted, adhesions outside the pericardium make pericardiectomy difficult.

We have found that systolic function is compromised in some of these patients. Echocardiography and angiocardiography have demonstrated low left ventricular ejection fractions, and thoracotomy or necropsy have confirmed the presence of dense adhesions that surround the heart and that attach it to the chest wall. Histological evidence of myocardial fibrosis or other abnormality does not preclude the possibility that the adhesions may have contributed to resisting systolic contraction during life.

We are convinced that a restrictive pericardium contributes importantly to complications occurring late after cardiac surgery and that interactions among cardiac chambers require more clarification and further study. Interruption of the cycle by a surgical correction of valve lesions, including tricuspid regurgitation (Fig. 8-30), may be indicated and is more likely to be successful than an attempt to remove the restricted pericardium or other adhesions.

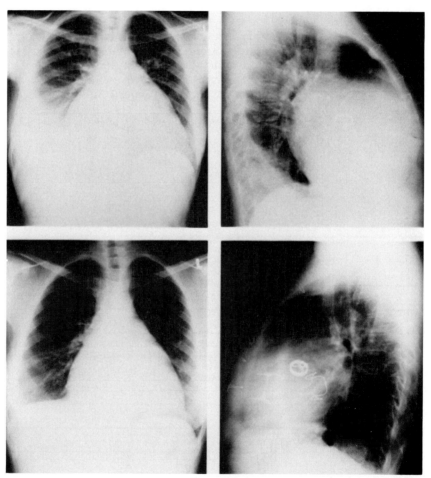

FIGURE 8-30. Posteroanterior (left panels) and lateral (right panels) chest radiographs before *(top)* and after *(bottom)* tricuspid valve replacement with an Ionescu-Shiley valve. The patient is the same as in Figure 8-28 and had severe tricuspid regurgitation with normal functioning aortic Björk-Shiley and mitral Carpentier-Edwards valves. There was considerable reduction in heart size after the tricuspid valve replacement.

TABLE 8-2. Outcome of Pregnancy with Mechanical Prosthetic Valves

| MODE OF THERAPY | NO. OF PATIENTS | FETAL WASTAGE | | MATERNAL COMPLICATIONS | | |
		ABORTION	STILL-BIRTH	THROMBO-EMBOLISM	POSTPARTUM HEMORRHAGE	DEATH
A. Warfarin only	14	4	2	0	0	0
B. Warfarin substituted by heparin at term	13	1	1	0	1	0
C. Heparin in first trimester, then warfarin; then heparin substituted for warfarin at term	4	1	1	0	0	0

MANAGEMENT OF PREGNANCY FOLLOWING MITRAL VALVE SURGERY

All our patients with mechanical prosthetic valves are receiving warfarin. Patients with large left atria and atrial fibrillation who have had a commissurotomy, valvuloplasty, or insertion of a tissue valve are also receiving anticoagulants, unless there is a specific contraindication such as peptic ulcer or the likelihood of poor compliance.

The hemodynamic overload of pregnancy in women who have been subjected to mitral valve surgery is seldom a problem. The principal problem relates to the management of anticoagulation. Anticoagulation is mandatory in all pregnant women with a mechanical prosthesis in the mitral position. Antithrombotic therapy with antiplatelet agents alone is inadequate, and this was recently confirmed by Salazar and co-workers[2] who observed cerebral embolism in 25 percent in pregnant women so treated. Moreover, 3 of 68 pregnant women who were treated with antiplatelet agents died only as a result of thrombosis of their mitral mechanical valve. Anticoagulation with coumarin derivatives was more effective, but 8 percent of infants (of 128 pregnancies) developed coumadin embryopathy.

Our advice to women who have undergone mitral valve replacement with a mechanical prosthesis is to avoid pregnancy. If a young woman is intent on pregnancy, is in sinus rhythm without a very large left atrium, and requires mitral valve replacement, it is our view that a tissue valve should be inserted. Salazar and co-workers[2] recently described 12 pregnant women with mitral bioprostheses who were not receiving coumarin anticoagulants, and who had no thromboembolic problems.

One of us (PS) has recently reviewed the outcome of 31 pregnancies in 31 Black women, 30 of whom were in sinus rhythm, and who had had mechanical prostheses inserted. Sodium warfarin was used in all but was combined with heparin as shown in Table 8-2. Although it was concluded that anticoagulation with warfarin, with or without heparin at term, provided adequate protection against maternal thromboembolic complications, the incidence of fetal wastage (32 percent) and perinatal fetal death (6 percent) was high. A possible solution to this would be to maintain these patients on heparin, administered by continuous subcutaneous infusion, throughout their pregnancy.

REFERENCES

SECTION 1

1. SPENCER, FC: *A plea for early open mitral commissurotomy.* Am Heart J 95:668–670, 1978.
2. HALSETH, WL, ELLIOT, DP, WALKER, EL, AND SMITH, EA: *Open mitral commissurotomy. A modern re-evaluation.* J Thorac Cardiovasc Surg 80:842–848, 1980.

3. SALERNO, TA, NEILSON, IR, CHARRETTE, EJP, AND LYNN, RB: *A 25-year experience with the closed method of treatment in 139 patients with mitral stenosis.* Ann Thorac Surg 31:300–304, 1980.

4. MONTOYA, A, MULET, J, PIFARRE, R, MORAN, J, AND SULLIVAN, HJ: *The advantages of open mitral commissurotomy for mitral valve stenosis.* Chest 75:131–135, 1979.

5. SCANNELL, JG: *Closed operation for mitral stenosis.* Ann Thorac Surg 31:299, 1981.

6. COMMERFORD, PJ, HASTIE, T, AND BECK, W: *Closed mitral valvotomy: Actuarial analysis of results in 654 patients over 12 years and analysis of preoperative predictors of long-term survival.* Ann Thorac Surg 33:473–479, 1982.

7. BONCHECK, W: *Indications for surgery of the mitral valve.* Am J Cardiol 46:155–158, 1980.

8. ANTUNES, MJ AND KINSLEY, RH: *Mitral valve annuloplasty: Results in an underdeveloped population.* Thorax 38:730–736, 1983.

9. CARPENTIER, A, DELOCHE, A, DAUPTAIN, J, SOYER, R, BLONDEAU, P, PINNICA, A, AND DUBOST, C: *A new reconstructive operation for correction of mitral and tricuspid insufficiency.* J Thorac Cardiovasc Surg 61:1–13, 1971.

10. KAY, JH AND EGERTON, WS: *The repair of mitral insufficiency associated with ruptured chordae tendineae.* Ann Surg 157:351–360, 1963.

11. RITTERHOUSE, EA, DAVIS, CC, WOOD, SJ, AND SAUVAGE, LR: *Replacement of ruptured chordae tendineae of the mitral valve with autologous pericardial chordae.* J Thorac Cardiovasc Surg 75:870–876, 1978.

12. CARPENTIER, A, CHAUVAUD, S, FABIANI, JN, DELOCHE, A, RELLAND, J, LESSANA, A, D'ALLAINES, C, BLONDEAU, P, PINNICA, A, AND DUBOST, C: *Reconstructive surgery of mitral valve incompetence: Ten-year appraisal.* J Thorac Cardiovasc Surg 79:338–348, 1980.

13. ROBERTS, WC: *Choosing a substitute cardiac valve: Type, size, surgeon.* Am J Cardiol 38:633–644, 1976.

14. EDMISTON, WA, HARRISON, EC, DUICK, GF, PARNASSUS, W, AND LAV, FYK: *Thromboembolism in mitral porcine valve recipients.* Am J Cardiol 41:508–511, 1978.

15. HETZER, KR, HILL, JD, KERTH, WJ, ANSBRO, J, ADDAPPA, MG, RODVIG, R, KAMM, B, AND GERBODE, F: *Thromboembolic complications after mitral valve replacement with Hancock xenograft.* J Thorac Cardiovasc Surg 75:657–658, 1978.

16. ANTUNES, MJ: *Bioprosthetic valve replacement in children. Long term follow-up of 135 isolated mitral valve implantations.* Eur Heart J 5:913–918, 1984.

17. ANTUNES, MJ AND SANTOS, LP: *Performance of glutaraldehyde-preserved porcine bioprosthesis as a mitral valve substitute in a young population group.* Ann Thorac Surg 37:387–392, 1984.

18. KINSLEY, RH, COLSEN, PR, AND ANTUNES, MJ: *Medtronic-Hall valve replacement in a third world population group.* Thorac Cardiovasc Surg 31:69–72, 1983.

SECTION 2

1. RIBEIRO, P, SAPSFORD, R, EVANS, T, PARCHARIDIS, G, AND OAKLEY, C: *Constrictive pericarditis as a complication of coronary artery bypass surgery.* Br Heart J 51:205–210, 1984.

2. SALAZAR, E, ZAJARIAS, A, GUTIERREZ, N, AND ITURBE, I: *The problem of cardiac valve prostheses, anticoagulants and pregnancy.* Circulation 70 (Suppl I):169–177, 1984.

BIBLIOGRAPHY

SECTION 1

ANTUNES, MJ: *Prosthetic heart valve replacement. Choice of prosthesis in a young, underdeveloped population group.* S Afr Med J 68:755–758, 1985.

ANTUNES, MJ, COLSEN, PR, AND KINSLEY, RH: *Mitral valvuloplasty: A learning curve.* Circulation 68 (Suppl II):70–75, 1983.

COBBS, BW, HATCHER, CR, CRAVER, JM, JONES, EL, AND SEWELL, CW: *Transverse midventricular disruption after mitral valve replacement.* Am Heart J 99:33–50, 1980.

KINSLEY, RH, ANTUNES, MJ, AND MCKIBBIN, JK: *Enlargement of the narrow aortic root and oblique insertion of a St Jude prosthesis.* Br Heart J 50:330–332, 1983.

LESSANA, A, HERREMAN, F, BOFFETY, C, COSMA, H, GUERIN, F, KARA, M, AND DEGEORGES, M: *Hemodynamic and cineangiographic study before and after mitral valvuloplasty (Carpentier's technique).* Circulation 64 (Suppl II):195–202, 1981.

LOUW, JWK, KINSLEY, RH, DION, RAE, COLSEN, PR, AND GIRDWOOD, RW: *Emergency heart valve replacement: An analysis of 170 patients.* Ann Thorac Surg 29:415–422, 1980.

RAHIMTOOLA, SH AND MURPHY, E: *Valve prosthesis—patient mismatch. A long-term sequela.* Br Heart J 45:331–335, 1981.

ROBERTS, WC: *The silver anniversary of cardiac valve replacement.* Am J Cardiol 56:503–506, 1985.

WESTABY, S, KARP, RB, BLACKSTONE, EH, AND BISHOP, SP: *Adult human valve dimensions and their surgical significance.* Am J Cardiol 53:552–556, 1984.

SECTION 2

BORTOLOTTI, U, MILANO, A, MAZZUCCO, A, VALFRE, C, RUSSO, R, VALENTE, M, SCHIVAZAPPA, L, THIENE, G, AND GALLUCCI, V: *Pregnancy in patients with a porcine valve bioprosthesis.* Am J Cardiol 50:1051–1054, 1982.

BUTLER, J: *The heart is in good hands.* Circulation 67:1163–1168, 1983.

COPANS, H, LAKIER, JB, KINSLEY, RH, COLSEN, PR, FRITZ, VU, AND BARLOW, JB: *Thrombosed Björk-Shiley mitral prostheses.* Circulation 61:169–174, 1980.

DE SWIET, M: *Pregnancy and heart valve replacement.* Int J Cardiol 5:741–743, 1984.

GOLDMAN, ME: *Emerging importance of the right ventricle.* J Am Coll Cardiol 5:925–927, 1985.

HESS, OM, BHARGAVA, V, ROSS, J, JR, AND SHABETAI, R: *The role of the pericardium in interactions between the cardiac chambers.* Am Heart J 106:1377–1383, 1983.

HORSTKOTTE, D, HAERTEN, K, SEIPEL, L, KÖRFER, R, BUDDE, T, BIRCKS, W, AND LOOGEN, F: *Central hemodynamics at rest and during exercise after mitral valve replacement with different prostheses.* Circulation 68 (Suppl II):161–168, 1983.

JOHN, S, BASHI, VV, JAIRAJ, PS, MURALIDHARAN, S, RAVIKUMAR, E, RAJARAJESWARI, T, KRISHNASWAMI, S, SUKUMAR, IP, AND SUNDAR RAO PSS: *Closed mitral valvotomy: Early results and long-term follow-up of 3724 consecutive patients.* Circulation 68:891–896, 1983.

KING, RM, SCHAFF, HV, DANIELSON, GK, GERSH, BJ, ORSZULAK, TA, PIEHLER, JM, PUGA, FJ, AND PLUTH, JR: *Surgery for tricuspid regurgitation late after mitral valve replacement.* Circulation 70 (Suppl I):193–197, 1984.

KING, SB III AND KUTCHER, MA: *Constrictive pericarditis following cardiac surgery; a complication that does exist.* Int J Cardiol 3:353–355, 1983.

KINGMA, I, TYBERG, JV, AND SMITH, ER: *Effects of diastolic transseptal pressure gradient on ventricular septal position and motion.* Circulation 68:1304–1314, 1983.

KINSLEY, RH, ANTUNES, MJ, AND COLSEN, P: *The St Jude medical valve replacement. An evaluation of valve performance.* J Thorac Cardiovasc Surg (in press).

KOTLER, MN, MINTZ, GS, PANIDIS, I, MORGANROTH, J, SEGAL, BL, AND ROSS, J: *Noninvasive evaluation of normal and abnormal prosthetic valve function.* J Am Coll Cardiol 2:151–173, 1983.

LINDERER, T, CHATTERJEE, K, PARMLEY, WW, SIEVERS, RE, GLANTZ, SA, AND TYBERG, JV: *Influence of atrial systole on the Frank-Starling relation and the end-diastolic pressure-diameter relation of the left ventricle.* Circulation 67:1045–1053, 1983.

MURPHY, ES AND KLOSTER, FE: *Late results of valve replacement surgery. II. Complications of prosthetic heart valves.* Mod Conc Cardiovasc Dis 48:59–66, 1979.

NISHIMURA, RA, FUSTER, V, BURGERT, SL, AND PUGA, FJ: *Clinical features and long-term natural history of the postpericardiotomy syndrome.* Int J Cardiol 4:443–450, 1983.

RAHIMTOOLA, SH: *Valvular heart disease: A perspective.* J Am Coll Cardiol 2:199–215, 1983.

TANI, M: *Roles of the right ventricular free wall and ventricular septum in right ventricular performance and influence of the parietal pericardium during right ventricular failure in dogs.* Am J Cardiol 52:196–202, 1983.

WEITZMAN, LB, TINKER, WP, KRONZON, I, COHEN, ML, GLASSMAN, E, AND SPENCER, FC: *The incidence and natural history of pericardial effusion after cardiac surgery—an echocardiographic study.* Circulation 69:506–511, 1984.

9

INFECTIVE ENDOCARDITIS

with WENDY A. POCOCK and ROBIN H. KINSLEY

Because of the prevalence of rheumatic heart disease in South Africa, infective endocarditis is commonly encountered and we have observed virtually all manifestations of the condition. The description of classic bacterial endocarditis is that of a patient with an abnormal heart, protracted fever, anemia, systemic embolism, splenomegaly, clubbing of the fingers, and positive blood cultures. For a number of reasons this clinical presentation has altered in the Western world. These reasons include the considerable decline in prevalence of rheumatic heart disease, improved oral hygiene, the widespread use of antibacterial agents, open heart surgery, a rising incidence of drug addiction, and a greater awareness of the clinical entity. Infective endocarditis is reputedly now observed more frequently in older patients in whom presenting clinical features may be nonspecific and atypical. The clinical presentation of infective endocarditis in White patients in South Africa is similar to that encountered in the Western world. On the other hand, the majority of our Black patients present when they are extremely ill with severe hemodynamic lesions.

WHICH PATIENTS ARE AT RISK?

Virtually all forms of congenital and valvular heart disease (Fig. 9-1) should be regarded as potential sites for infective endocarditis. Secundum atrial septal defect is a notable exception provided the mitral valve is normal. We cannot recall having ever encountered infective endocarditis in a patient with an atrial septal defect of the secundum type, whether or not mitral valve prolapse or other mitral valve disease was associated. Nor have we encountered infective endocarditis on a calcified mitral anulus. We have seen two cases only, both caused by Staphylococcus aureus, on ventricular septal defect with a short (so-called atypical) systolic murmur. Infective endocarditis is uncommon in patients with hypertrophic cardiomyopathy, but, in our experience, infection is more likely to occur when mitral regurgitation is associated. A middle-aged man treated by one of us (JBB) for severe hypertrophic cardiomyopathy, mitral regurgitation, atrial fibrillation, cerebral embolism, and congestive heart failure had vegetations at necropsy on both the interventricular septum and the

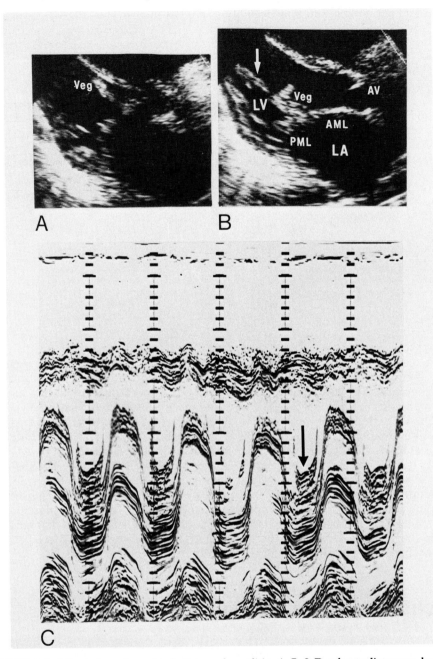

FIGURE 9-1. Mitral stenosis and infective endocarditis. *A, B,* 2-D echocardiograms, long-axis view, diastole (*A*) and systole (*B*). The large vegetation (Veg) on the anterior mitral leaflet (AML) and thickened chordae tendineae *(arrow)* are shown. *C,* M-mode echocardiogram. Both leaflets are thickened. The vegetation *(arrow)* is visible in the anterior leaflet. PML = posterior mitral leaflet; AV = aortic valve; LA = left atrium; LV = left ventricle.

mitral valve. It is accepted policy to give antimicrobial drugs to patients with known heart disease at times of risk. In 1973, Hayward[1] commented that the value of antibiotic prophylaxis in preventing infective endocarditis had yet to be confirmed. To our knowledge, such confirmation is still lacking, although a decrease in bacteremia after dental scaling has been demonstrated in subjects given antibiotics prior to the procedure.[2] Prophylaxis against infective endocarditis causes inconvenience to both dentist and patient, and the practicability as well as the possible advantages of such measures are relevant. The recommendations of the American Heart Association on dental prophylaxis are complicated and mostly entail the use of parenteral antibiotics. It is not surprising that compliance with these regimens, even in the United States, is apparently only 15 percent. It is our policy not to recommend prophylaxis in patients with hypertrophic cardiomyopathy, calcified mitral anulus, or secundum atrial septal defect, unless mitral regurgitation is associated. Similarly, we have reservations about advising prophylaxis in patients with small muscular ventricular septal defects and early nonpansystolic murmurs. We are aware that infective endocarditis has been encountered in patients with mitral valve billow without prolapse, as reflected by an isolated nonejection systolic click. There are many such subjects, most of whom are completely asymptomatic, and we think it is neither justifiable nor practicable to administer prophylaxis at times of risk to subjects with auscultatory or echocardiographic evidence of mitral billowing unless definite mitral regurgitation is associated.

The most common lesion predisposing to infective endocarditis is probably mitral regurgitation (Fig. 9-2). It is important to remember that infective endocarditis

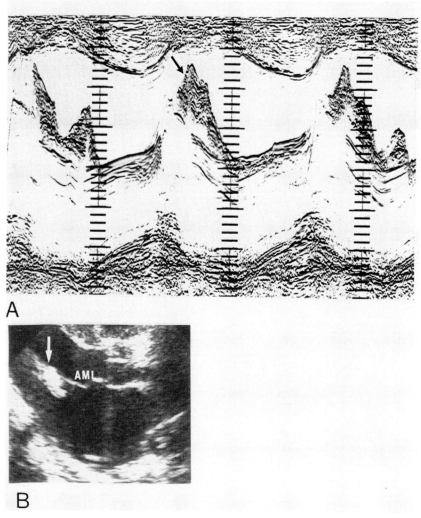

FIGURE 9-2. M-mode echocardiogram (*A*) and 2-D echocardiogram (long-axis view) (*B*) of a patient with infective endocarditis, severe mitral regurgitation, and chordal rupture. The large vegetation (*arrow*) is on the anterior mitral leaflet (AML).

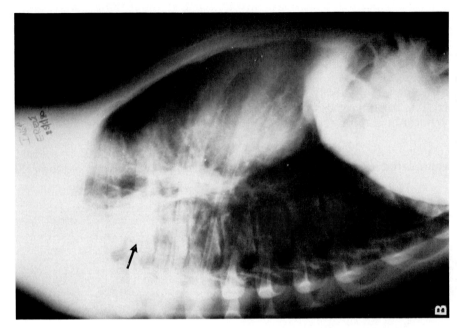

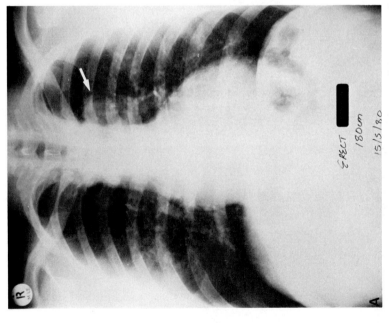

FIGURE 9-3. An 18-year-old young man with coarctation of the aorta who presented with a mycotic aneurysm (*arrow*) distal to the coarctation. Posteroanterior (*A*) and lateral (*B*) chest radiographs.

may supervene irrespective of the underlying cause of the regurgitation. Although rheumatic heart disease and primary mitral valve prolapse are the most common pathologies encountered, papillary muscle dysfunction, usually a result of myocardial ischemia, may also predispose to infective endocarditis. Patients with patent ductus arteriosus and coarctation of the aorta (Fig. 9-3) may present, for the first time and at virtually any age, with infective endocarditis. Infective endocarditis seldom if ever occurs after surgical closure of a ductus arteriosus, and we have not to date encountered infection on a repaired coarctation of the aorta. A patient with a small ventricular septal defect and a pansystolic murmur is susceptible to infective endocarditis, but this risk alone is not high enough to justify closure of the defect. In our experience, medical therapy has been successful in the large majority of those patients in whom infection has supervened. We have had several patients with ventricular septal defect in whom the aortic valve also became infected, resulting in significant regurgitation. Replacement of that valve as well as closure of the septal defect had later to be undertaken. Many elderly patients have atherosclerotic degeneration of their aortic valve leaflets without significant stenosis, and such valves are a potential site for infection. An aortic ejection systolic murmur, even when isolated, indicates that the valve is abnormal; and we repeat that aortic ejection murmurs are never "innocent" (see Chapter 4, Section 2). A congenital bicuspid aortic valve with no regurgitation and minimal stenosis may become infected, but this is uncommon in our experience. Any patient with aortic regurgitation, irrespective of the underlying cause or the hemodynamic significance, is a potential candidate for infective endocarditis.

With the possible exception of right-sided endocarditis as a consequence of intravenous drug abuse (of which we have no experience), it is difficult to assess the incidence of infective endocarditis on valves that are both anatomically and functionally normal. When left-sided endocarditis is encountered clinically, invariably a cardiac lesion is detectable even in the early stages. Patients who reputedly had no cardiac abnormality detected on previous clinical examination may have had mild abnormalities such as mitral valve prolapse or a bicuspid or atherosclerotic aortic valve. Since valves examined at necropsy or during surgery are necessarily severely damaged by the infection, the original underlying abnormality is not always apparent. Although right-sided endocarditis, especially when due to a virulent organism such as Staphylococcus aureus, almost certainly does occur on anatomically normal valves, it is possible that functional tricuspid regurgitation resulting from pulmonary disease, pulmonary embolism, and other causes of pulmonary hypertension may have preceded the infective endocarditis. We have observed several patients with infective endocarditis of the pulmonary valve associated with infection on a patent ductus arteriosus and have suspected that the pulmonary valve was anatomically normal before the infection. In such instances, however, functional pulmonary regurgitation may have preceded the infection on the pulmonary valve. Some patients with right-sided endocarditis encountered by us have had rheumatic tricuspid disease or a congenital pulmonary valve anomaly (Fig. 9-4).

Infection on prosthetic valves, including tissue valves, remains an important problem. Although we had achieved satisfactory results with homograft valve replacement in the aortic position, we abandoned their use more than a decade ago, because of difficulty in procuring them and because degeneration with time seemed to be inevitable. Those valves were sterilized with antibiotics and, unlike the experience of others, we rarely encountered fungal endocarditis. For reasons outlined in Chapter 8, we have largely reduced our use of porcine valves after having inserted approximately 500. We seldom use the Ionescu-Shiley pericardial valve, except for tricuspid valve replacement, but that operation is also rare in our unit and we have inserted less than 40. To date we have not encountered infection on an Ionescu-Shiley valve. Prosthetic valve endocarditis may occur at any time after insertion. Improved sterilization techniques of the pump oxygenator and of the prosthetic valve, perioperative antibiotic therapy, avoidance of infection of intravenous lines

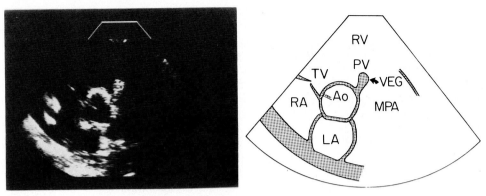

FIGURE 9-4. 2-D echocardiogram (short-axis, parasternal view) of a patient with mycosis fungoides and infection on an apparently normal pulmonary valve.

and aggressive treatment of skin, sternal or other sepsis have ensured that the incidence of early-onset prosthetic endocarditis is reduced. It is our current policy to favor either the St. Jude or Medtronic-Hall prosthesis for left-sided valve replacement, and we estimate that the incidence of early (within two months of insertion) infective endocarditis is less than 1 percent provided that infection is not present at the time of operation. Even when infection is present prior to surgery, ongoing postoperative sepsis remains rare if antibiotic treatment is appropriate and adequate. Contrary to a generally stated view, we have found late-onset endocarditis to be rare with a Björk-Shiley, Medtronic-Hall, or St. Jude valve, provided there was no ring leak on careful auscultation at least two months after surgery but before onset or detection of infection. Porcine valves, on the other hand, may become infected at any time, but especially after they have started to degenerate (Figs. 9-5, 9-6). Despite our favorable experience regarding infection on the mechanical prosthetic valves mentioned, our policy is to recommend prophylaxis against infective endocarditis at times of risk for all patients who have had any type of prosthetic valve inserted.

CAUSES OF TRANSIENT BACTEREMIA AND INFECTIVE ENDOCARDITIS

There are numerous causes of transient bacteremia, but these should be seen in perspective as to the likelihood of their resulting in infective endocarditis. The risk relates not only to the nature of the heart disease but also to the magnitude of the bacteremia and the organism likely to be involved. It is therefore difficult to generalize regarding prophylaxis. In many instances of infective endocarditis, the portal of entry of the organism is not known. Life is full of hazards, but it is often not practicable, desirable, or indeed possible to take precautions against all risks. We have not, to our knowledge, encountered infective endocarditis after upper respiratory tract viral infection, rectal examination, sigmoidoscopy, or cardiac catheterization. Provided obvious bacterial infection is not apparent, we do not recommend antibiotic prophylaxis under those circumstances. We have observed infective endocarditis following an infected insect bite, a septic skin abrasion, and the squeezing of a large pimple. It is difficult to know whether the endocarditis could have been avoided. We have treated severe Staphylococcus aureus endocarditis on a reputedly normal mitral valve in an upper social class woman in whom the organism was also cultured from an infected intrauterine device (Fig. 9-7). We do not favor this method of contraception in patients at risk of infective endocarditis. Infective endocarditis after a normal delivery is rare, but we nevertheless recommend antibiotic prophylaxis, especially when an episiotomy is performed. We practice prophylaxis for induced or spontaneous abortion, instrumention of the urinary tract, and gastrointestinal surgery. Prolonged use of the same intravenous line should be avoided in all patients but especially in those who are at risk of infective endocarditis.

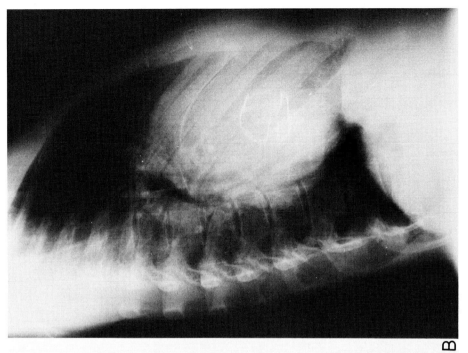

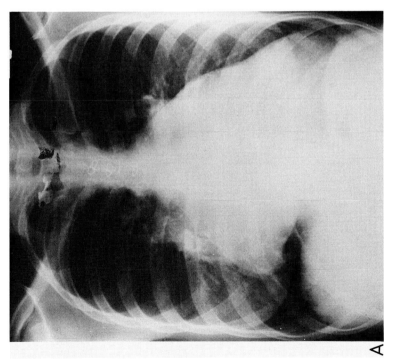

FIGURE 9-5. Posteroanterior (*A*) and lateral (*B*) chest radiographs of a patient with severe mitral regurgitation and a degenerated, infected Carpentier-Edwards valve. There is gross cardiomegaly and a giant left atrium.

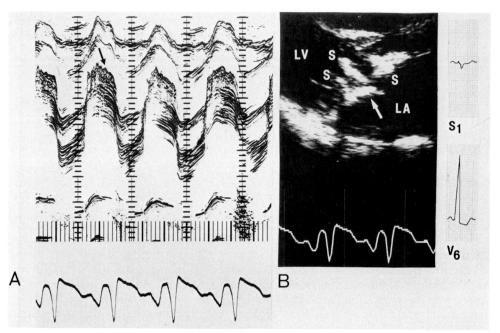

FIGURE 9-6. M-mode echocardiogram (*A*) and 2-D echocardiogram (*B*) of the same patient as in Figure 9-5. *A*, The leaflets are thickened with rounded edges. *B*, Long-axis view, systolic frame. Degenerated Carpentier-Edwards mitral prosthesis with thickened struts (S) and leaflets, one of which *(arrow)* is prolapsing into the left atrium (LA).

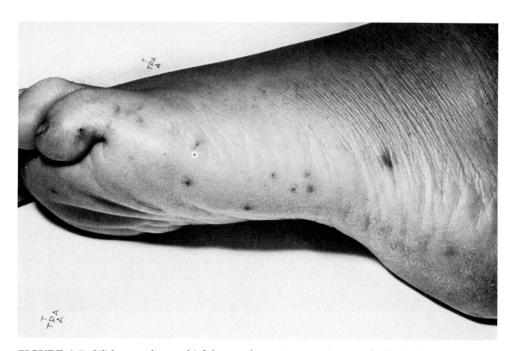

FIGURE 9-7. Widespread petechial hemorrhages in a patient with Staphylococcus aureus endocarditis on the mitral valve. The same organism was cultured from an infected intrauterine device.

The most important and common causes of bacteremia are dental procedures (including scaling), gingival infections, and tooth infections. Good dental hygiene and antibiotic prophylaxis prior to any form of dental therapy are mandatory for patients known to be at risk. Although rare, infective endocarditis may occur in edentulous subjects, sometimes as a result of gingival trauma from poorly fitting dentures.

Prophylactic procedures vary depending on whether the patient requires a general anaesthetic and is in hospital or is receiving outpatient treatment. The choice of antimicrobial agents is influenced by their bactericidal activity against the most likely pathogens, their relative toxicity, and the preferred route of administration. Patient factors, such as known allergy to certain antibiotics, therapy within the previous month and the nature of the cardiac condition are also of importance. Recommendations based on those of the British Society for Antimicrobial Chemotherapy[3] for antibiotic prophylaxis of infective endocarditis are provided in Table 9-1.

CLINICAL PRESENTATION

As has been mentioned, the clinical presentation of infective endocarditis in the Western world has altered. In our experience, the diagnosis is often overlooked or delayed, and many patients presenting with "pyrexia of unknown origin" are inadequately treated or given inappropriate antibiotics before infective endocarditis has been excluded. Infective endocarditis should be suspected in any patient with pyrexia, albeit low grade, and a pathological murmur. The diagnosis will be missed for weeks, or even months, if the clinician awaits signs such as anemia, systemic embolism, splenomegaly, clubbing of the fingers, positive blood cultures, or echocardiographic evidence of vegetations. *All patients with congenital or valvular heart disease who have an elevated temperature, albeit low grade and intermittent, should be suspected of having infective endocarditis and be fully investigated.* If the diagnosis remains in doubt after at most 10 days of observation and investigation, a therapeutic trial of appropriate antibiotics should be given.

The clinical features of infective endocarditis depend on the organism involved, the nature of the cardiac abnormality, and the length of time during which the patient has been infected. Some patients infected with an organism of low virulence, such as Staphylococcus epidermidis (albus), may have had symptoms of general malaise, sweating, anorexia, and weight loss for many months. Others, infected with a virulent organism such as Staphylococcus aureus, may have had a pyrexial illness of a few days' duration before they presented with a catastrophic event, such as subarachnoid hemorrhage or acute heart failure due to rupture of a valve. The nature of the cardiac abnormality is equally important: patients with right-sided endocarditis or infection associated with a left to right shunt, notably ventricular septal defect and patent ductus arteriosus, will frequently have a pyrexial illness accompanied by pulmonary symptoms and signs. They then present with pneumonitis as a result of infected pulmonary embolism. Several areas of lung may be involved (Fig. 9-8). More rarely, a radiological picture simulating miliary tuberculosis is encountered.

The prevalence of some important clinical features, based on an analysis of 70 White patients treated in the Johannesburg Hospital,[4,5] is shown in Figure 9-9. These patients reflect only a fraction of our total clinical experience but exemplify the pattern of presentation of infective endocarditis in that population group. Some of the presenting features require emphasis.

PYREXIA

Pyrexia, often low grade, is by far the single most important physical sign of infective endocarditis in a patient with a pathological cardiac murmur. We believe that any

TABLE 9-1. Recommendations for Antibiotic Prophylaxis of Infective Endocarditis

PROCEDURE	LA/GA	REMARKS	PENICILLIN ALLERGY		ANTIBIOTIC REGIMEN
DENTAL: Scaling Extraction Surgery to gingival tissues	LA			**A.** adults	: amoxicillin 3.0 g orally 1 hour prior to procedure
			–	children 5–10 years	: ½ adult dose
				children <5 years	: ¼ adult dose
			+ or penicillin in previous month	**B.** adults	: erythromycin 1.5 g orally 1–2 hours prior to procedure and : 0.5 g 6 hours later
				children 5–10 years	: ½ adult dose
				children <5 years	: ¼ adult dose
	GA	No special risk*	–	**C.** adults	: amoxicillin 1 g IMI immediately before induction and 0.5 g orally 6 hours later
				children <10 years	: ½ adult dose
			–	**D.** adults	: amoxicillin 1 g IMI plus gentamycin 120 mg IMI before induction or procedure and amoxicillin 0.5 g orally 6 hours later
				children <10 years	: amoxicillin ½ adult dose gentamycin 2 mg/kg body wt
		Special risk*	+	**E.** adults	: vancomycin 1 g slow IV infusion (20–30 minutes) followed by gentamycin 120 mg IVI before induction
				children <10 years	: vancomycin 20 mg/kg slow IVI infusion followed by gentamycin 2 mg/kg IVI

Procedure	Anaesthesia	Notes		Regimen	
GENITOURINARY SURGERY OR INSTRUMENTATION: Cystoscopy Urethral dilatation Prostatectomy Transrectal biopsy of prostate	GA	Routine prophylaxis not indicated for urethral catheterization unless infection present and procedure difficult	−	D	(Oral amoxycillin if LA)
			+	E	
OBSTETRIC AND GYNECOLOGICAL: Uncomplicated vaginal delivery	LA/GA	(NB: Reference 3 recommends prophylaxis for special risk* patients only)	−	D	(Oral amoxycillin if LA)
Cervical dilatation Insertion of intrauterine devices			+	E	
SURGERY TO UPPER RESPIRATORY TRACT: Tonsillectomy Adenoidectomy	GA	Prophylaxis not indicated for fiberoptic bronchoscopy	−	C D	for special risk* patients
			+	E	
GASTROINTESTINAL: Gastroscopy Colonoscopy Sigmoidoscopy Proctoscopy Barium enema	LA/GA	No routine prophylaxis except for special risk* patients	−	D	(Oral amoxycillin if LA)
			+	E	

GA = General anaesthesia

LA = Local anaesthesia

*Special risk patients comprise:
1. Patients who received penicillin in previous month
2. Patients with prosthetic valves
3. Patients who have had previous attack of infective endocarditis

Modified from British Society for Antimicrobial Chemotherapy,[3] 1982.

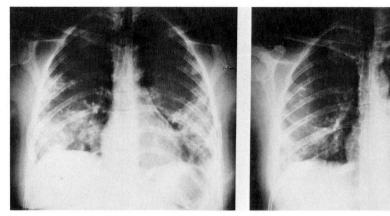

FIGURE 9-8. Posteroanterior chest radiograph of a patient with a ventricular septal defect who presented with a pyrexial illness and bilateral patchy areas of pneumonitis *(left)*. Blood cultures were positive for Staphylococcus aureus. Multiple septic pulmonary emboli, originating from infection on the septal defect, were diagnosed. Six weeks after antibiotic treatment *(right)*, there has been considerable clearing.

temperature above 37°C (98.4°F) is sufficient to warrant careful exclusion of bacterial endocarditis. The diagnosis may be unnecessarily delayed because of the reluctance of physicians to accept minor elevation of temperature as abnormal. Some patients are unaware of their pyrexia. The pyrexia may not be detected every day and may be partially masked by previous inadequate antibiotic therapy. It is a prevalent practice for doctors to treat a pyrexial illness early with antibiotics. Most White

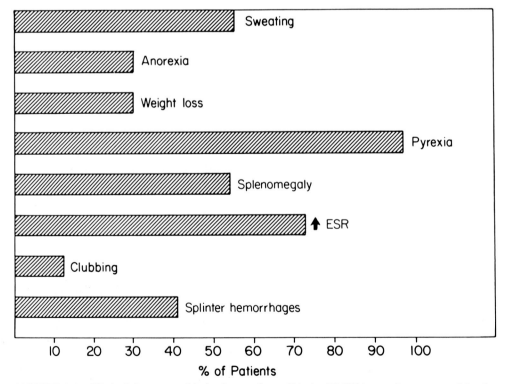

FIGURE 9-9. Clinical features of infective endocarditis in 70 White patients treated in the Johannesburg Hospital.

patients we encounter in hospital practice have received inappropriate antibiotic therapy without a definitive diagnosis having been made and without blood cultures having been taken. We have found that this practice is not confined to South Africa. Several of our patients were visiting Western countries when they first developed their pyrexia and received inadequate treatment, without a diagnosis having been reached. Presumably all medical students are taught not to prescribe antibiotics for a pyrexial illness until a diagnosis has been made, provided that the patient is not extremely ill. Nonetheless, this unnecessary practice prevails. The majority of patients with pyrexial illnesses present with clinical features that should make the diagnosis readily apparent. This is particularly true of viral infections. In other instances, a detailed history will often contribute to the nature of the illness. When the diagnosis is not apparent from the history and thorough clinical examination, blood cultures, agglutination, and other blood tests should be performed before antibiotic therapy is commenced.

It cannot be emphasized too strongly that an abnormal cardiac murmur and pyrexia may be the only evidence of infective endocarditis. Patients, including the elderly, are seldom truly apyrexial! It may be necessary to take the temperature frequently and carefully before an elevation is recorded. If the patient is dyspneic, pyrexia may be detected only by measuring the rectal temperature. In all instances, the thermometer should be left in situ for at least three minutes and then read by a responsible nurse or doctor.

GENERAL MALAISE

Many patients may not be aware of pyrexia but complain of tiredness, weakness, or of generally feeling unwell. On direct questioning, they may admit to anorexia and to have observed a weight loss. Abnormal sweating is a common symptom, occurring in 56 percent of our 70 patients but was seldom volunteered. The sweating may be accompanied by rigors and is noticed particularly at night. Arthralgia or myalgia occurs in about 15 percent of patients, but arthritis is unusual.

NEUROLOGICAL MANIFESTATIONS

Neurological manifestations have been reported in 10 percent to 50 percent of patients with infective endocarditis and carry a significant morbidity and mortality. Twenty percent of our 70 patients had neurological manifestations. Important presenting features include strokes, subarachnoid hemorrhage, and meningitis. Less ominous manifestations are mental confusion, psychiatric disturbances, headache, and mild encephalitis.

SYSTEMIC EMBOLI

Splinter hemorrhages are common and occurred in 41 percent in our series. Large emboli, especially those to the brain or to a mesenteric or coronary artery (Fig. 9-10) are a serious manifestation of infective endocarditis. A ruptured cerebral mycotic aneurysm, presenting as a stroke or subarachnoid hemorrhage, carries a very high mortality and may occur several weeks after the infective endocarditis has been cured. Small systemic emboli, reflected by petechial hemorrhages, Roth spots, and Osler's nodes, usually occur in longstanding cases when the diagnosis should already be obvious. Microscopic hematuria, observed in 25 percent of our patients, may be due to renal emboli or diffuse glomerulonephritis.

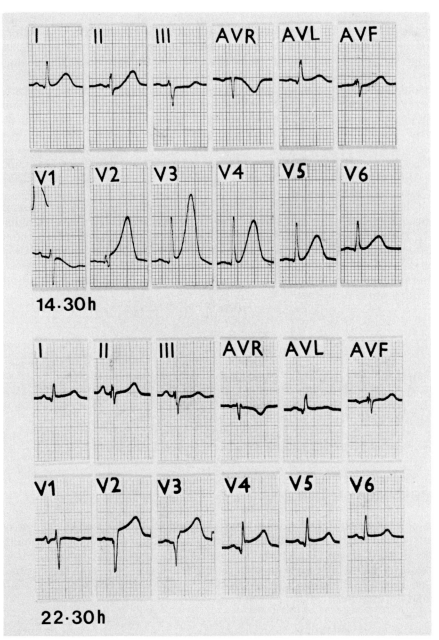

FIGURE 9-10. Evolving anteroseptal myocardial infarction in a 25-year-old man who sustained a coronary artery embolus during the course of infective endocarditis.

OTHER PHYSICAL SIGNS

An enlarged spleen was palpable in 54 percent of our patients, but clubbing of the fingers occurred in only 13 percent. Abnormally profuse sweating can commonly be detected, especially over the back in a subject who has been supine in bed. Persistent tachycardia, often out of proportion to the pyrexia or to the extent of cardiac decompensation, is a frequent finding.

LABORATORY FEATURES

It is meaningful to emphasize that the erythrocyte sedimentation rate remains normal in about 30 percent of patients. C-reactive protein may be a more sensitive indicator of infection, but we have not yet had the opportunity to confirm that. A high titre of circulating immune complexes and a depressed level of serum complement may be helpful to diagnosis, but the incidence and pertinence of these features require clarification. It is likely that these abnormalities will be absent early in the course of the disease. Normocytic normochromic anemia would be expected in the majority of patients who have been ill for more than four weeks, but this was present in only about 20 percent of our patients. The hemoglobin is seldom less than 10 g% unless there is associated blood loss, iron deficiency, or infection with an organism that causes hemolysis. A leukocytosis is not invariable and occurred in approximately 50 percent of our patients.

Although Staphylococcus epidermidis (albus) is widely regarded as an organism that is commonly responsible for early prosthetic valve endocarditis, it is not generally accepted as the offending organism in patients with infective endocarditis outside of the context of surgery. We cannot understand this reluctance to accept Staphylococcus epidermidis, especially when cultured repeatedly, as the cause of native valve infective endocarditis. We have cultured it as the sole organism in at least 20 percent of our White patients. The portal of entry into the bloodstream may be through abrasions in the skin or the gums.

The reported incidence of "culture-negative" patients varies from 5 percent to 30 percent and depends partly on the enthusiasm and efficiency of bacteriologists. We obtain positive cultures in about 80 percent of patients with infective endocarditis in the Johannesburg Hospital, but this figure is considerably lower in the other hospitals with which we are involved. Culture-negative infective endocarditis has been attributed to previous courses of antibiotics, infection with cell wall deficient bacteria (L-forms), infection with fastidious organisms and possibly sequestration of organisms within vegetations. A diagnosis of infective endocarditis is not excluded nor should therapy be delayed because of failure to culture an organism.

MANAGEMENT

When a positive blood culture is obtained, and the organism deemed to be pathological, sensitivity tests are undertaken and appropriate antibiotics started. Consultation with the bacteriologist is contributory and should always be sought. When we diagnose or strongly suspect infective endocarditis but have failed to culture an organism, we treat with parenteral penicillin, 12 million units intravenously. We add cloxacillin (2 g intravenously daily) and an aminoglycoside (tobramycin 2 g by intramuscular injection daily) if the response after five days' treatment is unsatisfactory. Should the patient fail to respond to this combined therapy or relapse after an initial response, the penicillin and cloxacillin are withdrawn and either a cephalosporin or clindamycin is added to the tobramycin.

There are two crucial questions to ask oneself when treating any patient with infective endocarditis. The first is "How is a satisfactory response to the antibiotics assessed?" Response to medical therapy is assessed primarily by its effect on the pyrexia. This should show improvement within 48 hours and the patient should be apyrexial, or very nearly so, after five days. Pyrexia in patients with infective endocarditis is a reflection of the bacteremia. If the organism is sensitive to the antibiotics that are being administered, bacteremia will be absent or mild and brief after five days' therapy. In addition, patients are often aware of a diminution of sweating and an increase in appetite. They generally "feel better." These latter features are largely

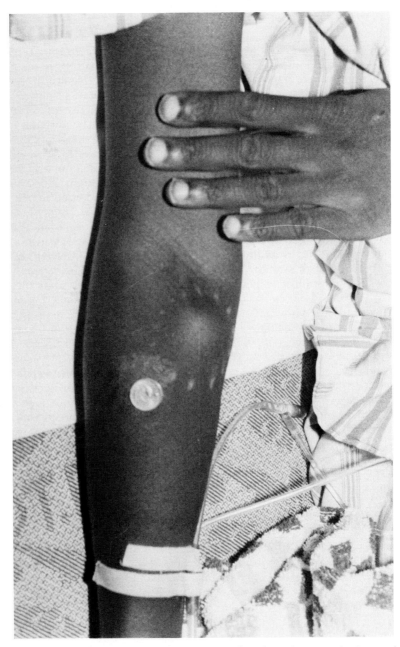

FIGURE 9-11. A 28-year-old man with gross mitral and aortic regurgitation and infective endocarditis who presented with a swelling of his right arm, diagnosed as a mycotic aneurysm of the right brachial artery. The marks around the mass represent scarification by a witchdoctor. The size is shown relative to a 5-cent coin (comparable to the size of a nickel).

subjective, and it is the response of the fever that is all important. Unabated pyrexia implies that the antibiotics are ineffectual or, much more rarely, that they are unable to reach the offending organisms; splenic, subphrenic, or other sites of abscess formation would be rare explanations for that occurrence.

The second question is "How long should antibiotic therapy be continued?" Many textbooks and scientific articles state a time period of four to six weeks. But four to six weeks after *what*? It is irrational to treat for this period of time if the patient has remained pyrexial. The essential decision that has to be made is the duration of treatment *after* the patient's temperature has returned to normal. There are no hard and fast rules, but we seldom treat for more than three weeks after the patient has become apyrexial. There may be an indication to treat for a longer period in patients with prosthetic endocarditis, infection on a rigid or calcified valve, recurrent endocarditis, or when a large vegetation has been demonstrated echocardiographically.

The response of laboratory tests to medical therapy is reassuring but is essentially an adjunct to the apyrexia, which must be attained before such therapy can be regarded as effectual. Erythrocyte sedimentation rate and serum globulin and complement levels may take several weeks to normalise. A rapid return to normal of C-reactive protein could be anticipated, but, as previously stated, we have not yet had extensive experience with that. A normochromic, normocytic anemia may persist for several weeks or even months after clinical cure of the infection.

Relevant dental therapy, including extractions, should be undertaken during the medical therapy, preferably immediately after the patient has become apyrexial. This is particularly important if the teeth are suspected of being the portal of entry of the infecting organisms.

Complications of infective endocarditis occurring either as presenting features or during treatment are managed on their merits. Renal impairment usually improves after successful antibiotic treatment, but temporary dialysis may be required. Large peripheral (Fig. 9-11) or mesenteric emboli may need surgery. The opinion of a neurosurgeon should be sought in the event of a subarachnoid hemorrhage, as surgery may be indicated. In our experience, subarachnoid hemorrhage carries an extremely high mortality with or without surgical intervention. Systemic emboli may be an indication for urgent cardiac surgery. However, if that is not favored, we advocate starting anticoagulant therapy to try to prevent further emboli. We have introduced sodium warfarin three days after a cerebral infarction, despite the possible danger of hemorrhage, but are uncertain whether such therapy has been of definite benefit. We favor prescribing warfarin derivatives to all patients with atrial fibrillation, including those with infective endocarditis, provided there is not a specific contraindication, such as peptic ulceration. We are aware of the hazards of anticoagulants, especially after cerebral infarction, but in our view further systemic emboli are the greater danger. Coronary embolism is responsible for the deaths of a few patients with endocarditis, but apart from that entity, a significant "myocardial factor" is extremely rare and probably never the principal cause of cardiac failure. Patients with right-sided endocarditis or with infection on lesions associated with a left-to-right shunt may die as a result of infective pulmonary thromboembolic disease. Overwhelming or intractable infection despite antibiotic therapy is rarely a cause of death. The majority of patients who die from infective endocarditis do so because of heart failure. Such heart failure is almost invariably caused by a severe cardiac work overload, which usually arises from an incompetent valve or valves or, more rarely, from an infected valve that becomes stenosed.

SURGICAL MANAGEMENT

Although the management of infective endocarditis is primarily medical, the most common cause of death is heart failure. As mentioned earlier, the heart failure is invariably due to a hemodynamic load and, provided severe pulmonary thromboembolic disease is not the causative factor (as in right-sided infective endocarditis), surgical correction is the only effective therapy. On theoretical grounds, it is preferable if a medical cure has been attained or at least that effective antibiotics have been administered for a few days prior to surgery. However, excellent results can be achieved with virtually no prior antibiotic treatment, and surgery should never be delayed in order for this to be given when the patient's life is at stake owing to heart failure. The timing of operation may be difficult. On the whole, it should be performed too early rather than too late. If a patient dies of heart failure before surgery, then the judgement of the cardiologist was invariably at fault. The overall mortality from infective endocarditis should be well under 20 percent, but that figure will be attained only when cardiologists adopt a more aggressive approach to surgical management.

The overall mortality of the 70 White patients analyzed by us was 13 percent. Eleven of the last 40 of those patients were subjected to surgery for hemodynamic reasons, with no resultant mortality. Over the last six years (1980 through 1985) during which a total of 1041 White patients in our unit were subjected to valve replacement, the indication for operation in 53 patients was infective endocarditis on mitral or aortic valves with severe hemodynamic overload. Ten patients had mitral valve, 34 aortic, and 9 double valve replacement. There were two hospital deaths (3.8 percent), both from "multiorgan failure" in men who had had aortic valve replacements as emergency procedures.

The majority of our Black patients present late in the course of their disease. Many are in severe heart failure or are moribund. These patients are therefore subjected to surgery without prior antibiotic treatment or having had antibiotics for less than a week. In an analysis from this unit by Lewis and co-workers[6] of 94 Black patients with active infective endocarditis, the overall operative mortality was only 16 percent, despite the fact that 61 of the 94 patients (64.8 percent) were operated on as emergencies. Only 11 patients were subjected to surgery as an elective procedure, and 22 were regarded as semiemergencies. More than half of the patients had received inadequate or no antibiotic treatment before surgery. More recently, we analyzed the operative results on 25 Black patients with active infective endocarditis, severe aortic regurgitation, and heart failure who required emergency surgery. Six of the 25 patients also required mitral valve replacement. All patients were operated on within 24 hours of admission. Antibiotic treatment was started within 12 hours of, or immediately after, operation. Vegetations were present on the aortic valve in all 25 patients and on the mitral valve in five. Five patients had aortic anular abscesses. There was only one operative death and two late deaths, neither of which was related to infection. These two series provide convincing evidence of the favorable results of surgery for patients with infective endocarditis who are in heart failure, regardless of whether medical therapy has been started, let alone having been shown to be effective or completed.

The indications for and timing of surgery in patients with infective endocarditis will now be discussed.

CARDIAC FAILURE

Aortic and mitral regurgitation are the most common lesions to be exacerbated by infective endocarditis and to subsequently result in heart failure. Patients with severe aortic regurgitation who develop left ventricular failure should be regarded as surgical emergencies or semiemergencies. Diuretic and vasodilator therapy will temporarily improve the heart failure, but surgery should be undertaken as soon as the diagnosis is made and certainly within 48 hours. Infective endocarditis involving the aortic valve is occasionally complicated by rupture of a sinus of Valsalva into the right atrium, right ventricle, or occasionally the left atrium. The associated aortic regurgitation is invariably hemodynamically significant, and surgery should not be postponed.

Pulmonary edema resulting from acute-onset mitral regurgitation is somewhat different. Fairly mild mitral regurgitation that is acutely produced, such as from rupture of a chorda tendinea, may result in pulmonary edema (Fig. 9-12), which is not necessarily a reflection of true left ventricular failure and should respond well to medical therapy. Severity of the mitral regurgitation is easier to assess after the pulmonary edema has subsided, and assessment can usually be accomplished by clinical

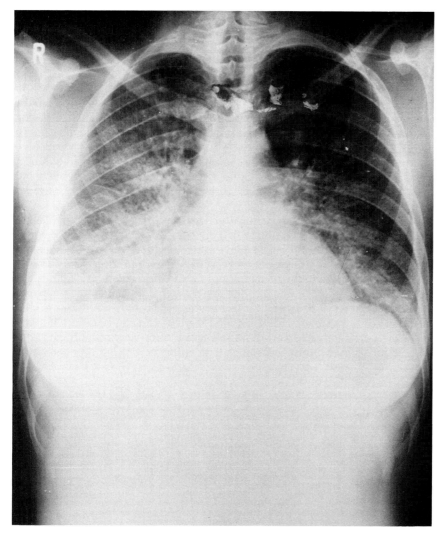

FIGURE 9-12. Pulmonary edema in a patient with acute mitral regurgitation secondary to chordal rupture in infective endocarditis.

examination alone. Surgery often may not be required or can be postponed for months or years.

Patients with pure or dominant mitral or aortic stenosis may develop increased stenosis of their valves during the course of infective endocarditis as a result of infected thrombus or vegetations—so-called Oslerian endocarditis.[7] Surgery is indicated once these changes have been detected because the lesions are invariably hemodynamically severe.

Patients with valvular lesions and mild heart failure, well controlled on medical therapy, may develop infective endocarditis. An example is a patient with a mixed mitral lesion, mildly symptomatic on diuretic therapy, for whom it had been judged that mitral valve surgery could be postponed. Such a patient must be observed for signs of increasing cardiac failure but is a somewhat different problem from one who was not in failure before the onset of the infective endocarditis. A more rapid ventricular rate, especially with atrial fibrillation, may result from the pyrexia; pulmonary infection may be associated; or pulmonary embolism may supervene because of the bed rest and immobility. Heart failure would be aggravated by all such factors, but in those circumstances the failure per se would not be an indication for immediate surgery.

ECHOCARDIOGRAPHIC DEMONSTRATION OF VEGETATIONS AND SYSTEMIC EMBOLI

Since the observations of Dillon and associates,[8] the value of echocardiography in demonstrating vegetations in patients with infective endocarditis has been confirmed by many workers. A minimum size of 5 mm is required before these vegetations can be identified with certainty. The demonstration of vegetations is not absolute proof of active infective endocarditis, as they do not always decrease in size or change in appearance after cure of the infection: as long as 12 months later they may remain unchanged. It is therefore important to be aware of previous bouts of infective endocarditis in the individual patient. In a patient with suspected infective endocarditis, vegetations not only confirm the diagnosis but also influence decisions regarding management. Vegetations greater than 10 mm are cause for concern because of the possibility of systemic embolism.

Unless stenosis is hemodynamically significant or the dominant lesion, large vegetations on the aortic valve (Fig. 9-13) are almost always associated with severe regurgitation, which in itself would be an indication for aortic valve replacement. We regard the presence of a large aortic valve vegetation as an indication for immediate surgery, regardless of whether the patient is in left ventricular failure. It is our impression that aortic valve vegetations are more liable than mitral vegetations to embolize, the greatest danger being coronary artery embolization and occlusion. In the absence of tight stenosis with thickened leaflets, the combination of a large vegetation on the aortic valve with only mild regurgitation is extremely rare, because a large vegetation is invariably associated with important valve damage, leaflet pro-

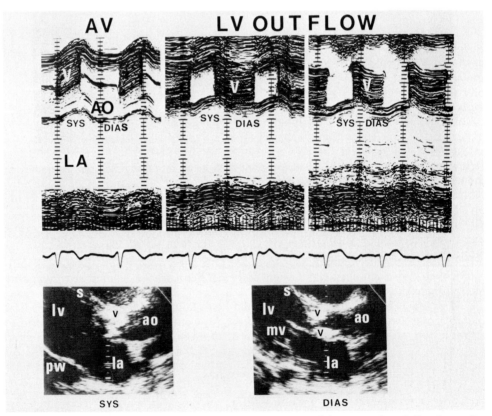

FIGURE 9-13. *Upper tracing,* M-mode echocardiogram; and *lower tracing,* 2-D echocardiogram. These show the large vegetation (V) on the aortic valve (AV), which prolapses into the left ventricular (LV) outflow tract during diastole.

lapse, and hence severe aortic regurgitation. In one instance, we elected to treat medically infective endocarditis in a middle-aged man with moderate aortic regurgitation, good left ventricular function, and a 20 mm vegetation on the aortic valve. Twenty-four hours later, he died suddenly from obstruction of his left coronary artery by the vegetation. Since the aortic regurgitation was hemodynamically significant, the large vegetation should have been an indication for immediate surgery, despite the absence of left ventricular failure.

Vegetations on the mitral valve are less ominous. Because of the different functional anatomy of that valve, mitral vegetations may be large yet the degree of mitral incompetence remain mild. In such cases, we favor medical management including anticoagulant drugs. In most instances, a satisfactory result can be anticipated without major systemic embolism or much progression of the mitral regurgitation supervening. If the regurgitation is hemodynamically significant, we refer patients for valve replacement after appropriate therapy for pulmonary venous congestion and, if possible, some effective antibiotic therapy. Thus, in summary:

1. We seldom regard a large vegetation detected echocardiographically on a mitral valve as a sole indication for immediate surgical intervention.
2. When the mitral valve lesion is hemodynamically significant, a large vegetation influences us to operate sooner rather than later.
3. Large vegetations on the aortic valve are almost always accompanied by a significant hemodynamic lesion. In such cases, there is probably a greater risk of major systemic embolism and there is certainly a greater risk of coronary occlusion, which may be fatal. Our policy is to operate as soon as possible when a large aortic valve vegetation is detected echocardiographically.

The occurrence of major systemic emboli may also influence the decision concerning early surgery. If the mitral valve is clinically normal and if it is strongly suspected that a major embolus arose from infective endocarditis on the aortic valve, the aortic lesion will invariably be hemodynamically significant and echocardiography will usually confirm a vegetation. In such a case, surgery is indicated. A major embolus from a hemodynamically severe mitral valve lesion would again be an indication for early surgery, especially if a large vegetation was detected echocardiographically. If the mitral lesion is not hemodynamically severe enough to warrant surgery, a decision to operate after a major systemic embolus has occurred would be influenced by other factors and it is difficult to generalize about this situation. In most cases, such embolism occurs as a presenting or early feature and effective antibiotic therapy should be started or continued even if a large vegetation is observed on an echocardiogram. It would be unusual for another embolus to occur once effective antibiotic therapy has been instituted. A second systemic embolus, progressive mitral regurgitation, a very large vegetation, and an unsatisfactory response to antibiotic therapy would be indications for early surgery.

PERICARDITIS AND CONDUCTION DEFECTS

In the context of infective endocarditis, a pericardial rub or pericardial effusion is occasionally a manifestation of an infected coronary embolus, but usually results from subanular infection in a patient with aortic valve endocarditis. The conduction system may then be involved, with resultant fascicular, first-degree, or more severe heart block. These signs are probably an indication for immediate surgery provided the aortic regurgitation is severe and warrants valve replacement. When the regurgitation is relatively mild, uncommon in our experience, we do not subject such patients to immediate cardiac surgery, and we have had satisfactory results with effectual antibiotic therapy. Electrical pacing is rarely indicated. The conduction defect often improves, suggesting that inflammatory edema is a causal factor. Cardiac rupture is a potential hazard in such cases, but we have encountered that complication in only one instance. Occasionally, a pericardial effusion that develops rapidly or is very large impairs the circulation and may cause cardiac tamponade. Pericardial paracentesis should not be delayed once hemodynamically significant pericardial effusion is detected. It is important to remember that cardiac tamponade will not cause pulsus paradoxus in the presence of moderate or severe aortic regurgitation.

INFECTION REFRACTORY TO MEDICAL THERAPY

Native valve endocarditis refractory to treatment should initially never be the sole indication for surgical intervention. For infection to persist without a hemodynamically significant valvular lesion supervening is extremely rare. Correction of the hemodynamics is then good reason for surgery. We recently treated unsuccessfully a man with Staphylococcus aureus septicemia, aortic endocarditis, and mild regurgitation. Necropsy confirmed that the infection was uncontrolled and widespread, with numerous abscesses in many organs. Aortic valve replacement would clearly not have been significantly advantageous. We have a large experience, particularly among our Black patients, of infective endocarditis that persisted despite antibiotic therapy, but it has always been associated with a hemodynamically significant lesion. Correction of the hemodynamics has been the indication for cardiac surgery, and cure of the infection has almost always been achieved. Removal of infected tissue is probably a factor in curing such cases. In general, however, the management of infective endocarditis is primarily medical. The crucial role of surgery is to prevent death from heart failure and not to cure the infection.

PROSTHETIC VALVE ENDOCARDITIS

Infection on a mechanical prosthetic valve may occur early (within two months of surgery) or late. It is our experience that late infective endocarditis, as with infection and a left-to-right shunt, on a Björk-Shiley, Medtronic-Hall, or St. Jude valve is rare in the absence of an antecedent paravalvular leak. The pertinence of careful auscultation about two months after prosthetic valve replacement is thus readily apparent. The management of mechanical prosthetic valve endocarditis is primarily medical, provided there is no major paravalvular regurgitation or valve obstruction. A leaking aortic prosthetic valve is reliably detected by the early diastolic murmur, wide pulse pressure, positive Duroziez's sign, and other evidence of aortic regurgitation. A leaking mitral prosthetic valve may be more difficult to diagnose. Contrary to the experience of others, we have never encountered a mitral prosthetic ring leak that is silent. The systolic murmur may be very soft, Grade 1, or at most Grade 2; but it should be audible on careful auscultation including that with the patient in the left lateral position. Not infrequently, the radiation of the murmur would be highly unusual for native mitral valve regurgitation, and the murmur may be loudest well medial to the apex or even over the back. A severe ring leak may be suspected or confirmed by other signs of mitral regurgitation such as a sustained apex beat, left atrial lift, wide splitting of the second sound, left atrial enlargement on the ECG, and pulmonary venous hypertension on chest roentgenogram. Screening of the valve may reveal "rocking" when it is detached from the valve ring for at least one third of its circumference. Immediate surgery is then indicated.

Obstruction of a mechanical prosthetic valve by infected material and thrombus is a surgical emergency. Once present, it progresses rapidly until the orifice is completely obstructed and death in intractable pulmonary edema or shock ensues.

The degree of impairment of the opening and closing sounds of the prosthesis varies with the type of valve and may not be marked, even when the obstruction is severe (see Chapter 8, Section 2). Echocardiography may be very contributory in confirming obstruction or paravalvular leak and is also discussed in Chapter 8.

Early postoperative infective endocarditis on a bioprosthetic valve should be treated medically, unless severe regurgitant lesions develop. Late infective endocarditis has only supervened, in our experience, on leaflets that have degenerated with hemodynamically significant stenosis or regurgitation. We then replace the tissue valve with a mechanical prosthesis after one or two weeks of appropriate antibiotic therapy.

RICKETTSIAL ENDOCARDITIS

For ill-understood reasons, Q fever (rickettsial) endocarditis is rare in South Africa; but the mortality has been about 50 percent in the few cases (less than 10) in which we have made or strongly suspected that diagnosis. Medical therapy may control the infection but is seldom curative. We have used tetracycline 2 g daily, but co-trimoxazole and rifampicin have also been recommended.[9] Treatment should be continued for months or even years in the hope that the positive agglutination titres will return to normal levels, implying control or even cure of the infection. Surgery is indicated if the hemodynamics warrant it.

FUNGAL ENDOCARDITIS

Fungal endocarditis carries a grave prognosis and has fortunately been rare in our experience. We have recognized four cases only. Two occurred after aortic homograft valve replacement and one after aortic Björk-Shiley prosthetic valve replacement. The fourth involved the mitral valve of a young woman who had had an indwelling intravenous line for a prolonged time. Large vegetations and major systemic embolism characterized the clinical course. Despite early valve replacement, all the patients died.

RIGHT-SIDED ENDOCARDITIS

A major problem in patients with right-sided endocarditis is infected pulmonary emboli, which manifest as fleeting and multiple areas of pneumonitis. Common sequelae are abscesses, pleural effusions, and empyemas for which surgery may be required. Numerous small infected pulmonary emboli may cause a radiological picture resembling miliary tuberculosis (Fig. 9-14). Mycotic pulmonary artery aneurysms (Fig. 9-15) may leak, causing recurrent hemoptysis or fatal hemorrhage. Similar to our experience in left-sided endocarditis, we are strongly opposed to cardiac surgery on a patient with right-sided endocarditis in order to attain a cure of the infection. Other investigators have advocated removal of the tricuspid valve in order to eradicate the infection. We find it difficult to understand how the pulmonary infection but not the associated right-sided endocarditis can be controlled by antibiotics. An illustrative example is that of a 9-year-old boy with staphylococcal endocarditis of the tricuspid valve and regurgitation due to a flail leaflet, who developed severe bilateral staphylococcal pulmonary infection (Fig. 9-16) and empyema requiring drainage. Infection of the valve and lungs was eradicated with appropriate antibiotic treatment. We have not regarded large right-sided vegetations as an indication for

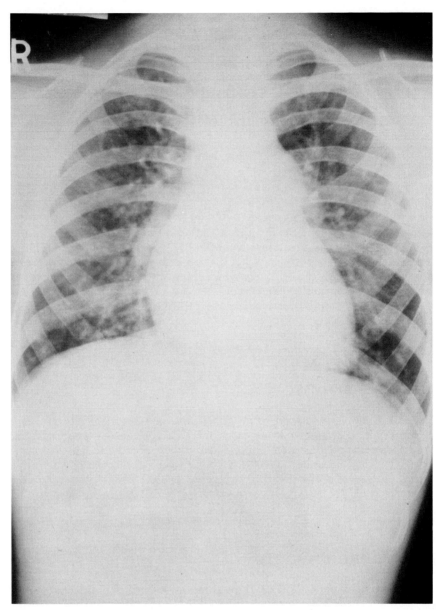

FIGURE 9-14. Posteroanterior chest radiograph resembling miliary tuberculosis in an 11-year-old girl with an infected patent ductus arteriosus and multiple pulmonary emboli. Existing pulmonary hypertension increased during the course of the illness.

cardiac surgery. One of our patients had gross isolated organic tricuspid regurgitation but no serious hemodynamic problems, because very early antibiotic therapy prevented significant pulmonary embolization causing her pulmonary vascular resistance to remain low. Another patient, a 24-year-old man with tetralogy of Fallot, developed infective endocarditis on the pulmonary valve but had had numerous infected pulmonary emboli before the diagnosis was made. After cure of the infection and subsequent surgical closure of the ventricular septal defect, he developed severe right ventricular failure, with a pulmonary artery pressure of 90/10 mmHg and gross pulmonary regurgitation. He improved considerably after pulmonary valve replacement with an Ionescu-Shiley valve and remains on anticoagulant therapy.

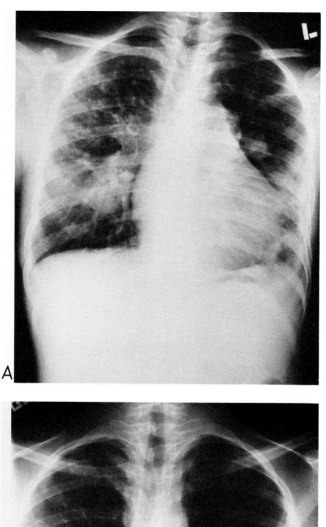

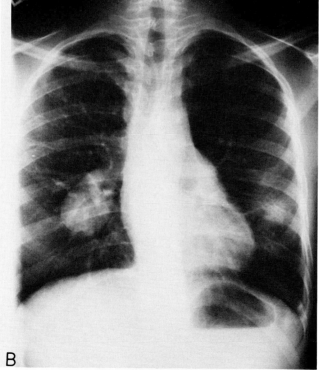

FIGURE 9-15. Posteroanterior chest radiographs of a 12-year-old boy who presented with bilateral pulmonary emboli from infection on a patent ductus arteriosus (*A*). The ductus was ligated after antibiotic treatment. The large mass in the right lung, noted postoperatively (*B*), was shown to be a pulmonary artery aneurysm.

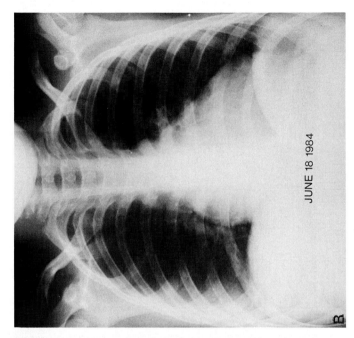

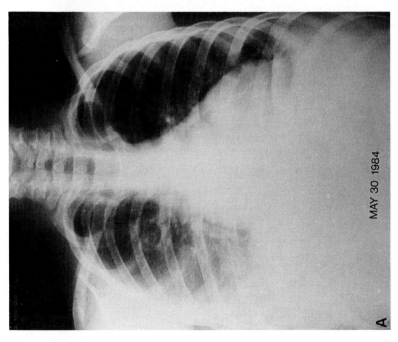

FIGURE 9-16. A 9-year-old boy with Staphylococcus aureus tricuspid endocarditis, tricuspid regurgitation, multiple pulmonary emboli, and right-sided empyema (*A*). After antibiotic therapy (*B*), there has been considerable improvement.

CONCLUDING REMARKS

The prevalence of infective endocarditis may decrease with improved oral hygiene and effective antibiotic prophylaxis at times of risk. It seems unlikely that this disease will occur in the immediate future, especially in Third World countries. We are convinced that the mortality can be significantly decreased and should not be higher than 20 percent, irrespective of the severity of the condition. The major cause of death is cardiac failure, which should be avoided by appropriate cardiac surgery. Definitive antibiotic treatment would be more effective if antibiotics were not indiscriminately prescribed for patients with a "pyrexia of unknown origin." Moreover, the possibility of infective endocarditis should always be kept in mind in any patient with a pyrexial illness. If clinical examination reveals a pathological murmur, then infective endocarditis must be carefully excluded. Early diagnosis and effective antibiotic treatment of infective endocarditis would markedly reduce the overall morbidity and mortality. Finally, response to appropriate antibiotic therapy is assessed primarily by its effect on the pyrexia. The patient should be apyrexial, or very nearly so, within five days of beginning such therapy.

REFERENCES

1. HAYWARD, GW: *Infective endocarditis: A changing disease.* Br Med J 2:706–709, 764–766, 1973.
2. BALTCH, AL, SCHAFFER, C, HAMMER, MC, SUTPHEN, NT, SMITH, RP, CONROY, J, AND SHAY-EGANI, M: *Bacteremia following dental cleaning in patients with and without penicillin prophylaxis.* Am Heart J 104:1335–1339, 1982.
3. BRITISH SOCIETY FOR ANTIMICROBIAL CHEMOTHERAPY: *The antibiotic prophylaxis of infective endocarditis. Report of a working Party.* Lancet 2:1323–1326, 1982.
4. MAZANSKY, C, LAKIER, JB, AND BARLOW, JB: *Aspects of bacterial endocarditis in the Johannesburg General Hospital. An analysis of 30 cases.* S Afr Med J 47:413–417, 1973.
5. CASSEL, GA, HAITAS, B, LAKIER, JB, AND BARLOW, JB: *Infective endocarditis at the Johannesburg Hospital. A retrospective analysis of 40 patients.* S Afr Med J 55:624–627, 1979.
6. LEWIS, BS, AGATHANGELOU, NE, COLSEN, PR, ANTUNES, M, AND KINSLEY, RH: *Cardiac operation during active infective endocarditis. Results of aortic, mitral, and double valve replacement in 94 patients.* J Thorac Cardiovasc Surg 84:579–584, 1982.
7. WITCHITZ, S, REGNIER, B, WOLFF, M, ROUVEIX, E, AND LAISNE, MJ: *Surgery in infective endocarditis.* Eur Heart J 5:87–91, 1984.
8. DILLON, JC, FEIGENBAUM, H, KONECKE, LL, DAVIS, RH, AND CHANG, S: *Echocardiographic manifestations of valvular vegetations.* Am Heart J 86:698–704, 1973.
9. GEDDES, AM: *Q Fever.* Br Med J 287:927–928, 1983.

BIBLIOGRAPHY

ALSIP, SG, BLACKSTONE, EH, KIRKLIN, JW, AND COBBS, CG: *Indications for cardiac surgery in patients with active infective endocarditis.* Am J Med 78:138–148, 1985.
BAYLISS, R, CLARKE, C, OAKLEY, C, SOMERVILLE, W, AND WHITFIELD, AGW: *The teeth and infective endocarditis.* Br Heart J 50:506–512, 1983.
BAYLISS, R, CLARKE, C, OAKLEY, CM, SOMERVILLE, W, WHITFIELD, AGW, AND YOUNG, SEJ: *The bowel, the genitourinary tract, and infective endocarditis.* Br Heart J 51:339–345, 1984.
DE LEON, SP AND WENZEL, RP: *Hospital-acquired bloodstream infections with Staphylococcus epidermidis.* Am J Med 77:639–644, 1984.
DURACK, DT: *Current issues in prevention of infective endocarditis.* Am J Med 78:149–156, 1985.
GUNTHEROTH, WG: *How important are dental procedures as a cause of infective endocarditis?* Am J Cardiol 54:797–801, 1984.

KAYE, D: *Infective endocarditis. An overview.* Am J Med 78:107–109, 1985.

LOWENTHAL, DT, PENNOCK, RS, LIKOFF, W, AND ONESTI, G: *Management of infective endocarditis in chronic renal failure.* In LOWENTHAL ET AL: *Management of the Cardiac Patient with Renal Failure.* FA Davis, Philadelphia, 1981, pp 173–190.

MISHELL, DR, JR: *Current status of intrauterine devices.* N Engl J Med 312:984–985, 1985.

MORRIS, GK: *Infective endocarditis: A preventable disease?* Br Med J 290:1532–1533, 1985.

O'BRIEN, JT AND GEISER, EA: *Infective endocarditis and echocardiography.* Am Heart J 108:386–394, 1984.

PROUDFIT, WL: *Skin signs of infective endocarditis.* Am Heart J 106:1451–1453, 1983.

RAHIMTOOLA, SH: *Infective Endocarditis. Clinical cardiology monographs.* Grune & Stratton, New York, 1978.

SIDDLE, N: *Risks of intrauterine contraceptive devices.* Br Med J 288:1554–1555, 1984.

TANDBERG, D AND SKLAR, D: *Effect of tachypnea on the estimation of body temperature by an oral thermometer.* N Engl J Med 308:945–946, 1983.

10

CONDITIONS RELEVANT TO ASSESSMENT OR FUNCTION OF THE MITRAL VALVE

SECTION 1: PULMONARY ARTERIAL HYPERTENSION

Every clinical cardiologist has an experience with pulmonary arterial hypertension, and the entity is of particular importance to one who encounters a large number of cases of mitral valve disease. Before the advent of echocardiography, it was a major challenge to the clinician to exclude that severe pulmonary arterial hypertension was not produced by a left-sided heart lesion amenable to surgical treatment, such as mitral stenosis and left atrial myxoma.

There is extensive scientific literature on all aspects of pulmonary arterial hypertension, a review of which is beyond the scope of this book. My observations and conclusions are based on investigation of a large number of cases and are now correlated with, or sometimes differentiated from, the current literature or dogma.

Some of the physical signs of pulmonary arterial hypertension may be modified by the underlying condition causing the hypertension. Clinical signs of pulmonary arterial hypertension comprise one or more of the following:

1. Tachycardia, small volume pulse, and peripheral cyanosis
2. Prominent a waves in the jugular venous pulse
3. A forceful right ventricular heave at the sternal area
4. Forceful pulmonary arterial pulsation and palpable pulmonary valve closure in the second left intercostal space
5. Right-sided gallop sound (usually atrial), tricuspid regurgitant murmur, early systolic pulmonary sound, loud pulmonary component of second sound, a pulmonary ejection murmur, and a pulmonary early diastolic murmur

The causes of pulmonary arterial hypertension fall into five main groups, which will be discussed separately.

PULMONARY THROMBOEMBOLIC DISEASE

This is the most prevalent cause of pulmonary arterial hypertension in our adult patients of all population groups. The diagnosis is frequently overlooked, especially when thromboembolic disease is associated with other conditions such as chronic obstructive airways disease, mitral valve disease, or left ventricular dysfunction from any cause. Isolated pulmonary thromboembolic disease is often misdiagnosed as "primary pulmonary hypertension," Eisenmenger's syndrome, or, less commonly, dilated cardiomyopathy. Reasons for clinicians underdiagnosing this condition include lack of awareness of its prevalence, the frequent absence of past or current thrombophlebitis or phlebothrombosis, the patient's inability to recall previous symptoms suggestive of acute pulmonary emboli, and, probably because the condition is almost always diffuse and bilateral, the lack of specific findings on ventilation-perfusion lung scans.

PAST HISTORY AND PATHOGENETIC MECHANISMS

We encounter chronic pulmonary thromboembolic disease at any age over 15 years, and it is more common in women. The past history may be unimpressive but direct questioning may elicit information relating to an initial predisposing factor and to the onset of the condition. Questions should be asked regarding previous operations, illnesses diagnosed (such as pneumonitis or pneumonia), unilateral swelling of a calf, trauma to a lower limb, pulmonary events after a pregnancy or after pelvic sepsis, pleurisy, and previous episodes of breathlessness. Previous or current hemoptysis is unusual in our experience. Although we encounter the condition in persons from all walks of life, factors of obesity and sedentary occupations (for example, bus drivers) are probably relevant.

The two principal presenting features are increasing dyspnea and symptoms of right ventricular failure, commonly swelling of the ankles or pain in the right hypochondrium owing to hepatic distension. Some patients present with pneumonitis with or without pleuritic pain. Previous syncope or dizziness is uncommon, and exertional angina-like chest pain is rare in our experience. Pathogenetic mechanisms are not understood, but it should be emphasized that this is a disease involving the proximal pulmonary arteries. The entity of multiple "microemboli" has not been encountered, and I do not believe that it exists. It would seem to me that the essential feature of chronic pulmonary thromboembolic disease is an initial thrombus, either in situ or embolic, in a pulmonary artery branch. Any cause of stasis in the pulmonary arterial system is probably pertinent. The condition is therefore prevalent in association with mitral valve or other left heart disease, chronic obstructive airways disease, or any other cause of pulmonary arterial hypertension. Possibly an initial

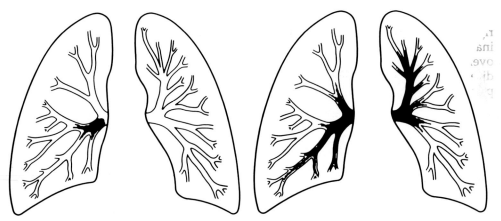

FIGURE 10-1. Diagrammatic representation of extension of an initial pulmonary thrombus or embolus to involve more distal branches as well as proximal vessels of the same and opposite lungs.

thrombus may develop in situ during a lung infection involving parenchymal tissue. Likely sites of origin of pulmonary emboli are well known, as are such predisposing factors as surgery, pelvic sepsis, deep vein thrombosis, and peripheral venous stasis. Although most cases of acute pulmonary embolism spontaneously recanalize within six or eight weeks, it is possible that lysis is not always complete and that residual clotting forms the nidus for subsequent extension of thrombosis. Once a thrombus has formed or lodged, spread to other branches of the pulmonary tree is understandable (Fig. 10-1). It would seem that this mechanism of progression of pulmonary thromboembolic disease is far more prevalent than the commonly emphasized "recurrent" pulmonary emboli arising from the systemic venous system.

PHYSICAL SIGNS

The obvious physical signs, already listed, of severe pulmonary arterial hypertension are almost always easily detected. A right atrial sound which becomes earlier and louder on inspiration may be audible over the lower sternum or epigastric area. Functional pulmonary regurgitation is common, and an early diastolic murmur is a prominent feature in about 10 percent of cases. In such instances, P2 is relatively softer and a tricuspid mid-diastolic murmur, possibly analogous to the left-sided Austin-Flint murmur, is usually present. In some cases, especially if the functional tricuspid regurgitation is mild and the pulmonary hypertension severe, the pansystolic murmur of tricuspid regurgitation may be as loud as Grade 3. Occasionally, a long systolic murmur, or even a continuous murmur, may be detected at any site over the precordium or back and arises from a partially obstructed pulmonary artery branch. Examination of the lungs is often unremarkable, but decreased air entry and crepitations may be detected. It is unusual to hear a pleural rub in chronic pulmonary thromboembolic disease.

Central cyanosis is variable and may range from being clinically undetectable to severe. It does not necessarily correlate with the severity of the pulmonary hypertension or right heart failure, and the degree is determined by perfusion defects, the opening of pulmonary arteriovenous shunts, and right-to-left shunting through a stretched patent foramen ovale. This latter mechanism has been the explanation for fairly severe central cyanosis in some of our patients.

ELECTROCARDIOGRAPHIC FEATURES

The ECG of "isolated" pulmonary thromboembolic disease is seldom normal; and right-axis deviation, prominent right atrial P waves, clockwise rotation, and a dominant R wave, or QR, in leads V_1 and V_{4R} are usually seen. T waves may be inverted r the right precordial leads (Fig. 10-2). When chronic pulmonary thromboembolic disease is associated with other conditions, there are wide variations in the different patterns.

RADIOLOGICAL FEATURES

The posteroanterior chest radiograph is all important in the diagnosis of chronic pulmonary thromboembolic disease (Figs. 10-3, 10-4). The features have to be specifically sought, and more than a decade ago we showed that assessment can be very accurate and observer error very small.[1] The main pulmonary artery may be prominent, but that is a nonspecific finding and may be present in patients with pulmonary hypertension from any cause, as well as in those with conditions of increased pulmonary flow (for example, atrial septal defect), with pulmonary stenosis, and with

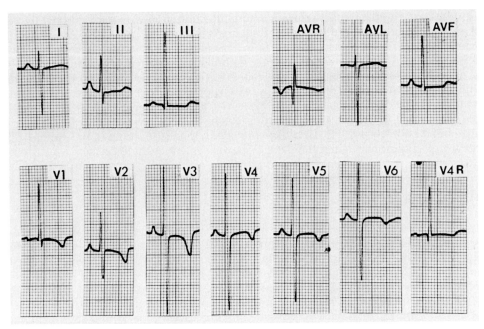

FIGURE 10-2. ECG of a 40-year-old woman with isolated pulmonary thromboembolic disease. There is marked right ventricular hypertrophy with inverted T waves in V_1–V_4 and right atrial enlargement.

"idiopathic dilatation of the pulmonary artery." The important radiological features of pulmonary thromboembolic disease are as follows:

1. *Prominence and increased opacity of the right pulmonary artery.* This is due to organized and old thrombus. The left pulmonary artery often has similar pathology but is not well seen in the posteroanterior view.
2. *Oligemia, distal to the right or left branches of the main pulmonary artery.* Because of lack of blood flow distal to the proximal pulmonary artery branches and because of decreased cardiac output, the pulmonary vessels are underfilled and a diminution of vascular markings may exist. Some of the vessels just distal to the right pulmonary artery may be abnormally opaque because of organized thrombus. Vessels in the left lung can be similarly assessed and compared with other areas in the left and the right lung.
3. *Inequality of vascular shadows.* Chronic pulmonary thromboembolic disease seldom involves both lung fields in an entirely symmetrical way, and thus areas in either lung field may be compared with other areas. Blood flow is diverted from occluded to patent vessels, and the area of lung supplied may appear relatively plethoric. When chronic pulmonary thromboembolic disease involves one lung considerably more than the other (Fig. 10-4), evaluation of the posteroanterior radiograph is easier.

The extent of cardiomegaly is variable, but it may be gross (Fig. 10-5). The right ventricle and right atrium are the chambers that dilate.

PULMONARY ANGIOGRAPHIC FEATURES

Pulmonary angiography is reputedly dangerous in patients with "primary pulmonary hypertension." We have not had a death in approximately 100 patients with pulmonary thromboembolic disease. Most of these cases had severe pulmonary

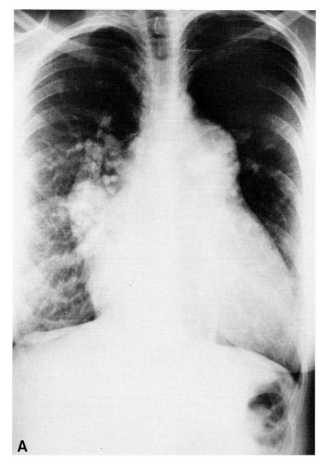

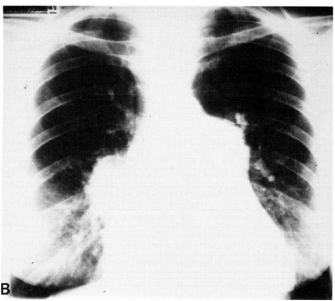

FIGURE 10-3. *A,* Posteroanterior chest radiograph of the same patient as in Figure 10-2. There is marked cardiomegaly with a very prominent main pulmonary artery segment and right pulmonary artery. The vascular markings in both upper lung fields and the left mid zone are diminished. *B,* Posteroanterior chest radiograph of a 48-year-old woman with pulmonary hypertension due to isolated chronic pulmonary thromboembolic disease. The heart is enlarged with a very prominent main pulmonary artery segment and large opaque right pulmonary artery branch. Apart from both lower zones, there is marked pulmonary oligemia.

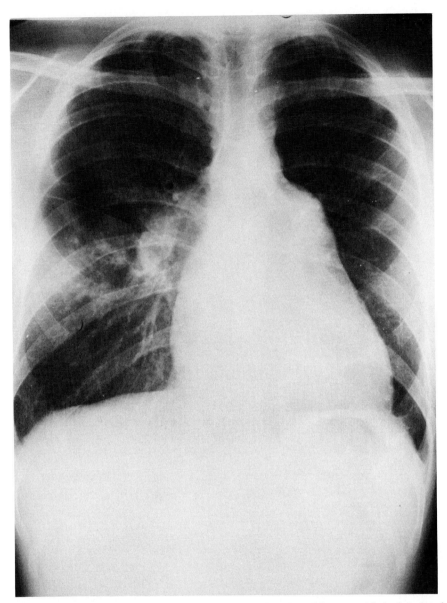

FIGURE 10-4. Posteroanterior chest radiograph of a 20-year-old man with isolated pulmonary thromboembolic disease and pulmonary artery pressure of 100/60 mmHg. The heart is enlarged and the main pulmonary artery segment prominent. The right pulmonary artery is prominent and vascular markings are diminished throughout both lungs except for the right mid and lower zones.

hypertension, and at least half had associated conditions such as an atrial septal defect or mitral valve disease.

In most instances we inject radio-opaque dye into the main pulmonary artery in the anteroposterior view. More recently, we have often repeated the injection into the right and then the left pulmonary arteries. The following features are sought:

1. *Rate of opacification of the arterial system.* Techniques vary, but we generally take at least four films per second. It is important to compare films taken before, during, and after the radio-opaque dye is injected. The rate of opacification of the main pulmonary artery branches is assessed (Fig. 10-6); those of the more distal vessels are assessed in later films. Vessels that

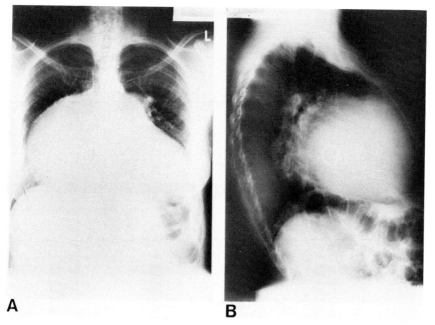

A **B**

FIGURE 10-5. Posteroanterior (*A*) and lateral (*B*) chest radiographs in a 48-year-old woman who had a mitral Starr-Edwards valve inserted 12 years previously. There is gross cardiomegaly due to enlargement of the right atrium and ventricle. (Rheumatic involvement of the atrial wall and of the anulus, as in this patient, would render the right atrium prone to a greater degree of dilatation than a non-rheumatic case with comparable pressures.) The main pulmonary artery is prominent, and the left pulmonary artery is more opaque than normal. The upper lung fields appear oligemic. Left-sided hemodynamics were normal at cardiac catheterization and angiography confirmed pulmonary thromboembolic disease.

    remain translucent or that have delayed opacification are sought. It is important to emphasize that vessels that are partially occluded will eventually opacify "normally." Thus, if they are not assessed in the early phase, they will be erroneously regarded as normal.

2. *Translucent areas.* Some areas will remain nonopacified throughout the observation period (Fig. 10-7). These are areas of lung supplied by completely occluded vessels. If one main pulmonary artery is considerably more involved than the other, this assessment is easier.

3. *Pulmonary venous phase.* This is assessed for the rate of filling as well as absence of filling in some areas. Although delayed filling is common, complete absence is unusual.

COMPUTERIZED TOMOGRAPHIC (CT) SCANNING

We have recent, albeit very limited, experience of this (Fig. 10-8). Kereiakes and coworkers[2] demonstrated the accuracy of this noninvasive technique in revealing occluding thrombus in proximal pulmonary arterial branches. This technique may be easier to interpret than pulmonary angiography and therefore possibly more reliable in establishing whether thrombus is present.

PROGNOSIS AND TREATMENT OF CHRONIC PULMONARY THROMBOEMBOLIC DISEASE

Patients with chronic thromboembolic disease almost always present when the disease is well established and the pulmonary artery systolic pressure is at least 90

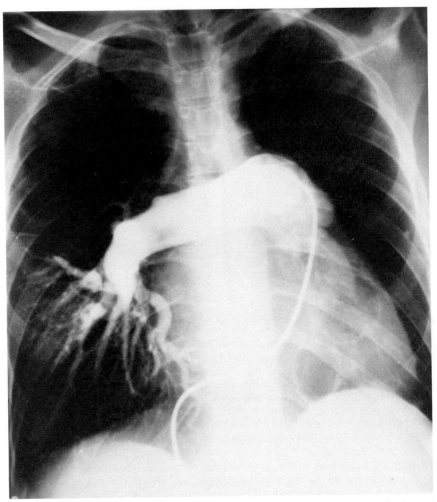

FIGURE 10-6. Pulmonary angiography in the same patient as in Figure 10-4. The injection of contrast material is mainly into the right pulmonary artery. There is cut-off of the major vessels to the right upper and mid zones and opacification of only some vessels supplying the lower zones.

mmHg. Patients who have had one or more acute pulmonary emboli may indeed have pulmonary artery pressures of only 60 mmHg or 70 mmHg, but this is because of the acute episode (Figs. 10-9, 10-10). Such patients nearly always do well on anticoagulant and other therapy. It is extremely rare, however, for a patient to present in the relatively early stage of *chronic* thromboembolic disease when the pulmonary artery pressure is 60 mmHg or 70 mmHg. All grades of severity of thromboembolic disease are observed at initial presentation, and the prognosis is necessarily variable. Central cyanosis and right ventricular failure are poor prognostic signs, and few patients survive more than five years thereafter. On the other hand, I have observed patients without failure or more than mild cyanosis survive for 10 and even 20 years on well-controlled anticoagulant therapy.

Patients with chronic thromboembolic disease have well-organized, even partially recanalized thrombi in their proximal and more peripheral pulmonary arteries. Surgical treatment is therefore seldom contributory and is not recommended. Management is principally that of well-controlled anticoagulation with sodium warfarin, which must be continued for life. It is possible that a few patients with chronic pulmonary thromboembolic disease have a vasospastic component to some of their normal or near-normal pulmonary vessels. In theory, these patients might improve on

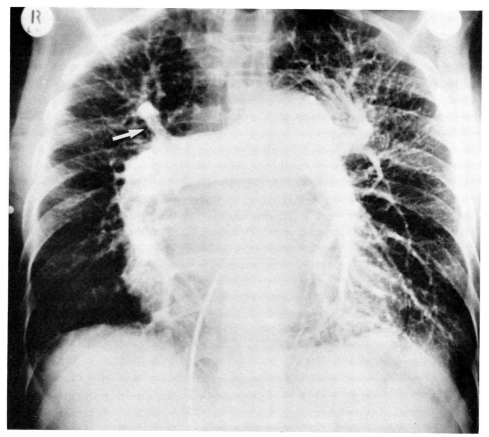

FIGURE 10-7. Frame from the late arterial phase of the pulmonary angiogram in a 30-year-old woman with mitral stenosis, pulmonary hypertension (RV 75 mmHg systolic) and associated thromboembolic disease. The systemic arterial oxygen saturation was ± 80 percent. The right mid and lower zones are less well opacified than the rest of the lung fields. A segment in the major vessel to the right upper zone *(arrow)* is partly translucent, compatible with partial occlusion of the lumen by thrombus.

vasodilator therapy, but this should be used with great caution, especially in the event of administration of captopril and other drugs that cause venous dilatation and hence decreased cardiac output. My experience with vasodilator therapy in chronic pulmonary thromboembolic disease has been disappointing. Diuretics are the mainstay of therapy for right ventricular failure.

PRIMARY PULMONARY HYPERTENSION

Primary pulmonary hypertension has been defined as "pulmonary arterial hypertension of unknown cause" and, according to Fuster and co-workers,[3] this remains the World Health Organization definition. The term is somewhat confusing; Oakley,[4] for example, uses "primary pulmonary hypertension" despite discussing some underlying conditions that cause pulmonary hypertension or are associated with it. There is a lot of literature, some of which is reviewed by Oakley, on the effects of various vasodilator drugs in patients with primary pulmonary hypertension. Authors seem able to collect at least 10 such cases suitable for study. I have not encountered such cases, although I have looked for them for over nearly two decades. What I do see, about once every one or two years, is severe pulmonary arterial hypertension in

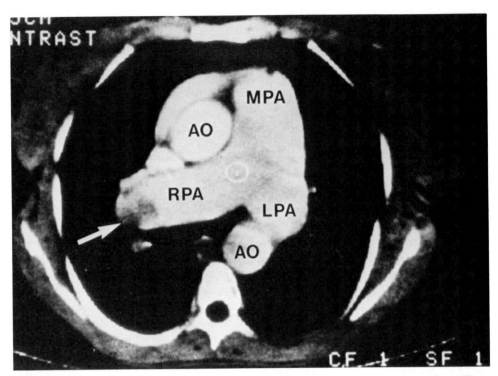

FIGURE 10-8. Contrast computed tomography (CT) of a 30-year-old woman with an Eisenmenger patent ductus arteriosus and pulmonary thromboembolic disease. The scan demonstrates a filling defect in the right pulmonary artery (RPA) *(arrow)*. The main pulmonary artery (MPA) and both right and left branches are enlarged. AO = aorta (ascending aorta anterior, descending posterior); LPA = left pulmonary artery.

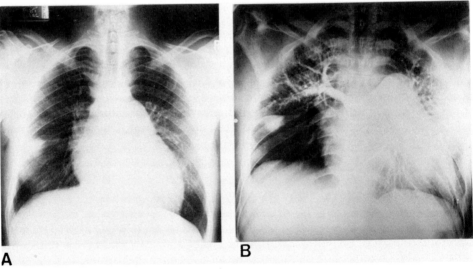

A　　　　　　　　　　　　　　　　**B**

FIGURE 10-9. Posteroanterior (*A*) chest radiography and pulmonary angiogram (*B*) in a 28-year-old man with chronic pulmonary thromboembolic disease who presented with an acute pulmonary embolus. *A,* There is cardiomegaly and a prominent pulmonary artery segment. The right pulmonary artery is opaque with distal oligemia in the area of supply. The right atrium is enlarged. The right lung appears undervascularized as compared to the left. The peripheral opacity is compatible with a recent pulmonary infarction. *B,* The angiogram demonstrates complete obstruction of arteries to the right mid and lower zones.

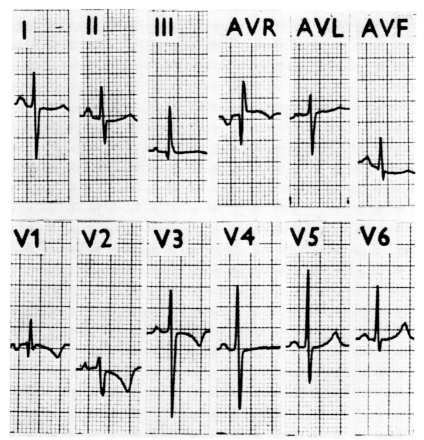

FIGURE 10-10. ECG of the same patient as in Figure 10-9 demonstrates moderate right ventricular hypertrophy and "strain," in keeping with pulmonary hypertension and superimposed acute on chronic pulmonary thromboembolic disease.

young subjects, predominantly female, who have progressive pulmonary hypertension and invariably die within two years. I call that condition "idiopathic pulmonary hypertension." These patients complain of increasing tiredness, central chest pain simulating angina, dizziness, and less commonly, syncope on exertion. They are seldom centrally cyanosed, unless a stretched patent foramen ovale is present. The pulmonary artery pressure ranges from 100 mmHg to more than 160 mmHg, and there are no radiological features of pulmonary thromboembolic disease (Fig. 10-11). The main pulmonary artery may be enlarged, but the remainder of the pulmonary vasculature is unimpressive. The lung fields are generally oligemic especially the peripheral one third. A large dense right pulmonary artery is not seen unless there is associated secondary thrombosis. Cardiomegaly may be marked on roentgenogram, and the ECG invariably shows considerable right ventricular hypertrophy (Fig. 10-12) and sometimes "strain." Severe right ventricular failure may supervene but patients often die suddenly before that. Pulmonary arteriography is dangerous in this condition, and I have encountered at least two fatalities.

I have no experience with patients with pulmonary hypertension due to anorectics or other drugs. I have encountered patients with severe pulmonary hypertension simulating "idiopathic pulmonary hypertension;" but the hypertension was associated with lupus erythematosus, schistosomiasis, or previous surgical closure of a ventricular septal defect. In the latter, the rise in pulmonary artery pressure usually occurs during adolescence, despite considerable reduction of pulmonary artery pressure after closure of the defect during infancy or early childhood. It is possible that

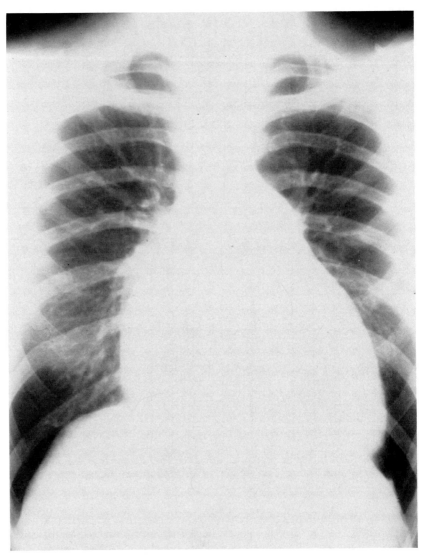

FIGURE 10-11. Posteroanterior chest radiograph of a 17-year-old boy with "idiopathic pulmonary hypertension," who presented with a two-month history of dyspnea, "faintness," syncope, and palpitations. The lung fields are generally oligemic. The heart is enlarged with a prominent main pulmonary artery segment. Pulmonary artery pressure at cardiac catheterization was 107/60 mmHg.

some adult patients with "idiopathic pulmonary hypertension" had an Eisenmenger ventricular septal defect that was not diagnosed and that underwent spontaneous closure many years previously.

On the general principle of attempting to prevent or delay secondary thrombosis, I recommend anticoagulation in patients with "idiopathic pulmonary hypertension." This is appropriate not only because the correct diagnosis in many instances of primary pulmonary hypertension is thromboembolic disease but also because the Mayo Clinic group[3] showed benefit from anticoagulant therapy in its review of patients with "primary pulmonary hypertension." Although Fuster and co-workers were, in my view, correct for reasons that were partially wrong, they concluded that "anticoagulant therapy is recommended for patients with primary pulmonary hypertension."[3]

Many studies on primary pulmonary hypertension followed the work of Wagenvoort and Wagenvoort in 1970.[5] This study is regarded as a "classic" in that the

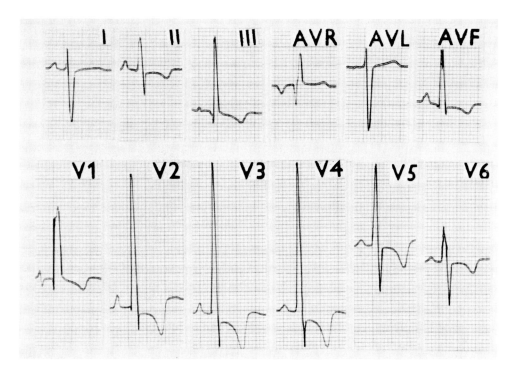

FIGURE 10-12. ECG of the same patient as in Figure 10-11 demonstrates marked right ventricular hypertrophy and "strain." The right atrium is enlarged.

authors claimed to differentiate *by histological studies* pulmonary thromboembolic disease from primary pulmonary hypertension, which, they postulated, had a dominant "vasoconstrictive" component. It is our understanding that the authors were not supplied with accurate clinical data for their case material, and we believe their conclusions to be fallacious. Chronic pulmonary thromboembolic disease is essentially a condition in which proximal vessels are obstructed. Histological examination of arterioles distal to an obstruction will not reveal the same changes as in similar-size vessels distal to a nonobstructed artery or to an artery that becomes obstructed relatively later. The situation is analogous to the Goldblatt kidney. Wagenvoort and Wagenvoort[5] attempted to formulate histological criteria for primary pulmonary hypertension, which have influenced clinicians. In my view, when clinicians have learnt to differentiate chronic pulmonary thromboembolic disease from "idiopathic pulmonary hypertension," then they may receive meaningful assistance from the histopathological reports.

EISENMENGER'S SYNDROME OR REACTION

Since the classic paper by Wood[6] in 1958, the term "Eisenmenger's syndrome" or "reaction" is used to indicate balanced or predominant right-to-left shunting, secondary to marked elevation of the pulmonary vascular resistance, in patients with congenital defects that allow free communication between the pulmonary and systemic circulations. Almost three decades later, aspects relating to when, why, or how the pulmonary vascular resistance increases in different congenital cardiac defects remain unsolved. A crucial question is whether the pulmonary vascular resistance will decrease, remain unchanged, or increase if the defect is surgically closed. This question sometimes has no answer that is certain to be correct, and clinicians will not always agree whether or not the defect should be closed. Cardiologists must evaluate *all* features of the individual case, including age, clinical examination, ECG, chest radiograph, and cardiac catheterization data (including, when relevant, the response to oxygen, and the lung biopsy). The decision regarding surgery must take into account that patients with Eisenmenger's syndrome are liable to live until at least 30 years of age and that there is a probability of successful total heart-lung transplants being practicable well within that time. Another factor to be borne in mind is that the pulmonary vascular resistance and pulmonary artery pressure may rise, occasionally precipitously, when the child reaches adolescence.

I am a clinician and have very limited knowledge of lung histology, but one lesson I have learned is that a child should neither be regarded as inoperable nor subjected to surgery solely on the basis of the pathologist's assessment of the pulmonary vascular disease. Virmani and Roberts[7] emphasized the limitations of the widely used classification of Heath and Edwards[8] and pointed out that Grade 6 of that classification, which comprises necrotizing arteritis, may occur in the absence of pulmonary hypertension. Virmani and Roberts[7] therefore confined their observations in adult patients with congenital heart disease and pulmonary arterial hypertension to medial and intimal thickening and plexiform lesions. They concluded that plexiform lesions indicate "the irreversible nature of pulmonary hypertension." Plexiform lesions are thus not observed in patients with pulmonary arterial hypertension secondary to chronic pulmonary venous hypertension, which is potentially always completely reversible. Hoffman and co-workers[9] have studied pulmonary vascular disease with congenital heart lesions for many years and emphasize the role of a reduced number of intra-acinar arteries in contributing to the early increase in pulmonary vascular resistance in some congenital heart lesions. They comment that the growth potential of new vessels after corrective surgery "is reduced after 2 years of age and argues for early surgical relief of pulmonary vascular stresses."[9] With the notable exception of patients with atrial septal defect, it has been widely accepted that irreversible pulmonary vascular changes in Eisenmenger's syndrome invariably take place before three and usually before two years of age. I have never observed Eisenmenger's syndrome to develop between the ages of 3 and 12 years.

Patients with Eisenmenger's syndrome in childhood have usually been observed from birth and have the clinical signs of pulmonary hypertension associated with cyanosis and clubbing of the fingers. The cyanosis is classically more severe in the feet than in the hands, particularly the right hand, in patients with patent ductus arteriosus. A number of patients present in adulthood whose conditions have gone unrecognized and who have been apparently asymptomatic during infancy and childhood. They usually complain of increasing tiredness and may have noticed cyanosis themselves.

Eisenmenger's syndrome due to an underlying patent ductus arteriosus or a ventricular septal defect can be differentiated clinically from isolated pulmonary thromboembolic disease or from "idiopathic pulmonary hypertension." Clubbing of the fingers and toes is likely to be more marked in Eisenmenger's syndrome, and the presence of differential cyanosis is contributory in this differentiation. Heart failure is not a feature of uncomplicated Eisenmenger's syndrome, and only mild cardiac dilatation is detected clinically or radiologically. Sometimes a short, soft systolic murmur is present over the sternal area and the base, which may have vibrations arising from the ventricular septal defect or right ventricular outflow tract. More commonly, a systolic murmur is due to mild tricuspid regurgitation. This murmur may be Grade 2 or 3 in intensity, but signs of significant tricuspid regurgitation are absent. I have seldom detected a right ventricular gallop sound in patients with Eisenmenger's syndrome.

The reason for increased cyanosis during adulthood in some patients with Eisenmenger's syndrome due to a patent ductus or ventricular septal defect has not been clearly explained. In my view, secondary pulmonary arterial thrombotic disease is the probable explanation (Fig. 10-13). Radiological appearance of patients with Eisenmenger's syndrome without secondary pulmonary thrombotic disease is remarkably unimpressive. The main pulmonary artery may be slightly dilated, but

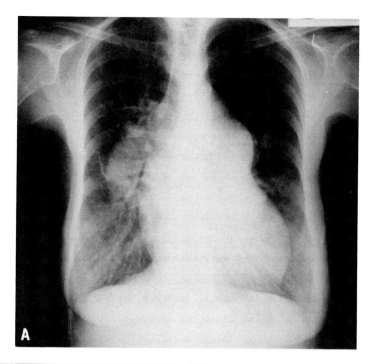

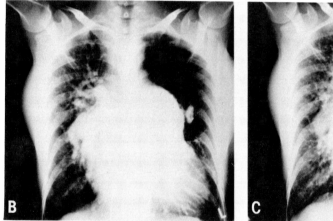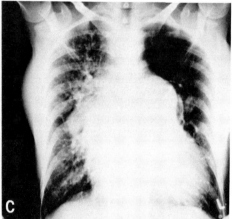

FIGURE 10-13. Posteroanterior chest radiograph (*A*) and pulmonary angiogram *(B, C)* of the same patient whose CT scan is shown in Figure 10-8. *A*, The heart is enlarged with marked prominence of the pulmonary artery segment. The right pulmonary artery is very prominent and dense. The left upper lung field is undervascularized as compared to the remainder of the lungs. *B, C,* Early (*B*) and later (*C*) arterial phases of the pulmonary angiogram demonstrate enlarged, tortuous proximal vesels, failure of opacification of major vessels to the left upper zone with distal oligemia, compatible with proximal occlusion on the left.

the pulmonary vasculature appears normal or slightly oligemic in the peripheral one third of the lung fields (Fig. 10-14). In our study[1] on observer error in the assessment of pulmonary vasculature, we were frequently unable to differentiate uncomplicated Eisenmenger's syndrome from idiopathic dilatation of the pulmonary artery or pulmonary stenosis.

There are two important aspects in the management of patients with Eisenmenger's syndrome. Because of secondary pulmonary thrombotic disease, all adult patients should receive sodium warfarin anticoagulant therapy, unless there is a specific contraindication. Pregnancy is contraindicated and should be terminated. Gen-

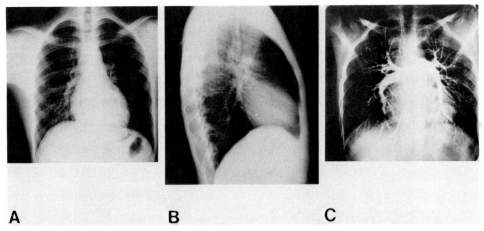

A   **B**   **C**

FIGURE 10-14. Posteroanterior (*A*) and lateral (*B*) chest radiographs and pulmonary angiogram (*C*) in a 30-year-old man with a ventricular septal defect and Eisenmenger's syndrome. The heart outline appears "bulky" owing to right atrial and right ventricular enlargement but the main pulmonary artery segment is not prominent and the lung fields are within normal limits, apart from peripheral oligemia. In *C*, there is no occlusion of major vessels and the pulmonary branches taper off gradually towards the periphery.

eral experience,[10] as well as our own, indicates that maternal mortality, which usually occurs during labor or within the first seven days postpartum, is approximately 27 percent.

EISENMENGER'S SYNDROME AND ATRIAL SEPTAL DEFECT

Many patients with secundum atrial septal defect remain asymptomatic until the third to fifth decades.[11-13] When symptoms develop, these usually relate to the development of congestive cardiac failure, arrhythmias, and pulmonary hypertension.[14,15] It is rare for severe pulmonary vascular disease to develop in infants with atrial septal defect.[9,16-18] Hoffman and colleagues[9] suggest that high pulmonary flows with atrial

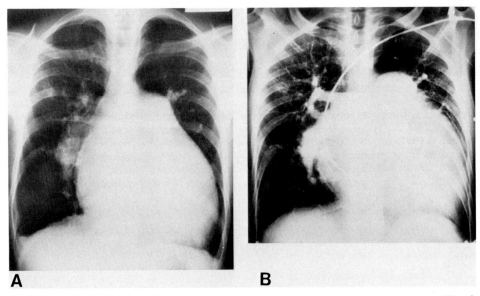

A   **B**

FIGURE 10-15. Posteroanterior chest radiograph (*A*) and pulmonary angiogram (*B*) of a patient with an atrial septal defect and pulmonary hypertension. Features of pulmonary thromboembolic disease are apparent, and there is marked cardiac enlargement.

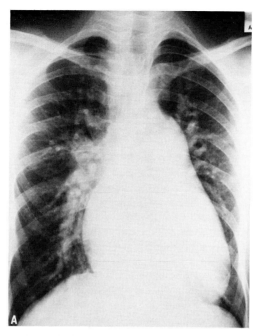

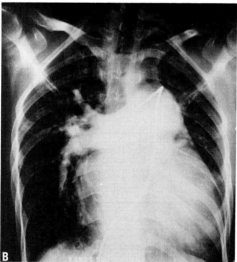
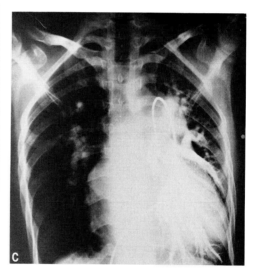

FIGURE 10-16. Posteroanterior chest radiograph (*A*) and pulmonary angiograms (*B, C*) of a 21-year-old man with a secundum atrial septal defect (left to right shunt 2.37:1), pulmonary hypertension (MPA 80/30, mean 50 mmHg) and thromboembolic disease, mainly confined to the right lung. *A*, The heart is enlarged with a prominent main pulmonary artery segment. The lung fields are plethoric, but there is cut-off of the proximal vessels on the right. *B*, Injection into the right pulmonary artery demonstrates large proximal vessels but almost complete absence of filling in the distal two thirds of the lung field. *C*, Injection into the left pulmonary artery outlines large vessels extending to the periphery, with the exception of the arteries to the upper zone, which do not opacify well.

septal defect are associated with *dilated* pulmonary arterial vessels, whereas the small pulmonary arteries in patients with large ventricular septal defects have a relatively small lumen. Thus, for any given volume flow, "the velocity of flow will be greater in large ventricular septal defects than in atrial septal defects, so that shearing forces and endothelial damage are likely to be more severe and progressive in the former."

It is widely accepted,[19,20] including by Hoffman and co-workers,[9] that pulmonary hypertension may supervene in adulthood in patients with atrial septal defect and that this is increasingly common in the older subject.[19] The pathogenesis has not been clarified. Pulmonary thrombotic disease involving the proximal pulmonary arteries has been cited in earlier literature as a factor.[11,21,22] Some children and young adults may have moderate pulmonary hypertension, but this is unusual. A relatively high prevalence was observed by Cherian and co-workers,[23] who considered the possibility of "ethnic variations." These investigators observed the Eisenmenger reaction in 7 percent of children in their first decade and in 8 percent in their second decade. They favored that the severe pulmonary hypertension in their young patients was related to "persistence of the fetal pulmonary vascular pattern."

Many adult patients with atrial septal defect have variable degrees of pulmonary hypertension. In some, the pulmonary artery pressure equals systemic pressure; the patients are desaturated because of the dominant right-to-left shunt; and there may be considerable disability. All such patients whom I have observed have obvious pulmonary thromboembolic disease with typical radiological appearances of proximal pulmonary artery thrombosis (Figs. 10-15, 10-16). The majority of adult patients with moderate pulmonary hypertension have similar appearances. I have never observed progression of pulmonary arterial hypertension in an adult with a secundum atrial septal defect in the absence of thromboembolic disease. Furthermore, when pulmonary hypertension increased after closure of an atrial septal defect, this was invariably due to progressive pulmonary thromboembolic disease. These observations were made in patients who failed to comply with anticoagulant therapy or were lost to follow-up for 5, 10, or more years after surgery.

More than a decade ago, I concluded that secondary pulmonary thromboembolic disease was invariably the cause of increasing pulmonary hypertension in adult patients with atrial septal defect. The radiological appearances are typical, and the prominent opaque main pulmonary arteries with immediate "cut-off" contrast with the radiological appearances of uncomplicated Eisenmenger's syndrome. Many examples of adults with "Eisenmenger's syndrome" in the literature clearly have pulmonary thromboembolic disease.

It is unlikely that the proximal pulmonary arterial thrombus formation in adult patients with secundum atrial septal defect results from emboli from systemic venous thrombosis. I have no explanation as to why proximal pulmonary artery thrombotic disease should develop in situ. It is easier to understand this occurring in patients after surgical closure because of decreased blood flow through a relatively dilated pulmonary arterial system.

Contrary to the generally accepted view, I am not convinced that all adult patients with left-to-right shunts of less than 3:1 should be subjected to surgery. It has not been my experience that surgery prevents or improves supraventricular tachyarrhythmias. It would seem to me that many asymptomatic patients could be observed but that anticoagulant therapy with sodium warfarin is indicated in those who have evidence of thromboembolic disease. Moreover, very careful observation is essential in all patients who have been subjected to surgical closure, with anticoagulant therapy if required.

Perloff[24] recently reflected the variable prognosis of secundum atrial septal defect in his report of two patients who survived to the ages of 87 and 94 years, respectively. One patient had acute pulmonary emboli at necropsy and the other (Perloff's Fig. 2)[24] had obvious radiological evidence of pulmonary thromboembolic disease.

PULMONARY HYPERTENSION SECONDARY TO PARENCHYMATOUS LUNG DISEASE

Diffuse parenchymatous lung disease may cause right ventricular failure (cor pulmonale) almost entirely through the mechanism of hypoxia, which results in pulmonary arteriolar vasoconstriction and hence pulmonary hypertension. In my view, secondary pulmonary thrombotic disease not infrequently supervenes in many such cases. Where practicable, long-term anticoagulant therapy with sodium warfarin should be considered in all cases of cor pulmonale due to parenchymatous lung disease, irrespective of the underlying disease process.

PULMONARY HYPERTENSION SECONDARY TO PULMONARY VENOUS HYPERTENSION

It is important to reiterate that "uncomplicated" pulmonary arterial hypertension secondary to pulmonary venous hypertension is *always* potentially reversible. The most frequent "complication" of reactive pulmonary arterial hypertension is pulmonary thromboembolic disease, but pulmonary fibrosis, sometimes a result of repeated infections, may also occur. Surgery should never be denied to any patient with severe uncomplicated reactive pulmonary arterial hypertension because of a fear of "irreversibility."

Severe pulmonary arterial hypertension secondary to pulmonary venous hypertension is more marked and more common in infants, children, and young patients with pulmonary venous hypertension from any cause. It is readily reversed after successful surgery in infants with conditions such as congenital aortic stenosis and coarctation of the aorta. Congenital mitral stenosis, cor triatriatum, and other conditions causing pulmonary venous obstruction may either not be amenable to successful surgery or are complicated by an associated left-to-right shunt. Pulmonary hypertension in rheumatic mitral valve disease should revert to normal, but the left heart hemodynamics are seldom completely normal postoperatively. Prosthetic valves have an early diastolic gradient; left ventricular function may be abnormal; commissurotomy and valvuloplasty seldom result in "perfect" mitral valve function; and, finally, there are the effects of the "restrictive-dilatation syndrome," discussed in Section 2 of Chapter 8. Nevertheless, the preoperative ECG showing marked right ventricular hypertrophy in young patients with severe pulmonary arterial hypertension and mitral stenosis will invariably have returned to normal, or near normal, after a period of between a few months and two years. A relatively rare cause of

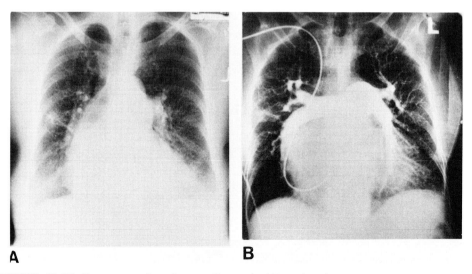

A   **B**

FIGURE 10-17. Posteroanterior chest radiograph (*A*) and pulmonary angiogram (*B*) in a patient with mixed rheumatic mitral valve disease and dominant stenosis. The pulmonary artery pressure was 110/38, mean 63. The lung fields exhibit features of thromboembolic disease and areas of fibrosis in the right lung.

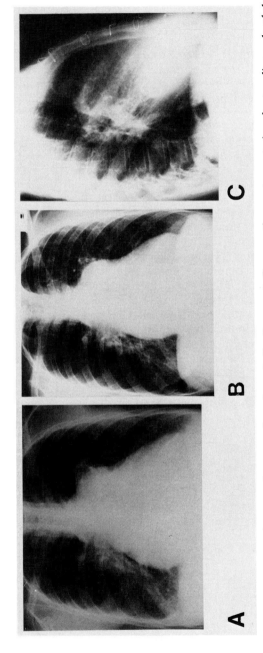

FIGURE 10-18. Mitral stenosis and chronic pulmonary thromboembolic disease. *A*, Preoperative posteroanterior chest radiograph of the same patient whose pulmonary angiogram is shown in Figure 10-7. *B*, Postoperative posteroanterior chest radiograph after replacing the mitral valve with a Medtronic-Hall prosthesis. *C*, Lateral view demonstrates the prosthesis. There has been considerable reduction in heart size despite the presence of thromboembolic disease.

severe reactive pulmonary arterial hypertension that may be "cured" by surgery is left atrial myxoma.

Although prolonged pulmonary arterial hypertension due to severe mitral stenosis may result in some medial and intimal thickening of the pulmonary arteries and arterioles, so-called plexiform lesions will presumably be encountered only when thromboembolic disease has supervened as a complication. The pulmonary artery pressure does not always drop immediately after successful mitral valve surgery, but temporary mild anoxia due to pulmonary atelectasis, edema, and infection complicate these assessments.

All patients with mitral stenosis who have more than mild chronic systemic desaturation must have some associated pulmonary thromboembolic disease (Fig. 10-17). But this, in itself, is certainly not always a contraindication to mitral valve surgery. We have observed patients with moderate to severe chronic pulmonary thromboembolic disease who have improved considerably after surgery for tight mitral stenosis (Fig. 10-18). It is impossible to generalize, but in most instances patients with a hemodynamically significant mitral valve lesion should be treated surgically despite associated moderate or even severe chronic pulmonary thromboembolic disease.

SECTION 2: TRICUSPID VALVE DISEASE

with THEO E. MEYER and WENDY A. POCOCK

TRICUSPID STENOSIS

By far the most common cause of tricuspid stenosis is rheumatic heart disease. Rheumatic involvement of tricuspid leaflets occurs in about 10 percent of patients with rheumatic heart disease. In an analysis of 525 patients with rheumatic heart disease, Yousof and co-workers[1] detected tricuspid stenosis, based on a mean diastolic gradient of 2 mmHg or more at cardiac catheterization, in about 9 percent. All their patients with tricuspid stenosis had associated hemodynamically significant tricuspid regurgitation. Rheumatic tricuspid stenosis, with no or very mild tricuspid regurgitation, is rare and, in our experience, is invariably accompanied by hemodynamically significant mitral or aortic valve lesions. Rheumatic tricuspid stenosis with no or minimal mitral or aortic valve disease is very unusual, and in these cases (Fig. 10-19) there is always hemodynamically significant tricuspid regurgitation as well.

Physical signs of rheumatic tricuspid stenosis include a prominent a wave in the jugular venous pulse, a mid-diastolic murmur at the sternal area that increases in intensity on inspiration or with abdominal compression, an opening snap that can be shown phonocardiographically to become earlier with inspiration, and an atrial systolic murmur that is crescendo-decrescendo in shape (Fig. 10-20). Because some organic tricuspid regurgitation is usually present, a pansystolic murmur, often Grade 2 or 3 in intensity, is heard over or to the left of the sternum (Fig. 10-20). This murmur may radiate towards the base of the heart, and it also becomes louder during inspiration or with abdominal compression. Some auscultatory features of rheumatic tricuspid stenosis have recently been studied by Wooley and co-workers.[2]

ECHOCARDIOGRAPHY

Extension of M-mode criteria for the diagnosis of mitral stenosis to the tricuspid valve has proved unreliable.[3] Two-dimensional echocardiography is more sensitive and specific for detecting tricuspid stenosis. Diastolic doming of the valve is the characteristic feature on 2-D echocardiogram.[3,4]

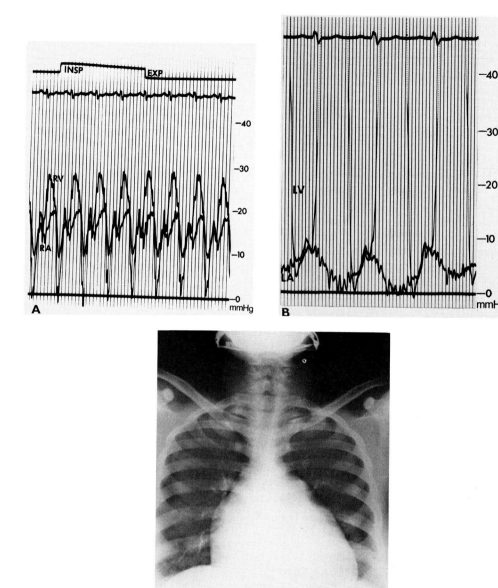

FIGURE 10-19. *A,* Simultaneous right atrial (RA) and right ventricular (*B*) pressures in a 19-year-old woman with significant tricuspid incompetence and stenosis. Kussmaul's sign is mildly positive. *B,* Simultaneous left atrial (LA) and left ventricular (LV) pressures demonstrate a normal LV end-diastolic pressure and absence of a gradient across the mitral valve. *C,* Posteroanterior chest radiograph demonstrates cardiac enlargement with a prominent right atrium. The lung fields appear oligemic.

MANAGEMENT

Dominant, or virtually "pure," tricuspid stenosis is a relatively benign lesion, and surgical intervention should not be undertaken if this will entail tricuspid valve replacement or leaving the patient with important tricuspid regurgitation. Because closed tricuspid commisurotomy invariably produces gross regurgitation, it should never be attempted.

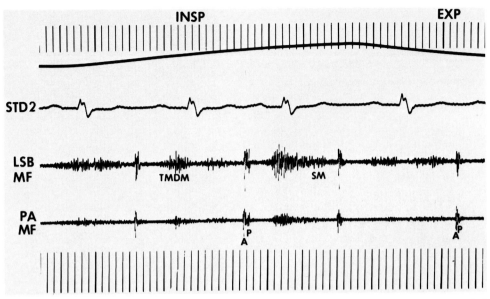

FIGURE 10-20. Phonocardiogram of the same patient as in Figure 10-19 recorded at the left sternal border (LSB) and pulmonary area (PA). The tricuspid mid-diastolic murmur (TMDM) is in fact an atrial systolic murmur and is crescendo-decrescendo in shape. Both it and the pansystolic regurgitant murmur are louder during inspiration. The tricuspid component of the first heart sound is soft.

Right ventricular inflow obstruction due to a nonrheumatic cause is commonly associated with other cardiac lesions. When patients present with a clinical picture suggesting isolated right ventricular inflow obstruction or tricuspid stenosis, conditions that should be considered include right atrial myxoma, constrictive pericarditis, hypertrophic cardiomyopathy, carcinoid syndrome, and the various forms of right ventricular hypoplasia, especially Ebstein's anomaly. All these entities may produce a right-sided mid-diastolic murmur. Libman-Sacks endocarditis may reputedly involve the tricuspid valve,[5] but no case of confirmed hemodynamically significant tricuspid stenosis has, to our knowledge, been described.[6]

TRICUSPID REGURGITATION

Any cause of pulmonary hypertension or raised pulmonary vascular resistance may result in functional tricuspid regurgitation. It is generally accepted that "functional" tricuspid regurgitation is caused by dilatation of the anulus without leaflet scarring or abnormality.[4] If this definition is used, the most common cause of severe functional tricuspid regurgitation is rheumatic heart disease. In our view, however, many such cases should be regarded as partially or entirely *organic* in that the tricuspid anulus is probably involved by the rheumatic process to produce dilatation in similar manner to the mitral anulus; this subject has been discussed in Chapters 7 and 8. Marked tricuspid regurgitation in cases of rheumatic heart disease is so often disproportionate to the severity of the mitral valve lesion or to the degree of pulmonary hypertension and raised pulmonary vascular resistance (from whatever cause, including pulmonary thrombotic disease) that an organic component contributing to the tricuspid anular dilatation must surely be incriminated. This concept has received scant attention in the literature. Functional tricuspid regurgitation resulting from nonrheumatic causes of pulmonary hypertension or a raised pulmonary vascular resistance is not usually hemodynamically severe unless the right ventricular myocardium is abnormal, as may occur in dilated cardiomyopathy or ischemic heart dis-

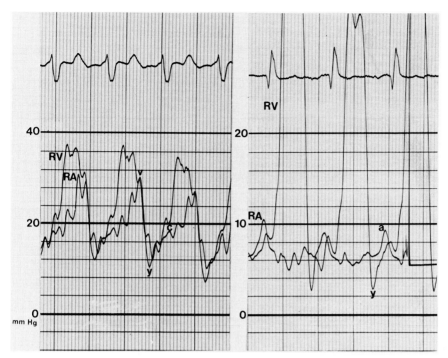

FIGURE 10-21. Preoperative *(left)* and postoperative *(right)* right atrial and right ventricular pressure tracings of a 45-year-old woman with severe isolated tricuspid regurgitation. Some chordae tendineae were absent, and part of the anterior tricuspid leaflet was markedly flail. The surgeon (M Antunes) favored a diagnosis of congenital anomaly. We consider it compatible with previous infective endocarditis. After valvuloplasty, the postoperative tracing shows a very small diastolic gradient.

ease. Functional tricuspid regurgitation resulting from marked pulmonary hypertension with normal or near-normal right ventricular myocardium is characterized by a fairly loud (Grade 2 or 3) systolic murmur, but there is no evidence of gross regurgitation such as prominent systolic waves in the jugular venous pulse and systolic pulsation of the distended liver.

"Organic" tricuspid regurgitation, as defined by leaflet involvement, is most commonly caused by rheumatic carditis; tricuspid stenosis may be associated; and the mitral valve is usually also involved. Causes of "isolated" tricuspid regurgitation are infective endocarditis, trauma, and congenital anomalies (Fig. 10-21),[7] including Ebstein's malformation, carcinoid heart disease, and so-called tricuspid valve prolapse.[8] The latter condition is seldom clinically manifest unless pulmonary arterial hypertension, from an unrelated cause, supervenes.

In our experience, infective endocarditis and trauma are the two most prevalent causes of isolated or near-isolated organic tricuspid regurgitation. Tricuspid regurgitation due to right-sided infective endocarditis is often complicated by a raised pulmonary vascular resistance following septic pulmonary emboli. Penetrating trauma, mainly from knife wounds, may be complicated by injury to other valves or by septal defects. Immediately after the stabbing, branches of coronary arteries may have been tied at emergency surgery and pericardial adhesions, which are an aftermath of the original hemopericardium and the thoracotomy, may also later affect the hemodynamics (Figs. 10-22 to 10-25). Nonpenetrating trauma may be complicated by myocardial contusion or other cardiac injury, including coronary cameral fistulae.[9] Patients are usually first seen by us years after the traumatic event (Figs. 10-26, 10-27).

We have had the opportunity to observe one patient who developed severe isolated tricuspid regurgitation from Staphylococcus aureus endocarditis and to fol-

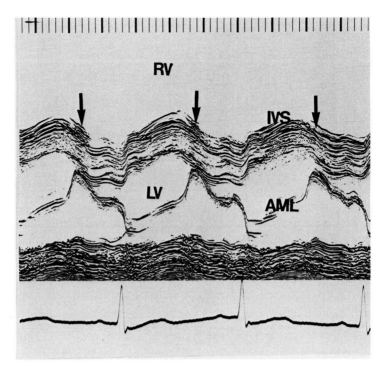

FIGURE 10-22. M-mode echocardiographic recording (paper speed 100 mm/sec) of the right ventricular cavity (RV), interventricular septum (IVS), left ventricular cavity (LV) and anterior mitral valve leaflet (AML) in a 28-year-old man with severe isolated tricuspid regurgitation and pericardial restriction following a stab wound, with hemopericardium necessitating thoracotomy, nine years previously. This is the same patient as in Chapter 8, Section 2, Figure 8-23. Note the marked early diastolic septal motion *(arrows)* which commences nearly concurrently with mitral valve opening.

low the course of that patient over a 14-year period. Because this woman had no complicating features, it is relevant to discuss her in some detail.

CASE REPORT

A 33-year-old Black woman was completely well until she developed a rigor on March 4, 1971. When admitted to hospital on the fifth day of her illness, she was pyrexial with a sinus tachycardia of 180 per minute. A Grade 1 blowing systolic murmur and a right-sided gallop rhythm were audible at the lower left sternal border; but the jugular venous pressure was not raised, the liver was not enlarged, and there was no clinical evidence of right ventricular hypertrophy. A soft spleen was palpable. The ECG showed a mean frontal plane QRS axis of +110°, clockwise rotation and inverted T waves in leads V_1–V_4. A chest radiograph was normal. The hemoglobin was 10.7 g percent, white blood cell count 19,000, and sedimentation rate (Westergren) 100 mm in the first hour. Coagulase-positive Staphylococcus aureus was cultured repeatedly from her blood. Despite careful investigation, including pelvic examination, no portal of entry for the staphylococcus was detected. Intravenous therapy of 2 million units of penicillin and 4 g of cloxacillin every four hours was started three days after admission and continued for six weeks. The pyrexia settled almost immediately and subsequent blood cultures were negative. Although the septicemia was cured, the signs of right ventricular "decompensation" increased. The patient had a sustained tachycardia of at least 120 per minute, prominent systolic waves developed in the jugular venous pulse, and the retrosternal impulse became forceful. The systolic murmur increased to Grade 3 in intensity, the right-sided gal-

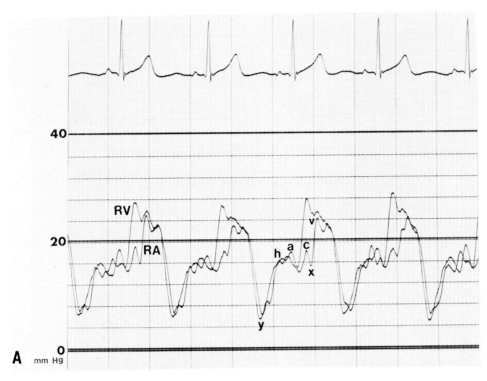

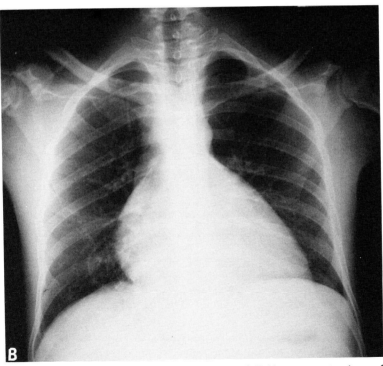

FIGURE 10-23. *A,* Right ventricular (RV) and right atrial (RA) pressure tracings of the same patient as in Figure 10-22 demonstrating prominent right atrial "systolic" waves of tricuspid incompetence as well as a rapid rise of pressures to the H wave after the y descent. The latter feature is compatible with "restriction." *B,* Posteroanterior chest radiograph demonstrates oligemic lung fields with cardiomegaly and a prominent right heart border due to an enlarged right atrium.

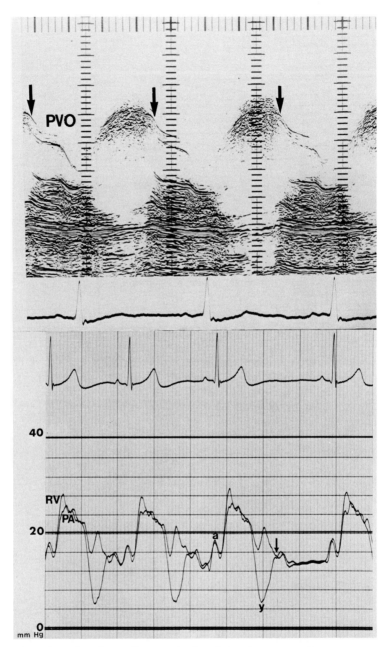

FIGURE 10-24. M-mode echocardiogram *(top)* and simultaneous pulmonary artery (PA) and right ventricular (RV) pressures *(bottom)* of the same patient as in Figure 10-23. The echo is technically poor, but pulmonary valve opening (PVO) is partial *(arrows)* in early ventricular diastole and more complete after atrial contraction. The equalization of pressures is also demonstrated *(arrow)* in early ventricular diastole.

lop persisted, and the second heart sound became clinically "single" owing to an inaudible pulmonary component. The chest radiograph remained normal, but the ECG showed a progressive decrease in QRS voltages.

Cardiac catheterization six weeks after admission demonstrated a mean pulmonary wedge pressure of 8 mmHg and right ventricular systolic pressure of 25 mmHg with an end-diastolic pressure of 18 mmHg (Fig. 10-28). Prominent V waves of 22 mmHg in the right atrial tracing were compatible with severe tricuspid regurgitation (Fig. 10-29). The pulmonary artery diastolic pressure rose from about 15

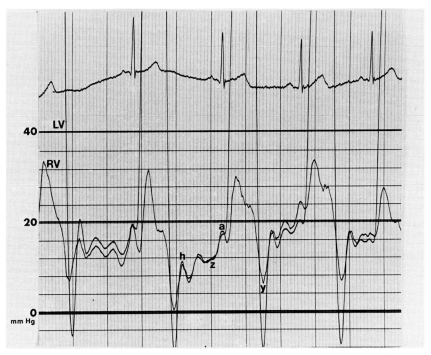

FIGURE 10-25. Left ventricular (LV) and right ventricular (RV) equalization of diastolic pressures in the same patient as in Figures 10-23 and 10-24 demonstrating the combined "restrictive" effect of tricuspid regurgitation and pericardial adhesions on the left ventricular hemodynamics.

mmHg in early diastole to 18 mmHg in end-diastole (see Fig. 10-28). Cineangiocardiography performed from the right atrium did not demonstrate any chamber enlargement, but prolonged opacification of the right heart was compatible with the considerable tricuspid regurgitation. A right ventriculogram was technically impossible, because the catheter tip could not be maintained in the ventricular cavity and

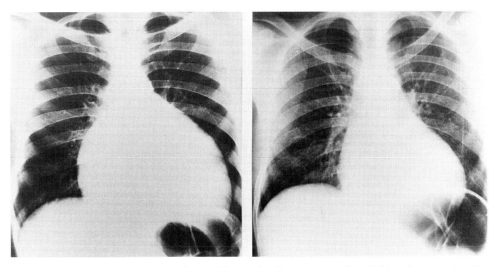

FIGURE 10-26. Posteroanterior chest radiographs. Before operation *(left)* and six weeks after operation *(right)* in a 34-year-old man with severe organic tricuspid regurgitation and a coronary artery–right ventricular fistula following severe nonpenetrating chest injury 10 years previously. (From Sareli et al,[9] with permission.)

Diastole Systole

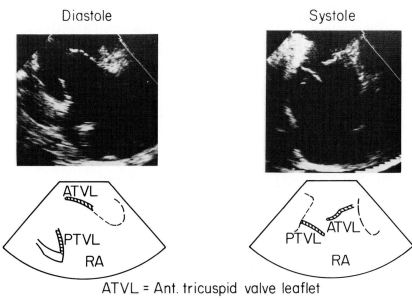

ATVL = Ant. tricuspid valve leaflet
PTVL = Post. tricuspid valve leaflet
RA = Right atrium

FIGURE 10-27. Two-dimensional echocardiograms, parasternal long-axis view, in the same patient as in Figure 10-26, demonstrating the flail posterior tricuspid valve leaflet (PTVL). ATVL = anterior tricuspid valve leaflet; RA = right atrium. (From Sareli et al,[9] with permission.)

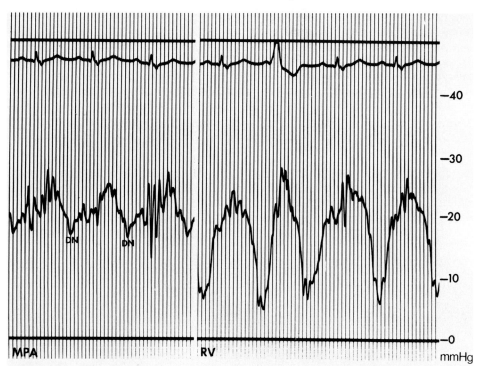

FIGURE 10-28. Immediately consecutive main pulmonary artery (MPA) and right ventricular (RV) pressures recorded in 1971 on a 33-year-old woman with recent-onset severe isolated tricuspid regurgitation. The elevated right ventricular end-diastolic pressure is demonstrated and is more apparent after the premature contraction. (From Bramwell-Jones et al,[11] with permission.)

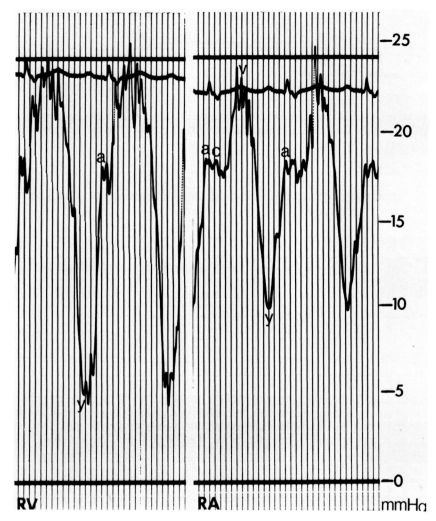

FIGURE 10-29. The same patient as in Figure 10-28 demonstrates the raised right ventricular (RV) end-diastolic pressure and the "ventricularized" right atrial (RA) pressure tracing. (From Bramwell-Jones et al,[11] with permission.)

was repeatedly forced back into the right atrium by the strong regurgitant stream. A pulmonary angiogram demonstrated an entirely normal vascular tree. A phonocardiogram, recorded two weeks later, showed a normally split second sound with a soft pulmonary component (Fig. 10-30).

She was discharged feeling well. Ten months after the onset of her illness the liver was pulsatile and palpable 3 to 4 cm below the right costal margin. The first heart sound was soft, and the tricuspid regurgitant murmur was barely audible and intermittent. The right-sided gallop was loud, and the second sound remained clinically single.

The presentation and subsequent course of this patient's illness was compatible with acute staphylococcal endocarditis causing destruction and severe incompetence of the tricuspid valve. It is probable that the valve was previously normal, but a mild anomaly such as tricuspid valve prolapse cannot be excluded. Unlike most cases of organic tricuspid regurgitation secondary to bacterial endocarditis, pulmonary embolism did not occur in our patient, and her hemodynamics were therefore unaffected by either a raised pulmonary vascular resistance or myocardial damage.

Because our patient's first ECG was recorded on the fifth day of her illness, when her tricuspid regurgitation was mild, we were able to observe the decrease in

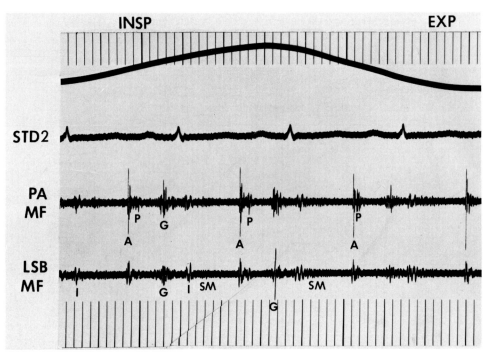

FIGURE 10-30. Medium-frequency (MF) phonocardiogram recorded at the left sternal border (LSB) and pulmonary area (PA) in the same patient as in Figures 10-28 and 10-29. The first heart sound (1) is soft. The second splits 0.04 second on inspiration and closes to 0.02 second on expiration. The pulmonary component (P) is decreased, while the aortic component (A) is of normal intensity. During inspiration, the right-sided gallop (G) increases in intensity. The soft systolic murmur (SM) and low-frequency vibrations surrounding the gallop sound are also slightly louder on inspiration. Time intervals 0.04 second. (From Bramwell-Jones et al,[11] with permission.)

her QRS voltages. Reduced QRS voltages, ascribed to an increase in cardiac volume[10] have been reported in congestive cardiac failure. Low-amplitude QRS complexes have also been recognized in isolated tricuspid regurgitation, without elevation of the right ventricular end-diastolic pressure but have not been explained. We believe that low myocardial contractile tension of the left ventricle, consequent on its small end-diastolic volume, is an important factor in the production of small voltages in isolated tricuspid incompetence. After replacement of the tricuspid valve, an increase in QRS voltages is often apparent.[11]

The rising pulmonary artery pressure during late diastole was a noteworthy finding in our patient. Provided that the pulmonary valve is competent, the usual fall in pulmonary arterial pressure after valve closure must result from forward flow of blood into the pulmonary capillary and venous systems. For the pressure in the pulmonary artery to rise during diastole, both a significant resistance to this forward flow as well as a volume displacement into the pulmonary arterial system must be present. The mean pulmonary wedge pressure of 8 mmHg would constitute resistance to forward flow, and we suspect that this level may well have been lower but for the "restrictive" effect of the stretched normal pericardium. A volume displacement would be provided by the forward flow of blood from the right ventricle after diastolic opening of the valve as the right ventricular diastolic pressure exceeded that in the pulmonary artery. Parry and Abrahams[12] and Somers and co-workers[13] observed similar pulmonary pressures in severe endomyocardial fibrosis of the right ventricle and concluded that the pulmonary valve must open in late diastole. Recently, our colleague P Manga has observed on echocardiography premature opening of the pulmonary valve in eight patients with severe constrictive pericardi-

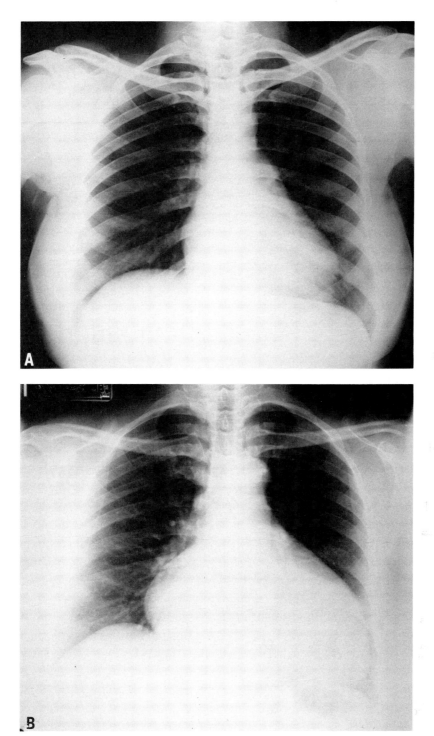

FIGURE 10-31. Posteroanterior chest radiographs of the same patient (see Figures 10-28 through 10-30) showing a cardiothoracic ratio (CTR) of 50 percent in 1973 (*A*) which increased to 70 percent in 1985 (*B*).

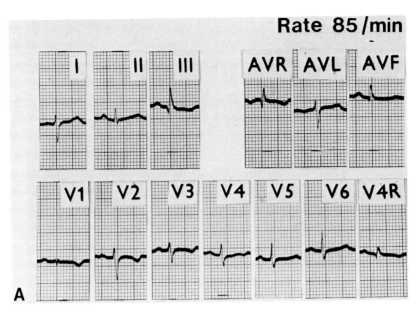

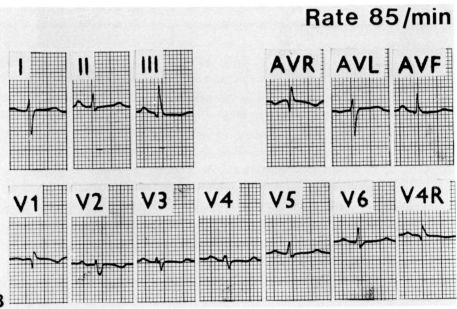

FIGURE 10-32. ECGs of the same patient as shown in Figures 10-28 through 10-31. Small voltages and QR waves in the right chest leads are shown in both the 1973 (*A*) and 1985 (*B*) tracings.

tis. Diastolic opening of the pulmonary valve has also been demonstrated echocardiographically after right ventricular infarction,[14] and we have demonstrated it (see Fig. 10-24) in other cases of severe tricuspid regurgitation.

Because isolated tricuspid regurgitation is a relatively benign condition with some patients remaining asymptomatic for as long as 30 years,[15,16] and also because we were not confident that a successful valvuloplasty could be performed, we elected to manage our patient conservatively. She has been followed regularly as an outpatient and remains asymptomatic but for several years has been treated for moderate systemic hypertension. A chest roentgenogram in 1973 (Fig. 10-31A) was unremarkable, with a cardiothoracic ratio (CTR) of 50 percent. An ECG at that time showed small voltages and a dominant, albeit small, R wave in V_{4R} (Fig. 10-32A).

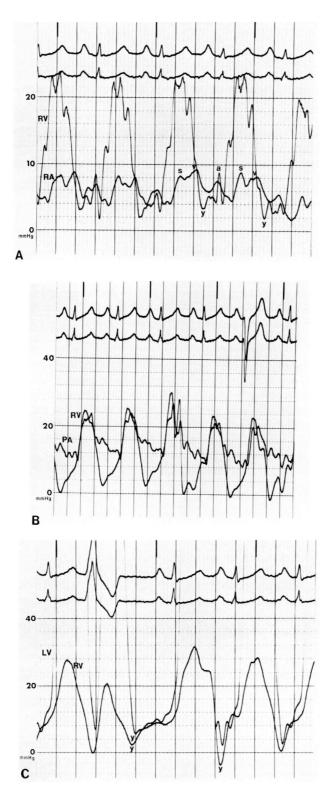

FIGURE 10-33. Repeat catheterization (see text) in 1985 of the patient who developed acute onset severe isolated organic tricuspid regurgitation in 1971 and whose pressure tracings in 1971 are shown in Figures 10-28 and 10-29. *A,* Right atrial and right ventricular pressures. The right atrial A, systolic (S), and V waves are prominent but are less than 10 mmHg. *B,* Pulmonary artery and right ventricular pressures. The right ventricular pulmonary artery pressure is now normal, and premature pulmonary valve opening does not occur. *C,* Simultaneous left ventricular and right ventricular pressures showing minimal evidence of "restriction." The y descent of the right ventricle precedes that of the left ventricle by 0.04 second or less.

The patient was examined by one of us (JBB) in November 1985. Her jugular venous pressure was raised about 8 cm, with discernible a and v waves. The liver was enlarged about 3 to 4 cm below the right costal margin, and hepatic pulsation was just detectable. Palpation of the precordium was not remarkable, but a systolic heave to the right of the sternum as well as systolic retraction to the left of the sternum and at the apex were present. On auscultation, both the first and second heart sounds appeared single. A Grade 2 pansystolic murmur of tricuspid regurgitation was audible at the left sternal border and apex and a prominent mid diastolic murmur was heard just inside the apex. Both systolic and mid-diastolic murmurs increased in intensity during natural inspiration. No gallop sounds were present.

M-mode and 2-D echocardiography demonstrated a flail anterior tricuspid leaflet, right atrial and right ventricular enlargement and early diastolic paradoxical movement of the interventricular septum. The ECG (Fig. 10-32B) showed small voltages with QR complexes in V_{4R} and V_1. A posteroanterior chest radiography confirmed considerable cardiac enlargement (see Fig. 10-31B) with a CTR of 70 percent. On cardiac catheterization, right atrial and right ventricular A-wave pressures varied but were usually less than 10 mmHg. Right atrial systolic waves were prominent (Fig. 10-33A). Pulmonary artery pressure also varied but the right atrial pressure was no longer reflected in the pulmonary artery tracing, and thus early pulmonary valve opening was not demonstrated (Fig. 10-33B). Right and left ventricular end-diastolic pressures nearly equalized at about 10 mmHg without evidence of significant restriction (Fig. 10-33C). Right ventricular cineangiography confirmed marked tricuspid regurgitation.

We conclude that this patient's originally raised right ventricular diastolic pressure and other evidence of "restriction" have subsided because of the dilation of her right atrial and right ventricular chambers and the stretching of her normal pericardium. She has considerable tricuspid regurgitation due to the flail anterior leaflet, but she remains asymptomatic and has no peripheral edema. Although we favor that a valvuloplasty could now be successfully performed, we do not see justification to attempt surgical intervention at this time.

CLINICAL SIGNS

Patients with severe tricuspid stenosis, or those with functional tricuspid regurgitation and a raised pulmonary vascular resistance, often have poor peripheral perfusion. This is reflected clinically by purplish discoloration of the cheeks (so-called tricuspid facies), cold and cyanosed extremities, and peripheral sores or scars due to delayed healing of minor abrasions (Fig. 10-34). Severe tricuspid regurgitation may be associated with suffused facies and even proptosis. Occasionally, central cyanosis may supervene if the foramen ovale is functionally patent.[17] The easily palpable systolic wave of the jugular venous pulse and the systolic expansion of the liver are characteristic features of severe tricuspid regurgitation. It has been previously mentioned (see Chapter 4) that severe mitral regurgitation may produce both a palpable systolic venous pulsation and a pulsatile liver in the absence of hemodynamically significant tricuspid regurgitation because of bulging of the interatrial septum towards the right atrium during ventricular systole. This is particularly likely to occur in the context of the "restrictive-dilatation" syndrome discussed in Chapter 8, Section 2.

In the absence of associated hemodynamically severe mitral regurgitation, palpation of the precordium in cases of severe tricuspid regurgitation reveals characteristic features especially when, for any reason, the pulmonary vascular resistance is raised. Some of these features were well described in 1937 by Dressler[18] and others have been confirmed on kinetocardiography by Armstrong and Gotsman in 1974.[19] Kinetocardiographic findings reflect precordial movements as detected by clinical inspection or palpation, preferably with the ball of the hand, and are not analogous

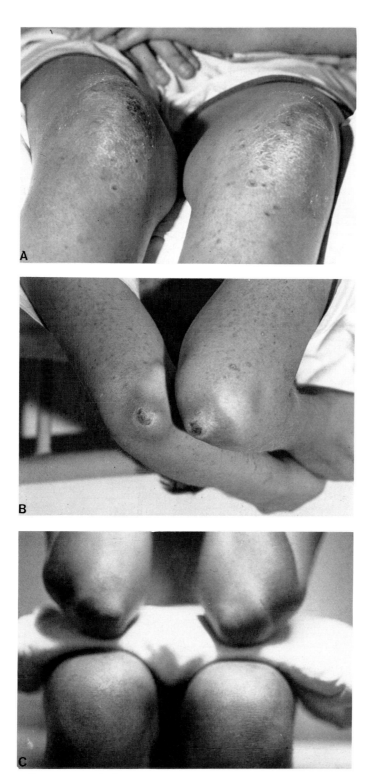

FIGURE 10-34. Knees (*A*) and elbows (*B*) of a 16-year-old boy with severe mixed mitral and aortic valve disease, pulmonary hypertension, and marked tricuspid regurgitation. The ulcerating skin and numerous small scars, particularly over the pressure points are demonstrated. (*C*) Two months after successful cardiac surgery, the skin appears normal.

to apex cardiography. Precordial pulsations detected by palpation also depend importantly on the site of palpation. Whereas Chesler[20] used the term "tricuspid rock" to describe systolic pulsation to the right of the sternum produced by rapid right atrial expansion and diastolic pulsation to the left of the sternum produced by right ventricular filling, Dressler emphasized a "see-saw movement" when comparing the systolic expansion to the right of the sternum with the synchronous systolic depression on its left. These terms may therefore be a little confusing. Nevertheless, precordial movements in severe tricuspid regurgitation, in the absence of associated mitral regurgitation, are characteristic and four components (Fig. 10-35) may be detected at three different sites. These are as follows:

1. Because the right ventricle is dilated and usually hypertrophied, a momentary thrust is felt over the lower sternum at the onset of systole and at the time of the first heart sound.
2. To the right of the sternum, there is a sustained expansile pulsation throughout ventricular systole, probably due to a combination of right atrial and right hepatic lobe expansion.
3. To the left of the sternum and towards the apex, there is retraction through-

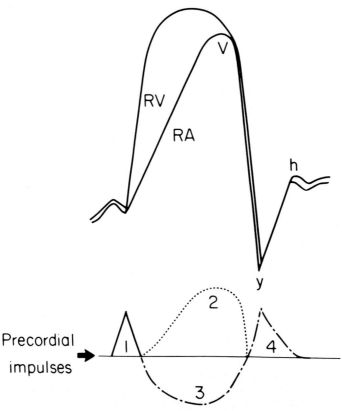

Precordial impulses and their hemodynamic correlates in tricuspid regurgitation

FIGURE 10-35. Schematic diagram of right ventricular and right atrial pressure tracings and synchronous precordial impulses in patients with severe tricuspid regurgitation. (1) the momentary positive impulse detected over the sternum at the beginning of ventricular systole; (2) the prolonged systolic expansion palpated to the *right* of the sternum; (3) the retraction throughout systole palpated at the *left* of the sternum and *apex*; (4) the diastolic impulse at the *left* of the sternum when the right ventricle fills rapidly in early ventricular diastole.

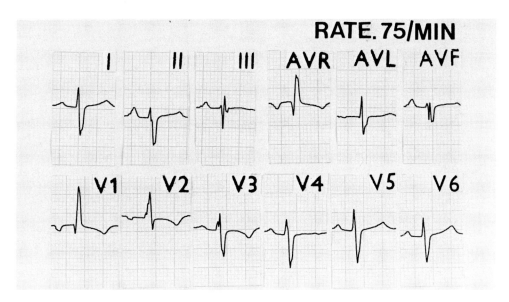

FIGURE 10-36. ECG of the 45-year-old woman (see Figure 10-21) with severe tricuspid regurgitation. The QRS voltages are relatively small, and there is clockwise rotation and a prominent QR complex in lead V_1.

out systole which presumably results from the rapid and complete right ventricular emptying because of the marked tricuspid regurgitation.

4. Also to the left of the sternum, the retraction during ventricular systole is replaced by a positive lift in early diastole at the time of a right ventricular third heart sound or the nadir of the y descent of the right atrial and right ventricular pressure tracings (Fig. 10-35; see also Fig. 10-25). This diastolic impulse results from rapid right ventricular filling and is similar to the diastolic lift encountered in constrictive pericarditis.

Just as there is systolic retraction to the left of the sternum with marked tricuspid regurgitation, it must be remembered that the apex beat, when it reflects a right ventricular impulse such as may occur in some cases of severe mitral stenosis, will sometimes retract at the beginning of systole. This must be borne in mind in timing the heart sounds under such circumstances. For practical purposes, a problem seldom arises because a sinus tachycardia of more than 120 per minute is rarely encountered in cases of chronic severe tricuspid regurgitation. It is also important to reiterate that chronic right ventricular pressure overload, as seen in pulmonary stenosis that causes right ventricular hypertrophy without dilatation, produces a barely palpable heave at the sternum. That impulse, as demonstrated by Armstrong and Gotsman,[19] will give only a small impulse at that site on a kinetocardiogram.

The systolic murmur of tricuspid regurgitation may be soft or absent when only minor turbulence is produced at the leaflets. This is common and occurs in many cases of rheumatic "functional" tricuspid incompetence. The pulmonary closing pressure is low or relatively low in severe tricuspid regurgitation, even when the pulmonary vascular resistance is raised. The intensity of the pulmonary component of the second sound is thus normal or decreased.

As has been stated, the QRS voltages on the ECG are relatively small and a QR complex may be recorded in leads V_{4R} and V_1 (Fig. 10-36).

ECHOCARDIOGRAPHY

Examination of the regurgitant tricuspid valve with 2-D echocardiography may demonstrate vegetations on the valve, flail leaflets following infective endocarditis or

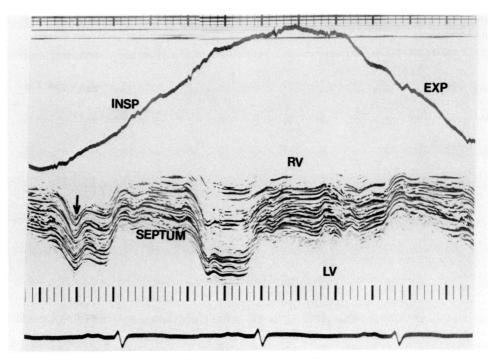

FIGURE 10-37. M-mode echocardiogram (paper speed 100 mm/sec) of the interventricular septum in a patient with severe constrictive pericarditis. The septum is flattened during systole, and there is early diastolic septal movement *(arrow)* that is more pronounced during inspiration (INSP).

trauma (see Fig. 10-27), anular dilatation, valve thickening, or prolapsing leaflets. Two forms of abnormal septal motion have been observed on M-mode echocardiography in patients with tricuspid regurgitation. The first is when the left ventricular posterior wall and septal echoes move in the same direction: anteriorly during systole and posteriorly during diastole.[21,22] The second is when the septal echoes are flattened during systole with posterior motion of the interventricular septum in early diastole (see Fig. 10-22).[22] These abnormal septal movements are not specific for tricuspid regurgitation and have been observed in right ventricular volume overload conditions and in pericardial constriction (Fig. 10-37).[22,23]

MANAGEMENT

Patients with significant tricuspid regurgitation and mitral valve disease can be managed medically for years, and it is difficult to generalize regarding the timing and indications for surgery. Aspects have been discussed in Chapter 8. Because of the "restrictive-dilatation" syndrome, tricuspid regurgitation should be eliminated by tricuspid anuloplasty at the time of mitral valve surgery. This is particularly pertinent when the anulus is very dilated and the pulmonary artery pressure normal or less than moderately raised. Patients with severe pulmonary arterial hypertension seldom have marked tricuspid anular dilatation, and the tricuspid regurgitation improves after restoration to normal or near-normal left heart hemodynamics. As discussed in Section 2 of Chapter 8, we nonetheless favor reduction by anuloplasty of any tricuspid anular dilatation at the time of surgery for mitral valve disease of rheumatic etiology. Surgery in patients with isolated organic tricuspid regurgitation should be delayed unless there is good reason to believe that a successful valvuloplasty can be performed or the patient continues to have peripheral edema or ascites despite adequate diuretic therapy. When surgery is indicated and insertion of a prosthetic valve unavoidable, we favor the use of a tissue valve. Degenerative changes in bioprosthetic valves in the tricuspid position are less extensive than in those in the mitral position.[24]

REFERENCES

SECTION 1

1. WEITZMAN, S, POCOCK, WA, HAWKINS, DM, AND BARLOW, JB: *Observer variation in radiological assessment of pulmonary vasculature.* Br Heart J 36:280–290, 1974.
2. KEREIAKES, DJ, HERFKENS, RJ, BRUNDAGE, BH, GAMSU, G, AND LIPTON, MJ: *Computed tomography in chronic thromboembolic pulmonary hypertension.* Am Heart J 106:1432–1436, 1983.
3. FUSTER, V, STEELE, PM, AND EDWARDS, WD: *Primary pulmonary hypertension: Natural history and the importance of thrombosis.* Circulation 70:580–587, 1984.
4. OAKLEY, CM: *Management of primary pulmonary hypertension.* Br Heart J 53:1–4, 1985.
5. WAGENVOORT, CA AND WAGENVOORT, N: *Primary pulmonary hypertension. A pathologic study of the lung vessels in 156 clinically diagnosed cases.* Circulation 42:1163–1184, 1970.
6. WOOD, P: *The Eisenmenger syndrome or pulmonary hypertension with reversed central shunt.* Br Med J 2:701–709, 755–762, 1958.
7. VIRMANI, R AND ROBERTS, WC: *Pulmonary arteries in congenital heart disease: A structure-function analysis.* In ROBERTS, WC (ED): *Congenital Heart Disease in Adults.* FA Davis, Philadelphia, 1979, pp 455–499.
8. HEATH, D AND EDWARDS, JE: *The pathology of hypertensive pulmonary vascular disease. A description of six grades of structural changes in the pulmonary arteries with special reference to congenital cardiac defects.* Circulation 18:533–547, 1958.
9. HOFFMAN, JIE, RUDOLPH, AM, AND HEYMANN, MA: *Pulmonary vascular disease with congenital heart lesions.* Circulation 64:873–877, 1981.
10. JONES, AM AND HOWITT, G: *Eisenmenger syndrome in pregnancy.* Br Med J 1:1627–1631, 1965.
11. CAMPBELL, M, NEILL, C, AND SUZMAN, S: *The prognosis of atrial septal defect.* Br Med J 1:1375–1383, 1957.
12. MARKMAN, P, HOWITT, G, AND WADE, EG: *Atrial septal defect in the middle-aged and elderly.* Q J Med 34:409–426, 1965.
13. GAULT, JH, MORROW, AG, GAY, WA, ROSS, J JR: *Atrial septal defect in patients over the age of 40 years. Clinical and hemodynamic studies and the effects of operation.* Circulation 37:261–272, 1968.
14. DEXTER, L: *Atrial septal defect.* Br Heart J 18:209–225, 1956.
15. COHN, LH, MORROW, AG, AND BRAUNWALD, E: *Operative treatment of atrial septal defect: Clinical and haemodynamic assessments in 175 patients.* Br Heart J 29:725–734, 1967.
16. HAWORTH, SG: *Pulmonary vascular disease in secundum atrial septal defect in childhood.* Am J Cardiol 51:265–272, 1983.
17. HAWORTH, SG: *Pulmonary vascular disease in different types of congenital heart disease. Implications for interpretation of lung biopsy findings in early childhood.* Br Heart J 52:557–571, 1984.
18. JOFFE, HS: *Effect of age on pressure-flow dynamics in secundum atrial septal defect.* Br Heart J 51:469–472, 1984.
19. GRAHAM, TP: *The Eisenmenger reaction and its management.* In ROBERTS, WC (ED): *Congenital Heart Disease in Adults.* FA Davis, Philadelphia, 1979, pp 531–542.
20. HAMILTON, WT, HAFFAJEE, CI, DALEN, JE, DEXTER, L, AND NADAS, AS: *Atrial septal defect secundum: Clinical profile with physiologic correlates in children and adults.* In ROBERTS, WC (ED): *Congenital Heart Disease in Adults.* FA Davis, Philadelphia, 1979, pp 267–277.
21. BEDFORD, DE, SELLORS, TH, SOMERVILLE, W, BELCHER, JR, AND BESTERMAN, EMM: *Atrial septal defect and its surgical treatment.* Lancet 1:1255–1261, 1957.

22. KELLY, JJ AND LYONS, HA: *Atrial septal defect in the aged.* Ann Intern Med 48:267–283, 1958.

23. CHERIAN, G, UTHAMAN, CB, DURAIRAJ, M, SUKUMAR, IP, KRISHNASWAMI, S, JAIRAJ, PS, JOHN, S, KRISHNASWAMI, H, AND BHAKTAVIZIAM, A: *Pulmonary hypertension in isolated secundum atrial septal defect: High frequency in young patients.* Am Heart J 105:952–957, 1983.

24. PERLOFF, JK: *Ostium secundum atrial septal defect—survival for 87 and 94 years.* Am J Cardiol 53:388–389, 1984.

SECTION 2

1. YOUSOF, AM, SHAFEI, MZ, ENDRYS, G, KHAN, N, SIMO, M, AND CHERIAN, G: *Tricuspid stenosis and regurgitation in rheumatic heart disease: A prospective cardiac catheterization study in 525 patients.* Am Heart J 110:60–64, 1985.

2. WOOLEY, CF, FONTANA, ME, KILMAN, JW, AND RYAN, JM: *Tricuspid stenosis. Atrial systolic murmur, tricuspid opening snap and right atrial pressure pulse.* Am J Med 78:375–384, 1985.

3. NANNA, M, CHANDRARATNA, PA, REID, C, NIMALASURIYA, A, AND RAHIMTOOLA, SH: *Value of two-dimensional echocardiography in detecting tricuspid stenosis.* Circulation 67:221–224, 1983.

4. DANIELS, SJ, MINTZ, GS, AND KOTLER, MN: *Rheumatic tricuspid valve disease: Two-dimensional echocardiographic, hemodynamic, and angiographic correlations.* Am J Cardiol 51:492–496, 1983.

5. LAUFER, J, FRAND, M, AND MILO, S: *Valve replacement for severe tricuspid regurgitation caused by Libman-Sacks endocarditis.* Br Heart J 48:294–297, 1982.

6. BARLOW, JB, FULLER, D, AND DENNY, M: *Case Report: A case of right atrial myxoma with special reference to an unusual phonocardiographic finding.* Br Heart J 24:120–125, 1962.

7. SAKAI, K, INOUE, Y, AND OSAWA, M: *Congenital isolated tricuspid regurgitation in an adult.* Am Heart J 110:680–681, 1985.

8. TEI, C, SHAH, PM, CHERIAN, G, TRIM, PA, WONG, M, AND ORMISTON, JA: *Echocardiographic evaluation of normal and prolapsed tricuspid valve leaflets.* Am J Cardiol 52:796–800, 1983.

9. SARELI, P, GOLDMAN, AP, POCOCK, WA, COLSEN, P, CASARI, A, AND BARLOW, JB: *Coronary artery–right ventricular fistula and organic tricuspid regurgitation due to blunt chest trauma.* Am J Cardiol 54:697–699, 1984.

10. ISHIKAWA, K, BERSON, AS, AND PIPBERGER, HV: *Electrocardiographic changes due to cardiac enlargement.* Am Heart J 81:635–643, 1971.

11. BRAMWELL-JONES, DM, POCOCK, WA, SALANT, DJ, AND BARLOW, JB: *Isolated tricuspid bacterial endocarditis resulting in severe tricuspid insufficiency.* Chest 62:749–752, 1972.

12. PARRY, EHD, AND ABRAHAMS, DG: *The function of the heart in endomyocardial fibrosis of the right ventricle.* Br Heart J 25:619–629, 1963.

13. SOMERS, K, BRENTON, DP, D'ARBELA, PG, FOWLER, JM, KANYEREZI, BR, AND SOOD, NK: *Haemodynamic features of severe endomyocardial fibrosis of right ventricle, including comparison with constrictive pericarditis.* Br Heart J 30:322–332, 1968.

14. LOPEZ-SENDON, J, GARCIA, AG, MARTI, JS, AND ROLDAN, I: *Complete pulmonic valve opening during atrial contraction after right ventricular infarction.* Am J Cardiol 56:486–487, 1985.

15. MORGAN, JR AND FORKER, AD: *Isolated tricuspid insufficiency.* Ciruclation 43:559–564, 1971.

16. CROXSON, MS, O'BRIEN, KP, AND LOWE, JB: *Traumatic tricuspid regurgitation: Long-term survival.* Br Heart J 33:750–755, 1971.

17. BARDY, GH, TALANO, JV, MEYERS, S, AND LESCH, M: *Acquired cyanotic heart disease secondary to traumatic tricuspid regurgitation. Case report with a review of the literature.* Am J Cardiol 44:1401–1406, 1979.

18. DRESSLER, W: *Pulsations of the wall of the chest III. Pulsations associated with tricuspid regurgitation.* Arch Int Med 60:441–448, 1937.

19. ARMSTRONG, TG AND GOTSMAN, MS: *The left parasternal lift in tricuspid incompetence.* Am Heart J 88:183–190, 1974.

20. CHESLER, E: *Schrire's Clinical Cardiology,* ed 4. John Wright & Sons, Bristol, 1981, p 15.

21. FEIGENBAUM, H: *Echocardiography.* ed 3. Lea & Febiger, Philadelphia, 1981, pp 284–286.

22. ASSOD-MORELL, JL, TAJIK, AJ, AND GIULIANI, ER: *Echocardiographic analysis of the ventricular septum.* Prog Cardiovasc Dis 17:219–237, 1974.

23. GIBSON, TC, GROSSMAN, W, MCLAURIN, LP, MOOS, S, AND CRAIGE, E: *An echocardiographic study of the interventricular septum in constrictive pericarditis.* Br Heart J 38:738–743, 1976.

24. COHEN, SR, SILVER, MA, MCINTOSH, CL, AND ROBERTS, WC: *Comparison of late (62 to 140 months) degenerative changes in simultaneously implanted and explanted porcine (Hancock) bioprostheses in the tricuspid and mitral valve positions in six patients.* Am J Cardiol 53:1599–1602, 1984.

BIBLIOGRAPHY

SECTION 1

DISESA, VJ, COHN, LH, AND GROSSMAN, W: *Management of adults with congenital bidirectional cardiac shunts, cyanosis, and pulmonary vascular obstruction: Successful operative repair in 3 patients.* Am J Cardiol 51:1495–1497, 1983.

FINCH, EL, MITCHELL, RS, GUTHANER, DF, FOWLES, RF, AND MILLER, DC: *Pulmonary artery surgical aneurysmorrhaphy: Where do we go from here?* Am Heart J 106:614–618, 1983.

GOLDHABER, SZ, HENNEKENS, CH, EVANS, DA, NEWTON, EC, AND GODLESKI, JJ: *Factors associated with correct antemortem diagnosis of major pulmonary embolism.* Am J Med 73:822–826, 1982.

GOLDMAN, L: *The autopsy versus the ostrich.* Int J Cardiol 5:550–553, 1984.

HALLIDIE-SMITH, KA, WILSON, RSE, HART, A, AND ZEIDIFARD, E: *Functional status of patients with large ventricular septal defect and pulmonary vascular disease 6 to 16 years after surgical closure of their defect in childhood.* Br Heart J 39:1093–1101, 1977.

KULIK, TJ, BASS, JL, FUHRMAN, BP, MOLLER, JH, AND LOCK, JE: *Exercise induced pulmonary vasoconstriction.* Br Heart J 50:59–64, 1983.

MCGREGOR, M AND SNIDERMAN, A: *On pulmonary vascular resistance: The need for more precise definition.* Am J Cardiol 55:217–221, 1985.

MARSH, JD, GLYNN, M, AND TORMAN, HA: *Pulmonary angiography. Application in a new spectrum of patients.* Am J Med 75:763–770, 1983.

STAHL, RL, JAVID, JP, AND LACKNER, H: *Unrecognized pulmonary embolism presenting as disseminated intravascular coagulation.* Am J Med 76:772–778, 1984.

UEDA, K: *Clinical profiles, pathologic spectrum and management of atrial septal defect in patients aged 50 or over: How should be treated?* J Cardiog 14:129–136, 1984.

SECTION 2

BOICOURT, OW, NAGLE, RE, AND MOUNSEY, JPD: *The clinical significance of systolic retraction of the apical impulse.* Br Heart J 27:379–391, 1965.

GLANCY, DL, MARCUS, FI, CUADRA, M, EWY, GA, AND ROBERTS, WC: *Isolated organic tricuspid valvular regurgitation. Causes and consequences.* Am J Med 46:989–996, 1969.

KING, RM, SCHAFF, HV, DANIELSON, GK, GERSH, BJ, ORSZULAK, TA, PIEHLER, JM, PUGA, FJ, AND PLUTH, JR: *Surgery for tricuspid regurgitation late after mitral valve replacement.* Circulation 70:193–197, 1984.

REED, GE, BOYD, AD, SPENCER, FC, ENGLEMAN, RM, ISOM, OW, AND CUNNINGHAM, JN: *Operative management of tricuspid regurgitation.* Circulation 54:96–98, 1976.

TEI, C, PILGRIM, JP, SHAH, PM, ORMISTON, JA, AND WONG, M: *The tricuspid valve annulus: Study of size and motion in normal subjects and in patients with tricuspid regurgitation.* Circulation 66:665–671, 1982.

WANN, LS, WEYMAN, AE, DILLON, JC, AND FEIGENBAUM, H: *Premature pulmonary valve opening.* Circulation 55:128–133, 1977.

EPILOGUE

Early in my professional career at Baragwanath Hospital in Johannesburg, I learnt from my chief, Dr. H. Grusin, the value of clinical observation and of interpreting physical signs. Shortly thereafter I was fortunate, while on the staff of the Royal Postgraduate Medical School in London, to be exposed to an environment nurtured by Professor (later Sir John) McMichael in which current dogma was never accepted as truth. My friend and compatriot Priscilla Kincaid-Smith and I were influenced by McMichael's philosophy, and we started to challenge concepts of auscultation, hypertension, and renal disease. Whereas her ongoing striving in Australia has justifiably brought her universal recognition as a leading authority in her field, I flatter myself that my own endeavours have directly or indirectly resulted in improved patient care and cardiological practice in my complex country. I am indebted to those colleagues for their roles in affecting my professional life. I hope that I, in turn, have favorably influenced others in similar vein.

Writing on any scientific matter enforces the author to clarify thoughts, concepts, and ideas. In this book, I have drawn conclusions or formulated opinions by correlating what I have read in the scientific literature with a long experience of a vast amount of clinical material. I have attempted to elucidate several issues that are apparently not always recognized or that continue to be disputed. Pulmonary arterial hypertension secondary to left-sided cardiac pathology (reactive pulmonary hypertension) is never, in the absence of an associated factor such as pulmonary thromboembolic disease or a left-to-right shunt, permanent. Thus, the severe pulmonary arterial hypertension resulting from mitral stenosis, left atrial myxoma, pulmonary venous obstruction, or a raised left ventricular end-diastolic pressure from any cause, is always potentially reversible.

Patients with virulent active rheumatic carditis die from heart failure because of a severe hemodynamic overload; thus, steroid therapy is neither indicated nor "life-saving"—surgical intervention is! Infective endocarditis will surely remain a fatal illness for some patients but the current mortality, sometimes still quoted as 30 percent, will only be drastically reduced by earlier diagnosis and by widespread recognition that the heart failure results from a hemodynamic factor that is invariably amenable to surgical treatment.

Most aspects of the prevalent hemodynamic conundrum that I have called the "restrictive-dilatation syndrome" have either not been recognized or have received scant attention. In fact, the inter-relationships of cardiac chambers require much further study. Comprehension of these inter-relationships explains a raised left ventricular end-diastolic pressure in some cases of mitral stenosis, the effects on the right atrial pulse form of a raised left atrial pressure in mitral regurgitation, and the role of the normal and abnormal pericardium on any heart that has reason to dilate. An appreciation of cardiac chamber inter-relationships also clarifies the important hemodynamic effects of tricuspid insufficiency and substantiates an aggressive surgical approach toward so-called functional tricuspid regurgitation.

Cardiologists and cardiac surgeons must continue to revise currently accepted concepts. I submit that we should be better observers of the objective data available to us, some of which have been looked at somewhat cursorily for many years, and not necessarily seek the development of new and higher priced technological diagnostic procedures. Intracardiac pressures, for example, should reveal many more secrets than an evaluation of a pressure difference across a valve or the conclusion that a large left atrial v wave may sometimes signify mitral regurgitation. More discerning observations of chest radiographs and pulmonary arteriograms should disclose an increased number of cases of pulmonary thromboembolic disease and far fewer of primary pulmonary hypertension. Evaluation of ST-segment and T-wave time-course behavior, and not only their configuration, should enhance the accuracy of stress electrocardiography and restore its status as the most practicable and cost-effective screening test for occlusive coronary artery disease.

Last, a comment on so-called mitral valve prolapse. I cannot envisage meaningful clinical, echocardiographic, or cineangiocardiographic criteria for "pathological prolapse" until there is universal agreement on terminology. This is more than a problem of semantics if it is realized that an anatomically normal leaflet may functionally be flail and that a floppy leaflet may not be prolapsed.

Certainly cardiac catheterization, echocardiography, ambulatory electrocardiographic monitoring, and other technological advances have assisted tremendously in our diagnoses and in our understanding of cardiac function; however, they should not obviate our ongoing consideration of cost-benefit and clinical context.

INDEX

An *italic* page number indicates a figure. A "t" following a page number indicates a table.

---

rheumatic, rheumatic fever and, epidemiology of, 227–228
Cardiac failure
late-onset
after mitral valve surgery, 275–277, *276, 277, 278*
left ventricular dysfunction or dilatation and, *278, 279*
mitral valve dysfunction and, 278
pericardial restriction or constriction and, 283–284, *283, 284*
pulmonary thromboembolic disease and chronic obstructive airways disease and, 279–281, *280*
tricuspid regurgitation and, 281–283, *281, 282*
surgical management of infective endocarditis and, 306–307, *307*
Cardiac murmur(s), timing of, in auscultation, 42–43. *See also* Murmur(s)
Cardiac sound(s). *See* Heart sound(s); Murmur(s)
Cardiomyopathy
dilated, as differential diagnosis of left atrial myxoma, 218
hypertrophic (HCM)
mitral valve mechanism and, 198–201, *199, 200, 201, 202*
auscultatory features of, 201
early diastolic murmurs, 208
first heart sound, 207
mid-diastolic murmurs, 208
second heart sound, 205–207, *206, 207*
systolic clicks, 207
systolic murmurs, *200,* 202–205, *203, 204, 205*
third and fourth heart sounds, 208
echocardiographic features of, 208, *209, 210, 211*
etiology of, 208
management of, 211
primary BML (Barlow's) syndrome and, 89–91, *89, 90, 91, 92*
Carditis
acute rheumatic, myocardial dysfunction in, 240–243, *241, 242*
rheumatic, 230
clinical features of, 230–234, *231,* 231t, *233,* 233t
histological findings of, 235
stage I: alterative (exudative-degenerative) phase, 235–236
stage II: granulomatous phase, 236
stage III: chronic (healing) phase, 236
operative findings of, 234–235, *234, 235*
Carpentier-Edwards mitral valve prosthesis, 259–260, *261*
Catheterization, cardiac
in mitral stenosis, *164,* 174–175, *174*
medical management of mitral regurgitation and, 118, 126–127

associated mitral stenosis, *123, 128, 129, 130*
circulating blood volume, 128
extent of mitral regurgitation, 129
left atrial cavity size and wall compliance, *127, 127, 128*
left ventricular end-diastolic pressure, 128
Chest pain, history taking and, 28–29
Chest radiography, in medical management of mitral regurgitation, 124–125, *125*
Chorda(e) tendinea(e), 4–6, *5, 6*
commissural, *6, 7*
leaflet, *4,* 6–8
ruptured, as cause of mitral regurgitation, 120–122, *121, 122, 123*
Chronic (healing) phase (stage III) of rheumatic carditis, 236
Chronic obstructive airways disease, after mitral valve surgery, 279–281, *280*
Click(s), systolic, hypertrophic cardiomyopathy and, 207
Clinical examination of cardiovascular system, 31–35, *31, 32, 33, 34*
auscultation of heart in
auditory acuity, 43–44
auscultator concentration, 41–42
choice of stethoscope for, 41
location and method of listening, 43
method for, 41
theoretical knowledge of cardiac sounds and murmurs, 42
timing of heart sounds and murmurs, 42–43
precordium and
inspection of, 39
palpation of, 39–40
percussion of, 40–41
pulse and, 35, *35*
jugular venous pulse, *21,* 37–39, *38*
pulse rate, 35–36
pulse volume and character, 36–37, *37, 38*
Clinical sign(s) of tricuspid regurgitation, 352–355, *353, 354, 355*
Closed commissurotomy, technique for, 248–250, *249, 250*
Closure, mitral valve
leaflets and, 9–11, *238*
left atrial wall and anulus and, 11–12
left ventricular free wall and, 12–13
papillary muscles and chordae tendineae and, 11–12
Commissural chorda(e), *6, 7*
Commissural fusion, mitral stenosis and, 151
Commissurotomy(ies)
closed, technique for, 248–250, *249, 250*

primary, mitral valve and, 325–329, *328,329*
"silent" mitral stenosis and, 166
pulmonary venous
   medical management of mitral regurgitation and, 131
   pulmonary arterial hypertension caused by, 335–337, *335, 336*
Hypertrophic cardiomyopathy (HCM)
   mitral valve mechanism and, 198–201, *199, 200, 201, 202*
   auscultatory features of, 201
      early diastolic murmurs, 208
      first heart sound, 207
      mid-diastolic murmurs, 208
      second heart sound, 205–207, *206, 207*
      systolic clicks, 207
      systolic murmurs, 200, 202–205, *203, 204, 205*
      third and fourth heart sounds, 208
   echocardiographic features of, 208, *209, 210, 211*
   etiology of, 208
   management of, 211
   primary BML (Barlow's) syndrome and, 89–91, *89, 90, 91, 92*

INCOMPETENCE
   mitral, as differential diagnosis of left atrial myxoma, 214–217, *217*
   prosthetic valve, as cause of mitral regurgitation, 123–124
Infarction, myocardial, primary BML (Barlow's) syndrome concurrent with, *58,* 84–89, *86, 87, 88*
Infection, after mitral valve surgery, 268
Infective endocarditis, 289
   causes of transient bacteremia and, 294–297, *296,* 298t–299t
   clinical presentation of, 297, *300*
      general malaise, 301
      laboratory features, 303
      neurological manifestations, 301
      other physical signs, 302
      pyrexia, 297–301
      systemic emboli, 301, *302*
   management of
      medical, 303–305, *304*
      surgical, 305–306
         cardiac failure and, 306–307, *307*
         echocardiography and, 308–309, *308*
         fungal endocarditis and, 311
         infection refractory to medical therapy and, 310
         pericarditis and conduction defects and, 309–310
         prosthetic valve endocarditis and, 310–311
         rickettsial endocarditis and, 311
         right-sided endocarditis and, 311–314, *312, 313, 314*

patients at risk, 289–294, *290, 291, 292, 294, 295, 296*
   prophylaxis against, medical management of mitral regurgitation and, 129
   refractory to medical therapy, 310
Infective endocarditis syndrome, atrial myxoma and, 213
Intracardiac pressure(s), cardiac catheterization and, *18,* 25–27, *26, 27, 28*
Ischemia, myocardial, primary BML (Barlow's) syndrome concurrent with *58,* 84–89, *86, 87, 88*
Ischemic heart disease, as differential diagnosis of left atrial myxoma, 217–218

JUGULAR venous pulse, examination of cardiovascular system and, *21,* 37–39, *38*

LEAFLET(S)
   billowing mitral (BML), mitral prolapse and, 45
      auscultatory features of, 49, *50, 51*
         early systolic murmurs, 51, *57*
         late systolic murmurs, 49–50, *52, 53, 54*
         musical systolic murmurs, 51, *54, 55, 56*
         nonejection systolic clicks, 50, *52–56, 57, 58*
      cineangiocardiographic and echocardiographic evidence and correlation of, 56–60, *58, 59, 60*
      historical background on, 45–46
      nomenclature for, 46–49, *48*
      primary
         asymptomatic
            isolated NESC and, 93–94, 93t
            nonpansystolic mitral murmur and, *60,* 94, *95*
            pansystolic mitral murmur and, *60,* 94–96
         prevalence of, 65–67, *67*
         symptomatic, 96
            anxiety and, 96
            arrhythmias and conduction defects and, 99–101, *99, 100*
            chest pain and, 96–97
            infective endocarditis and, 98–99
            progressive mitral regurgitation and, 98
            sudden death and, *53, 66, 69,* 101–107, *102, 103, 104, 105, 106*
            systemic emboli and, 97–98
      secondary, 61, 61t
         congenital heart disease, 61t, 64
         left atrial myxoma, 64
         left ventricular aneurysm, 64
         papillary muscle dysfunction, *62,* 63–64